Essentials of Physiotherapy

Essentials of Physiotherapy

Edited by Pete Edner

SYRAWOOD
PUBLISHING HOUSE

New York

Published by Syrawood Publishing House,
750 Third Avenue, 9th Floor,
New York, NY 10017, USA
www.syrawoodpublishinghouse.com

Essentials of Physiotherapy
Edited by Pete Edner

© 2017 Syrawood Publishing House

International Standard Book Number: 978-1-68286-481-4 (Hardback)

Cataloging-in-Publication Data

Essentials of physiotherapy / edited by Pete Edner.
    p. cm.
Includes bibliographical references and index.
ISBN 978-1-68286-481-4
1. Chiropractic. 2. Physical therapy. 3. Therapeutics, Physiological. I. Edner, Pete.
RZ232.2 .E87 2017
615.534--dc23

Printed in the United States of America.

TABLE OF CONTENTS

Preface..IX

Chapter 1 Guidelines for the practice and performance of manipulation under
anesthesia...1
Robert Gordon, Edward Cremata and Cheryl Hawk

Chapter 2 The correlation of radiographic findings and patient symptomatology
in cervical degenerative joint disease...11
Iris Sun Rudy, Alexandra Poulos, Laura Owen, Ashlee Batters,
Kasia Kieliszek, Jessica Willox and Hazel Jenkins

Chapter 3 Attitudes toward drug prescription rights: a survey of Ontario
chiropractors..18
Peter Charles Emary and Kent Jason Stuber

Chapter 4 Short term treatment versus long term management of neck and back
disability in older adults utilizing spinal manipulative therapy and
supervised exercise: a parallel-group randomized clinical trial
evaluating relative effectiveness and harms....................................30
Corrie Vihstadt, Michele Maiers, Kristine Westrom, Gert Bronfort,
Roni Evans, Jan Hartvigsen and Craig

Chapter 5 Evaluation of a modified clinical prediction rule for use with spinal
manipulative therapy in patients with chronic low back pain:
a randomized clinical trial...45
Paul E Dougherty, Jurgis Karuza, Dorian Savino and Paul Katz

Chapter 6 Indicating spinal joint mobilisations or manipulations in patients
with neck or low-back pain: protocol of an inter-examiner reliability
study among manual therapists..57
Emiel van Trijffel, Robert Lindeboom, Patrick MM Bossuyt,
Maarten A Schmitt, Cees Lucas, Bart W Koes and Rob AB Oostendorp

Chapter 7 Current preventative and health promotional care offered to
patients by chiropractors in the United Kingdom..........................68
Patricia E Fikar, Kent A Edlund and Dave Newell

Chapter 8 Chiropractic treatment approaches for spinal musculoskeletal
conditions...75
Mattijs Clijsters, Francesco Fronzoni and Hazel Jenkins

Chapter 9   **US chiropractors' attitudes, skills and use of evidence-based**
practice: A cross-sectional national survey.. 85
Michael J Schneider, Roni Evans, Mitchell Haas, Matthew Leach,
Cheryl Hawk, Cynthia Long, Gregory D Cramer, Oakland Walters,
Corrie Vihstadt and Lauren Terhorst

Chapter 10   **Sick leave and healthcare utilisation in women reporting pregnancy**
related low back pain and/or pelvic girdle pain at 14 months postpartum................. 97
Cecilia Bergström, Margareta Persson and Ingrid Mogren

Chapter 11   **The role of information search in seeking alternative treatment for**
back pain...108
Hoda McClymont, Jeff Gow and Chad Perry

Chapter 12   **Attitudes and beliefs of Australian chiropractors' about managing**
back pain...121
Stanley I Innes, Peter D Werth, Peter J Tuchin and Petra L Graham

Chapter 13   **Bladder metastasis presenting as neck, arm and thorax pain**....................................129
Clinton J. Daniels, Pamela J. Wakefield and Glenn A. Bub

Chapter 14   **Chiropractic identity, role and future: a survey of North American**
chiropractic students..134
Jordan A Gliedt, Cheryl Hawk, Michelle Anderson, Kashif Ahmad,
Dinah Bunn, Jerrilyn Cambron, Brian Gleberzon, John Hart,
Anupama Kizhakkeveettil, Stephen M Perle, Michael Ramcharan,
Stephanie Sullivan and Liang Zhang

Chapter 15   **The use of diagnostic coding in chiropractic practice**...142
Cecilie D Testern, Lise Hestbæk and Simon D French

Chapter 16   **Patients' experiences and expectations of chiropractic care: a national**
cross-sectional survey..151
Hugh MacPherson, Elizabeth Newbronner, Ruth Chamberlain and
Ann Hopton

Chapter 17   **Chiropractic care and the risk of vertebrobasilar stroke: results of**
a case–control study in U.S. commercial and Medicare Advantage
populations... 161
Thomas M Kosloff, David Elton, Jiang Tao and Wade M Bannister

Chapter 18   **Absence of low back pain to demarcate an episode: a prospective**
multicentre study in primary care...171
Andreas Eklund, Irene Jensen, Malin Lohela-Karlsson,
Charlotte Leboeuf-Yde and Iben Axén

Chapter 19   **The chiropractic profession in Denmark 2010–2014** 178
Orla Lund Nielsen, Alice Kongsted and Henrik Wulff Christensen

Chapter 20   **Does cervical lordosis change after spinal manipulation for non-specific neck pain? A prospective cohort study**..186
Michael Shilton, Jonathan Branney, Bas Penning de Vries and
Alan C. Breen

Chapter 21   **Chiropractors' perception of occupational stress and its influencing factors: a qualitative study using responses to open-ended questions**...................195
Shawn Williams

Chapter 22   **The simulated early learning of cervical spine manipulation technique utilising mannequins**..202
Peter D Chapman, Norman J Stomski, Barrett Losco and
Bruce F Walker

Chapter 23   **Spinal myxopapillary ependymoma in an adult male presenting with recurrent acute low back pain**...209
Dean Petersen and Reidar P. Lystad

Chapter 24   **Acute thoracolumbar pain due to cholecystitis**..214
Chris T. Carter

Chapter 25   **Match injuries in amateur Rugby Union: a prospective cohort study - FICS Biennial Symposium Second Prize Research Award**..........................219
Michael S. Swain, Reidar P. Lystad, Nicholas Henschke,
Christopher G. Maher and Steven J. Kamper

Permissions

List of Contributors

Index

PREFACE

The world is advancing at a fast pace like never before. Therefore, the need is to keep up with the latest developments. This book was an idea that came to fruition when the specialists in the area realized the need to coordinate together and document essential themes in the subject. That's when I was requested to be the editor. Editing this book has been an honour as it brings together diverse authors researching on different streams of the field. The book collates essential materials contributed by veterans in the area which can be utilized by students and researchers alike.

Physiotherapy primarily uses mechanical force and movements to treat impairments related to functioning and mobility of the body. It is mostly used as an added medical treatment to conventional medicine. This book provides significant information of this discipline to help develop a good understanding of this discipline and related fields. It includes some of the vital pieces of work being conducted across the world, on various topics related to physiotherapy. As this field is emerging at a rapid pace, the contents of this book will help the readers understand the modern concepts and applications of the subject. It will prove to be immensely beneficial to students and researchers in this field.

Each chapter is a sole-standing publication that reflects each author's interpretation. Thus, the book displays a multi-facetted picture of our current understanding of applications and diverse aspects of the field. I would like to thank the contributors of this book and my family for their endless support.

Editor

Guidelines for the practice and performance of manipulation under anesthesia

Robert Gordon[1], Edward Cremata[2,3] and Cheryl Hawk[4*]

Abstract

Background: There are currently no widely accepted guidelines on standards for the practice of chiropractic or manual therapy manipulation under anesthesia, and the evidence base for this practice is composed primarily of lower-level evidence. The purpose of this project was to develop evidence-informed and consensus-based guidelines on spinal manipulation under anesthesia to address the gaps in the literature with respect to patient selection and treatment protocols.

Methods: An expert consensus process was conducted from August-October 2013 using the Delphi method. Panelists were first provided with background literature, consisting of three review articles on manipulation under anesthesia. The Delphi rounds were conducted using the widely-used and well-established RAND-UCLA consensus process methodology to rate seed statements for their appropriateness. Consensus was determined to be reached if 80% of the 15 panelists rated a statement as appropriate. Consensus was reached on all 43 statements in two Delphi rounds.

Results: The Delphi process was conducted from August-October 2013. Consensus was reached on recommendations related to all aspects of manipulation under anesthesia, including patient selection; diagnosis and establishing medical necessity; treatment and follow-up procedures; evaluation of response to treatment; safety practices; appropriate compensation considerations; and facilities, anesthesia and nursing standards.

Conclusions: A high level of agreement was achieved in developing evidence-informed recommendations about the practice of chiropractic/manual therapy manipulation under anesthesia.

Keywords: Manipulation under anesthesia, Chiropractic, Spinal manipulation, Spine-related pain

Introduction

Spinal manipulation under anesthesia (MUA) is a procedure that was originally practiced by orthopedic surgeons and osteopathic physicians for the treatment of spinal pain since the late 1930's [1,2]. Since the 1960's, Doctors of Chiropractic (DC) have come to perform the majority of spinal MUA procedures [3]. Fibrosis Release Procedures is a term which includes MUA and perhaps better describes the comprehensive nature of the procedures used by DCs in performing MUA, since more than spinal manipulation is involved [4].

There are currently no widely accepted guidelines on standards for chiropractic MUA. The 1993 Guidelines for Chiropractic Quality Assurance and Practice Parameters considered MUA "equivocal", and these guidelines have

not been updated since 1993 [5]. In 2012, the American Association of Manipulation Under Anesthesia Providers (AAMUAP), a multidisciplinary panel of MUA experts, developed a set of guidelines for the practice, and educational parameters for MUA. Members of the organization undertook a further effort to develop a set of evidence-informed and consensus based guidelines developed by a panel of multidisciplinary experts, including MUA practitioners as well as experts who were not MUA practitioners. The results of this consensus process are presented in this article.

Although MUA has been said by some authorities to be "a reasonable method of treating certain patients with spinal pain", [2] evidence for its effectiveness is limited, with few controlled studies. However, the studies that exist, the majority of which are case series, have shown positive results [2,3,6]. In the absence of higher levels of evidence, or when the published literature does

* Correspondence: hawkcheryl@aol.com
[4]Logan University, 1851 Schoettler Rd 63017 Chesterfield, MO, USA
Full list of author information is available at the end of the article

not provide adequate detail about management parameters, formal consensus by experts can be useful [7,8].

Indications for MUA

A concern in providing MUA is the lack of standardized protocols for patient selection [6]. Selecting the patient who will benefit most from MUA is essential to the success of the procedure, yet selection criteria have not been investigated thoroughly [6]. Generally, spinal MUA is used for patients who suffer from chronic nonspecific mechanical spine-related pain who have been minimally responsive (not reaching the expected level of outcome) to previous conservative therapy; this is considered a treatment failure for conservative therapy [3,9,10]. Etiology of their pain may be disc bulge/herniation, chronic recurrent sprain/strain, failed back surgery, or myofascial pain syndromes. The procedure is considered by many practitioners to be beneficial for the patient who has muscle spasm accompanied with pain and loss of terminal joint range-of-motion. These types of patients typically respond well to manipulation/physical therapy/exercise, but their relief may only be temporary.

Hallmarks for choosing a patient for MUA are 1) the presence of intersegmental and/or global recalcitrant motion restrictions that are thought to be fibrosis maintained, and 2) the unsuccessful attempt at more conservative measures that have included in-office spinal manipulation [4].

Description of MUA procedures and follow up care

Another concern is the lack of standardization of MUA procedures and follow-up care [6]. It is well-established that MUA requires an interdisciplinary team which includes an anesthesiologist, an operating room (OR) nurse and a DC or other qualified manual therapy physician [4]. It is also generally accepted that the phases of MUA are 1) sedation; 2) manipulative procedures; 3) additional stretching/traction procedures; 4) follow-up in-office care without sedation [4].

Sedation

Monitored Anesthesia Care (MAC) is used, most frequently Diprivan (Propofol) and Versed [11].

Manipulative and additional procedures

The patient is taken through passive spinal, hip, shoulder, and extra spinal extremity ranges of motion, determined by the treating physician. Specific spinal manipulation is performed when the elastic barrier of resistance and segmental end range of motion is achieved. Stretching of the paraspinal and surrounding supportive musculature is performed to promote cervical, thoracic, lumbar, lumbopelvic and extra spinal flexibility in conjunction with attempting to restore proper kinetic motion. The patient is then awakened from the anesthesia which usually occurs minutes after the Diprivan (propofol) is stopped. They are then taken to recovery and monitored until full recovery has occurred. The patient is then discharged to rest until post MUA therapy is begun later the same day (or in as short a time as possible following MUA).

Follow-up care without sedation

Post MUA therapy is an essential part of the MUA procedure and is accomplished the same day, if possible. Post MUA therapy consists of warming up the involved areas, passive stretching as was accomplished in the MUA procedure, followed by interferential stimulation and cryotherapy. The patient is then sent home to rest. This procedure is repeated serially in most cases by having the patient return to the facility the next day and the following day(s). The average number of days for the MUA procedure to accomplish the desired outcome has been shown to be between 2-4 days [12,13]. The concept is that increasing movement each day in incremental amounts accomplishes the desired increase in range of movement and decreases pain far better than spending large amounts of time in one day to achieve the same result. This protocol for post MUA therapy is repeated 7-10 days after the final MUA followed by pre-rehabilitation and then formal rehabilitation for 3-6 weeks. Additional reduction in soreness and mild edema with an increase in range of motion has been noted when small, portable, multi-modality interferential/NMES/HVPC or TENS devices are applied in the OR immediately following the MUA and when the patients are sent home with these units as part of the post MUA therapy [12,13]. The rehabilitation program continues for 3-6 weeks following the MUA procedure to give the patient time to recover to pre-injury status. Marked improvement (80-97%) has been the general rule when the properly selected cases have received this procedure [14,15].

Evidence for MUA treatment effects

A PubMed literature search using the term "manipulation under anesthesia" found 2 systematic reviews (2002 [2] and 2008 [3]) and one narrative review, [6] and no articles that were not addressed in the reviews [2,3,6]. The secondary sources (reviews) [2,3,6] were the primary references used for evaluating the evidence related to MUA, with emphasis on the most recent review (2013) [6]. Although it did not claim to be a systematic review, it did evaluate the strength of the existing evidence on the topic [6]. The evidence was assessed using the scheme described in the 2003 *Journal of Bone & Joint Surgery,* [16] which is commonly used in musculoskeletal medicine [17]. Definitions of the levels of evidence in this scheme are summarized in Table 1.

The evidence for treatment effects of MUA consisted of Levels II, IV and V. Level II evidence included three

Table 1 Definition of levels of evidence for treatment results*

Level I	Level II	Level III	Level IV	Level V
high-quality RCT	Prospective cohort	CC	Case series	Expert opinion
SR of high-quality RCTs	Poor-quality RCT	Retrospective cohort		Case reports[1]
	SR of above study types	SR of above study types		

*Source: Wright JG, Swiontkowski MF, Heckman JD. Introducing levels of evidence to the journal. *J Bone Joint Surg Am.* Jan 2003;85-A(1):1-3.
Abbreviations: *RCT* randomized controlled trial, *SR* systematic review, *CC* case control study.
[1]For this project, case reports were classified as the same level as expert opinion.

prospective cohort studies and [18-20] three reviews (narrative review, 2013) [6] and (systematic reviews 2008 [3] and 2002) [2]. The remaining published literature on MUA consisted of Level IV studies (case series) and Level V studies (case reports and expert opinion) [6]. Overall, positive effects were noted for MUA in appropriately selected patients; however, the absence of control groups make it impossible to make a definitive assessment [2].

Evidence related to safety of MUA

No serious adverse effects were noted in any of the published studies of MUA treatment by chiropractors [3,4].

The purpose of this project was to develop evidence-informed and consensus-based guidelines on spinal MUA to address the gaps in the literature with respect to patient selection and treatment protocols in particular.

Methods

Preparation for Delphi panel

All three published reviews [2,3,6] were provided to the Delphi panel at the beginning of the project as background documents. The core committee, two of whom are experienced MUA practitioners who have been active in guideline development for MUA and one who is experienced in conducting consensus projects for guideline development, developed 43 seed statements, based on previous MUA guidelines and the background documents.

Delphi consensus panel

The project was determined to be exempt (P/N 2013-017) by the Institutional Review Board of Life Chiropractic College West prior to conducting the Delphi process. An expert consensus process was conducted using the Delphi method. Because a Delphi panel is made up of experts, we selected individuals on the basis of their established expertise in the area of spine-related care. We identified both individuals who practice MUA and those who provide spinal care without MUA, to avoid bias toward MUA practice. We also included laypersons familiar with spine-related care, such as insurance specialists and attorneys. A list of 24 panelists to be invited included healthcare providers who had published on MUA, were MUA practitioners, were experienced DCs who did not practice MUA but had a practice emphasis in chronic spinal pain and were familiar with guideline development, and several

laypersons with healthcare experience such as insurance specialists and attorneys. Medical doctors (MD) (anesthesiologists and other specialists), osteopathic and chiropractic physicians were included, as well as registered nurses (RNs). A total of 16 panelists accepted, of which 10 (63%) were DCs. Panelists included 1 MD anesthesiologist, 2 MDs in other medical specialties, 2 RNs who work on MUA teams, 6 DCs who practice MUA, 4 DCs who do not practice MUA, and 1 attorney. Of the DCs, all were practitioners and 5 were also on the faculty of 5 different chiropractic colleges. There were 13 (81%) male and 3 (19%) female panelists, with a mean of 23 years professional experience (median 25 years). States represented were CA (5), FL (4), TX (2) and 1 each from GA, NC, NY and RN; one panelist resides in Malaysia. Most of the DCs were broad-scope in terms of practice approach, meaning that they utilized a number of procedures in addition to manipulation [21].

Delphi process

The Delphi process was conducted by e-mail. Each set of seed statements to be rated was identified by an ID number. Only the project coordinator could link the ID to the panelist's names, for purposes of distribution and follow-up. The Delphi process was conducted in a blinded manner, so that neither the panelists nor the core committee knew the identity of the raters or those who had made any individual comments, during the development of consensus. We used the widely-used and well-established RAND-UCLA consensus process methodology in rating the seed statements [22]. We used an ordinal rating scale ranging from 1 (highly inappropriate) to 9 (highly appropriate). We explained that by "appropriateness" (as specified by RAND/UCLA) [22], "we mean that the expected health benefit to the patient exceeds the expected negative consequences by a sufficiently wide margin that it is worth doing, exclusive of cost" [22].

In scoring, ratings of 1-3 indicated "inappropriate"; 4-6 "undecided"; and 7-9 "appropriate". Panelists rating a statement as "inappropriate" were required to give a specific reason and, if possible, provide a reference from the peer-reviewed literature to support it. There was unlimited space provided for panelists to make comments, and the project coordinator entered all comments into a Word file, identified by ID number, rating and seed statement number. The project coordinator entered the numerical ratings into an SPSS v. 21.0 database and one of the investigators (CH) analyzed the results, computing the median rating and percentages of agreement for each statement. We considered consensus present when both the median rating was 7 or higher and at least 80% of the panelists gave a rating of 7 or higher. Rounds were to be repeated until consensus was reached.

The core committee reviewed all comments and revised the statements on which consensus was not reached, based on the panelists' comments. The project coordinator then circulated the revised statements, along with the de-identified comments, to the entire panel for the next round.

Delphi process and panelist summary

The Delphi process was conducted from August-October 2013. Fifteen panelists of the 16 participated in each of the two Delphi rounds, although one panelist of the 16 participated in only Round 1 and a different panelist only participated in Round 2. Consensus on all was reached on 38 of the 43 statements after one round, and consensus on the remaining 5 statements after the second round.

Results: consensus guidelines

The following section contains the consensus-based guideline statements. It provides the statements that are the result of the consensus process, which is therefore the complete guideline on for the practice and performance of manipulation under anesthesia.

General guideline disclaimer

This guideline is intended for practitioners, facilities, and other interested parties. Decisions to adopt particular courses of action must be made by trained practitioners on the basis of the available resources and the particular circumstances of the individual patient. This guideline is not to be applied to any specific patient, in any manner, and any decision requiring necessary testing, patient candidacy or follow-up procedures must be made by the individual doctor and determined by the needs of the patient. Safety and effectiveness should drive the doctor's decision when considering Manipulation Under Anesthesia protocols. This guideline is not intended for utilization review purposes. The American Association of Manipulation Under Anesthesia Physicians denies responsibility for any injury or damage resulting from actions taken by practitioners after considering this guideline.

Protocols and standards
Patient selection: clinical candidacy for MUA

The following factors qualify a patient for clinical candidacy for MUA.

- The patient has undergone an adequate trial of appropriate care, usually including spinal manipulation by a chiropractor, and often with medical co-management, and continues to experience intractable pain, interference to activities of daily living, and/or biomechanical dysfunction.
- Sufficient care has been rendered prior to recommending MUA. A sufficient time period is usually considered a minimum of 4-8 weeks, but exceptions may apply depending on the patient's individual needs. Most patients selected for MUA procedures have had longer courses of care, but those with more severe symptoms and little or no response to conservative management are best considered sooner than later to avoid unnecessary additional costs and increased suffering.
- Physical medicine procedures have been utilized in a clinical setting during the 6-8 week period prior to recommending MUA.
- The patient's level of reproduced pain interferes with activities of daily living or causes disability (that is, the inability to fully participate in work and other activities).
- Diagnosed conditions must fall within the recognized categories of conditions responsive to MUA. The following disorders are classified as acceptable conditions for utilization of MUA:
  1) Patients for whom manipulation of the spine or other articulations is the treatment of choice; however, the patient's pain threshold inhibits the effectiveness of conservative manipulation.
  2) Patients for whom manipulation of the spine or other articulations is the treatment of choice; however, due to the extent of the injury mechanism, conservative manipulation has been minimally effective during a minimum of 4-8 weeks of care and a greater degree of movement of the affected joint(s) is needed to obtain patient progress.
  3) Patients for whom manipulation of the spine or other articulations is the treatment of choice by the doctor; however, due to the chronicity of the problem and/or the fibrous tissue adhesions present, in-office manipulation has been incomplete and the plateau in the patient's improvement is unsatisfactory.
  4) When the patient is considered for surgical intervention, MUA is an alternative and/or an interim treatment and may be used as a

therapeutic and/or diagnostic tool in the overall consideration of the patient's condition.

5) When there are no better treatment options available for the patient in the opinions of the treating doctor and patient and in consideration of the cause of the patient's related pain, impairment, and/or disability.

Diagnosis
Establishing medical necessity
Every condition treated must be diagnosed and justified by clinical documentation in order to establish medical necessity. Documentation of the patient's progress and the patient's response to treatment are combined to confirm the working diagnosis. Those diagnoses which are most responsive to MUA include, but are not limited to the following:

- Sclerotogenous pain from the medial branch of the dorsal rami.
- Cervical, thoracic, lumbar, sacroiliac, and sacrococcygeal sprain/strain subluxations (neuromechanical dysfunctions) with or without resultant myofascial pain syndromes.
- Intervertebral disc syndromes without fragment, sequestration, or any contraindication to in-office manipulative procedures and with or without radiculopathy.
- Cervical brachial pain syndrome.
- Chronic recurrent cervicogenic headaches, after ruling out pathologic etiologies (for example, organic brain syndromes, or other vascular or neurological syndromes).
- Failed back surgeries with adhesion formation in a patient who has not adequately responded to clinical therapeutic trials of manipulation, traction, and soft tissue techniques (including but not limited to myofascial release).
- Adhesive capsulitis and/or soft tissue contractures relative to articular motion of the appendicular skeleton, e.g. shoulder and knee.
- Functional biomechanical dysfunction syndromes (including but not limited to sprain/strain with fixation and vertebral subluxation complex). Functional radiography and particularly lateral bending, weightbearing radiographs are recommended, as clinically indicated, to detect and characterize intersegmental motion restrictions in the spine.

Frequency and follow-up procedures
Determining the necessity and frequency of MUA
The following should be considered when determining the necessity and frequency of manipulation under anesthesia:

- Patient's response and progress to previous conservative care.
- Consideration of activities of daily living and disability.
- Patient's psychological acceptance of the MUA procedure, and psychosomatic response to overcoming chronic pain and discomfort.
- Prevention of additional gross deterioration.
- Prevention of possible surgical intervention.
- Chronicity.
- Length of current treatment and patient progress.
- Patient's age.
- Number of previous injuries to the same area.
- Level of pain considering standard 4-8 week minimum protocol parameters and deciding whether a variation from the guidelines may be appropriate for the individual patient's needs.
- Patient's tolerance of previous treatment procedures and their success or failures.
- Muscle contraction level (beyond splinting).
- Response to previous MUA's based on objective clinical documentation and protocols for determining patient progress.
- Fibrous adhesion from failed back surgery or prior injury.
- Patient willingness and availability to participate in appropriate post-procedures follow-up to optimize results.

Protocols for determining the frequency of the MUA procedure
A treatment plan of three consecutive days of treatment is recommended, on the rationale that serial procedures allow a gentler yet effective treatment plan with better control of biomechanical force resulting in increased safety, and more focused and effective subsequent procedures after monitoring the effects of those administered previously.

Ranges of motion should always be measured after an appropriate warm-up period for consistency and as recommended within the American Medical Association Impairment Guidelines.

- Single spinal MUA is most often recommended for younger patients; when the area to be treated has not been previously injured; and when the verifiable global and intersegmental motion restrictions are relatively mild.
- Single spinal MUA is most often recommended when conservative care has been rendered for a sufficient time (usually a 4-6 week minimum) and the patient's activities of daily living or work activities are interrupted in such a fashion as to warrant a more aggressive approach.

- If the patient is treated for intractable pain with a single MUA procedure and responds with 80% symptomatic and functional resolution, the necessity for future MUA's should be considered and depends in part on the objective parameters determined during and after the MUA procedures.
- Serial MUA is recommended when the patient's condition is chronic and when conservative care as described in this guideline has been rendered.
- Serial MUA is recommended when the injury is recurrent in nature and fibrotic tissue and articular fixation prevents a single MUA from being optimally effective.

Parameters for determining MUA progress

Parameters for determining MUA progress may include, but are not limited to:

- Subjective changes
- Patient's pain index, visual analogue scale, faces of pain.
- Patient's ability to engage in active range of motion.
- Patient's change in activities of daily living.
- Patient's change in job performance.
- Objective changes
- Change in measurable muscle mass, function, and strength.
- Change in muscle contractibility.
- Change in EMG and/or nerve conduction studies.
- Change in controlled measurable passive range of motion.
- Change in diagnostic studies (X-rays, CT, MRI), including functional radiography.

General post MUA therapy
Therapy following first MUA

- Repeat MUA stretching.
- Physiotherapeutic modalities as indicated by patient presentation.
- Patient to rest at home with walking and range of motion exercises encouraged to patient tolerance.

Therapy following subsequent MUAs

- Same as 1st day.
- No further manipulation should be required.
- May add proprioceptive neurofacilitation protocols. These can be incorporated during stretching if tolerated.

Therapy following last MUA

- Same protocol as above with proprioceptive neurofacilitation.

- Additional home instructions to include range of motion and strengthening exercises as condition permits and to patient tolerance can be provided to the patient at this time.

Follow-up therapy following MUA—one week after last MUA

Treatment frequency during the first week should be 3-4 days dependent on the individual patient's needs. These follow-up procedures should include all fibrosis release and manipulative procedures performed during the MUA procedure to help prevent re-adhesion.

Follow-up therapy following MUA—weeks 2 and 3 after last MUA

- Continue full protocols to include fibrosis release procedures, proprioceptive neurofacilitation, and manipulative procedures as needed to maintain global and intersegmental motion improvements obtained during the MUA procedure.
- Begin home rehabilitation exercises 2-3 times per week.

Follow-up therapy following MUA—weeks 7-8 after last MUA

- Continue full protocol (fibrosis release procedures, proprioceptive neurofacilitation and manipulative procedures).
- Patient treated 1-2 times per week for 4-5 weeks depending on patient needs.
- Active progressive resistive strength/stabilization exercises, supervised/unsupervised 2-3 times per week; optimal rehabilitative procedures should include attention to aerobic, flexibility, strength, and coordination considerations.

Safety
Physicians and co-attending doctors should be appropriately certified. Both patient and doctor safety are important factors to be taken into consideration.

Patient safety
MUA is performed using the anesthesia techniques determined by the anesthesiologist to be appropriate for the patient. MUA is performed with the patient in a sedated state as determined safe and effective by the attending anesthesiologist. The chiropractic providers do not make any decisions regarding the medical management nor do they direct or use any of the medications required by the anesthesiologist during his or her medical management.

The primary doctor and the co-attending doctor move the patient into specific ranges of motion to accomplish the procedure. In this capacity, the patient depends on the primary doctor and co-attending doctor to protect them from bodily injury. Since the patient is only minimally responsive to painful stimuli and does not have the ability to respond to immediate proprioceptive input, both the primary doctor and the co-attending doctor are key to a safe and successful procedure.

The co-attending doctor is responsible for patient stability, patient movement, patient observation, and completing portions of the procedure should the primary doctor need assistance or become unable to perform the procedure. Since there are several instances during the procedure when the primary doctor has to move the patient, stabilizing and working with the patient would be unsafe without assistance from another doctor competent and knowledgeable in MUA.

Doctor safety

Manipulation under anesthesia is a very physically demanding therapeutic procedure. Since the patient is in a sedated state, the doctor has the added responsibility of insuring that the patient's extremities and torso do not fall from the treating surface. The doctor must also be able to move the patient without the assistance of the patient.

The co-attending doctor is an integral part of this procedure and is responsible for helping the primary doctor move the patient through the prescribed ranges of motion. The co-attending doctor is present to insure that all movements are accomplished without injury to the patient or to the primary doctor performing the procedure. As a result of the added potential risk to the patient in a sedated state, there is a high risk of injury to the doctor and the patient if only one doctor were to attempt the complex techniques necessary for the MUA procedure. Inclusion of a co-attending doctor, who is a certified MUA practitioner, is the safest way to perform this procedure. It may be unsafe to perform an MUA without a competent and knowledgeable MUA doctor as the co-attending doctor and anything other than allowing another MUA certified doctor to act as a co-attending doctor imposes potential risks. By using a certified MUA practitioner as a co-attending doctor, optimal effectiveness and safety standards are maintained. This is proper standard of care policy for the MUA procedure and needs to be recognized as such by anyone recommending MUA, or reimbursing for MUA.

In the cervical spine, the co-attending doctor must secure the patient's shoulders and provide counterforce procedures to obtain the necessary traction for this part of the procedure. In the thoracic spine, the co-attending doctor turns the patient, stabilizes the patient and applies proper counter traction for the MUA maneuvers. In the lumbosacral area, the co-attending doctor coordinates movements with the primary doctor, assists with

the actual procedures, and can complete the MUA procedures as necessary. Procedure efficacy is enhanced when both doctors are trained and knowledgeable regarding the appropriate forces and counterforces required to perform safe and effective MUA procedures.

A certified MUA physician carries the appropriate malpractice insurance to perform MUA and so does his or her co-attending doctor. Since non-certified assistants may not carry malpractice insurance for MUA, utilization of ancillary staff to assist with the MUA procedure may potentially place the entire team and the facility at risk. Therefore, only a certified MUA practitioner should co-attend the MUA procedure.

Facilities

All MUA procedures should be performed in the highest quality facility available and within the parameters of state regulations. MUA should only be performed in hospitals, ambulatory surgery centers or other specialty centers that meet the American Society of Anesthesiology standards, and adhere to recognized standards of care.

Compensation

Fees must be reasonable and in relation to standards and relative values within each state. The CPT codes used for spinal MUA include but are not limited to 22505, 20999, 23700, 27275. It is recommended that chiropractic/medical necessity and authorization be obtained prior to scheduling the patient. Fees should be reasonable and in keeping with standard fee structures.

Anesthesia standards for outpatient MUA

- Anesthesia is provided under the direct supervision of a board-certified anesthesiologist or other osteopathic or medical physician based on applicable state law. The MUA certified chiropractors limit their involvement to procedures within their scope of practice which may vary from state to state.
- The anesthesia provided must adhere to guidelines and recommendations accepted in his/her community for delivering anesthesia to patients.

Pre-MUA anesthetics procedures

- Patients are appropriately evaluated by their chiropractic or MUA doctors to assess candidacy prior to the procedure. Anesthesiologists will typically perform a history and physical prior to the procedure and may elect to not go forward with and may cancel the procedure if they feel that the patient might be at risk from a medical standpoint.

- All appropriate clearance forms, laboratory results, imaging reports and other supported data are available for review in the patient's chart. Special testing should be provided only as deemed necessary and based on individual needs. Since the fibrosis release from manipulative procedures performed during MUA carries similar risks as chiropractic in-office procedures, the need for diagnostic tests is commonly determined using similar criteria as might be performed during in-office care with physical methods. Individual laboratory testing or special testing requirements may differ from state to state or from facility to facility.

Intra-MUA anesthetics procedures

- The anesthesiologist selects the anesthesia based on the patient's medical condition and is responsible for all medical decisions.
- The chiropractic doctor does not order or administer any medications.
- Blood pressure, oxygen saturation and EKG are recorded by the anesthesiologist, or at his/her direction, throughout the procedure.
- Supplemental oxygen is available in case it is needed.
- Resuscitate equipment and medications must be readily available at all times.
- An emergency facility must be available locally pursuant to state and accreditation agency requirements.

Post-MUA anesthetics procedures

- The anesthesia provider is responsible for the medical discharge of the patient.
- Once the patient is stable, the anesthesia provider may depart as long as there is a trained Advanced Cardiac Life Support (ACLS) provider present in the facility and pursuant to local regulations and patient needs.

Nursing standards—patient care responsibilities
Pre-MUA nursing patient care responsibilities

- Witness signature of procedure consent.
- Verify and document NPO compliance.
- Verify responsible adult driver or escort is available for the patient.
- Verify and document present medications and allergies.
- Direct and assist the patient with appropriate attire for procedure.
- Escort the patient and medical chart to procedure room.

Intra-MUA nursing patient care responsibilities

- Direct and assist patient in transferring to the procedure table.
- Maintain patient safety, privacy and dignity.
- Complete appropriate medical record forms.
- Be available to assist anesthesia provider as needed.
- Be available to assist MUA providers as needed.
- Assist in transferring the patient to a recovery bed.
- Raise the bed's side rails for patient safety as required.

Post-MUA nursing patient care responsibilities

- Transport patient to recovery room with anesthesia provider.
- Receive report from anesthesia provider including medications given, vital signs, IV history and any other pertinent information.
- Secure appropriate monitoring equipment.
- Record vital signs on admission to recovery area and every 15 minutes until stable and then every 30 minutes until discharge.
- When the patient is conscious and alert, oral fluids may be offered.
- When the patient is tolerating fluids, a light snack may be offered.
- When the patient is tolerating foods and fluids well and vital signs have remained stable for 15 minutes, the IV/heparin lock may be discontinued.
- The patient may then be discharged to their responsible adult escort/driver with written instructions for activity and follow-up care.

Discussion

Similar to many other treatments available for spinal conditions, MUA does not have the unequivocal support for effectiveness and efficacy that would be provided by multiple randomized controlled trials and meta-analyses. If proven alternatives that addressed these same conditions were available, other choices would be recommended prior to considering MUA.

However, there is a fair amount of lower-level evidence in regards to the safety and efficacy of this procedure. This led Dagenais et al. in their systematic review to state: "However, almost all studies to date on these procedures have reported positive results, indicating that patients who undergo their procedures have a reasonable prognosis" [3], p. 148.

In the absence of strong evidence, this guideline was designed to provide recommendations on best practices of MUA for interested and affected parties; namely, patients, doctors, and payers.

When a doctor or patient considers MUA, he/she is commonly comparing the appropriateness of this procedure to many other procedures with a similar evidence level for support. Kohlbeck, et al., in their systematic review expressed this consideration for practitioners:

"Medicine-assisted spinal manipulation therapies have a relatively long history of clinical use and have been reported in the literature for over 70 years. However, evidence for effectiveness of these protocols remains largely anecdotal, based on case series mimicking many other surgical and conservative approaches for the treatment of chronic pain syndromes of musculoskeletal origin. There is, however, sufficient theoretical basis and positive results from the case series to warrant further controlled trials on these techniques" [2], [p. 288].

Payers are also faced with challenges when considering reimbursement for MUA procedures. This is also summarized by Kohlbeck, et al. as follows:

"If a clinician recommends or offers, and a payer reimburses, surgery, injections, epidurals, and certain physical therapy approaches, to a patient without requiring substantial proof of effectiveness and safety, then it would be difficult to deny the use of medication-assisted manipulation or fail to reimburse for it... It would seem unreasonable, however, to hold medication-assisted manipulation to a higher standard of scientific rigor than that required of other treatment approaches" [2], [p. 301].

The Delphi panel who developed this guideline was composed of experienced physicians, nurses and educators, both practitioners of MUA and practitioners who do not practice MUA but are experienced in the treatment of spine-related pain. This group reached a high level (80%) of consensus on recommendations related to the practice of MUA. This lends clinical validity to the recommendations and therefore should guide MUA practitioners. This guideline is not intended to be prescriptive, or to suggest that MUA is the only therapy of choice when seeking relief for spinal dysfunction and pain. It is intended to provide practitioners with evidence-informed, consensus-based parameters guiding the use of MUA.

Competing interests
The American Association of Manipulation Under Anesthesia Providers provided consultant fees for Dr. Hawk's role on the project. She served as an independent contractor to the project, which is not associated with her position at Logan University. RG and EC have no financial interest in any part of the process and have not received any remuneration for their part in this project. Both RG and EC practice manipulation under anesthesia and teach it in post-graduate education. The authors declare that they have no competing interests.

Authors' contributions
RG developed the original seed statements, contributed to the literature search, participated in conducting the Delphi rounds, and was the primary author of the paper. EC also developed the original seed statements, contributed to the literature search, participated in conducting the Delphi rounds, and contributed to writing the paper. CH conducted the Delphi rounds, contributed to the literature search and contributed to writing the paper. All authors read and approved the final manuscript.

Acknowledgements
The authors thank Michelle Anderson for coordinating the conduct of the Delphi process, and the Delphi panelists for generously contributing their time and expertise to the consensus process: Donald Alosio, DC; E. Graham Baker, Jr, JD; Ulyss Bidkaram, DC; Ian Brown, MD; Charles Davis, DC; Sarb Dhesi, DC; Robert Francis, DC; Kathryn Hoiriis, DC; Michael Hubka, DC; Tom Hyde, DC; Rita Iwanski, RN; John LaFalce, DC; Ramses Nashed, MD; Michael Ramcharan, DC, MPH; Susan Rhodes, RN; Richard Skala, DC; Ronald Wellikoff, DC; David Wolstein, MD.

Author details
[1]Cornerstone Professional Education, Inc, 4002 Streamlet Way, 28110 Monroe, NC, USA. [2]Palmer College of Chiropractic West, San Jose, CA, USA. [3]Fremont Chiropractic Group, Fremont, CA, USA. [4]Logan University, 1851 Schoettler Rd 63017 Chesterfield, MO, USA.

Received: 21 November 2013 Accepted: 1 February 2014
Published: 3 February 2014

References
1. Greenman PE: Manipulation with the patient under anesthesia. *J Am Osteopath Assoc* 1992, **92:**1159–1160. 1167–1170.
2. Kohlbeck FJ, Haldeman S: Medication-assisted spinal manipulation. *Spine J* 2002, **2:**288–302.
3. Dagenais S, Mayer J, Wooley JR, Haldeman S: Evidence-informed management of chronic low back pain with medicine-assisted manipulation. *Spine J* 2008, **8:**142–149.
4. Cremata E, Collins S, Clauson W, Solinger AB, Roberts ES: Manipulation under anesthesia: a report of four cases. *J Manipulative Physiol Ther* 2005, **28:**526–533.
5. Haldeman S, Chapman-Smith D, Petersen DJ (Eds): *Guidelines for Chiropractic Quality Assurance and Practice Parameters.* Gaithersburg, Maryland: Aspen Publishers; 1993.
6. Digiorgi D: Spinal manipulation under anesthesia: a narrative review of the literature and commentary. *Chiropractic Man Ther* 2013, **21:**14.
7. Driever MJ: Are evidence-based practice and best practice the same? *West J Nurs Res* 2002, **24:**591–597.
8. Manchikanti L, Boswell MV, Giordano J: Evidence-based interventional pain management: principles, problems, potential and applications. *Pain Physician* 2007, **10:**329–356.
9. Francis R: Spinal manipulation under general anesthesia: a chiropractic approach in a hospital setting. *J Chiropr* 1989, **26:**39–41.
10. Kirkaldy-Willis W, Burton CV: *Managing low back pain.* New York: Churchill Livingstone; 1992.
11. Gordon R, Rogers A, West D, Mathews R, Miller M: Pain management: a practical guide for clinicians, 6th ed. In *MUA: an anthology of past, present, and future use.* Edited by Weiner RS. Sonora, CA: American Academy of Pain Management; 2001.
12. Gordon RC: An evaluation of the experimental and investigational status and clinical validity of manipulation of patients under anesthesia: a contemporary opinion. *J Manipulative Physiol Ther* 2001, **24:**603–611.
13. Francis R, Beckett RH: Spinal manipulation under anesthesia. In *Advances in Chiropractic. Volume 1.* Edited by Lawrence DL. St. Louis: Mosby; 1994:325–340.
14. Gordon R: Support for MUA: evidence-based research and literature review. In *Manipulation Under Anesthesia, Concepts In Theory and Application.* Edited by RC G. Boca Raton, FL: CRC Press/Taylor and Francis; 2005:113–122.
15. Russo F: Post-therapy MUA physical therapy and rehabilitation guidelines. In *Manipulation Under Anesthesia, Concepts In Theory and Application.* Edited by RC G. Boca Raton, FL: CRC Press/Taylor and Francis; 2005:211–225.
16. Wright JG, Swiontkowski MF, Heckman JD: Introducing levels of evidence to the journal. *J Bone Joint Surg Am* 2003, **85-A:**1–3.
17. Wright JG: A practical guide to assigning levels of evidence. *J Bone Joint Surg Am* 2007, **89:**1128–1130.
18. Kohlbeck FJ, Haldeman S, Hurwitz EL, Dagenais S: Supplemental care with medication-assisted manipulation versus spinal manipulation therapy alone for patients with chronic low back pain. *J Manipulative Physiol Ther* 2005, **28:**245–252.

19. Palmieri NF, Smoyak S: **Chronic low back pain: a study of the effects of manipulation under anesthesia.** *J Manipulative Physiol Ther* 2002, **25**:E8–E17.

20. Siehl D, Olson DR, Ross HE, Rockwood EE: **Manipulation of the lumbar spine with the patient under general anesthesia: evaluation by electromyography and clinical-neurologic examination of its use for lumbar nerve root compression syndrome.** *J Am Osteopath Assoc* 1971, **70**:433–440.

21. McDonald W, Durkin KF, Pfefer M: **How chiropractors think and practice: the survey of North American chiropractors.** *Semin Integr Med* 2004, **2**:92–98.

22. Fitch K, Bernstein SJ, Aquilar MS, Burnand B, LaCalle JR, Lazaro P, van het Loo M, McDonnell J, Vader J, McDonnell J: *The RAND UCLA Appropriateness Method User's Manual.* Santa Monica, CA: RAND Corp; 2003.

2

The correlation of radiographic findings and patient symptomatology in cervical degenerative joint disease: a cross-sectional study

Iris Sun Rudy, Alexandra Poulos, Laura Owen, Ashlee Batters, Kasia Kieliszek, Jessica Willox and Hazel Jenkins[*]

Abstract

Background: There are few known studies investigating the correlation of symptomatology with the specific subtypes of cervical spine degenerative joint disease demonstrated on radiograph. The aim of this study was to assess the correlation and diagnostic test accuracy of specific symptoms in determining the presence, type and severity of degenerative joint disease on radiograph.

Methods: A retrospective cross-sectional design was used to correlate cervical radiographic findings with neck pain and related symptomatology. Radiographs of 322 patients from April 2010 to June 2012 were assessed and evidence of radiographic cervical degenerative joint disease was extracted. Clinical data for each patient was obtained from their patient files including: pain using a VAS, presence of neck stiffness, presence of headaches, presence of shoulder referral, presence of hand radiculopathy and presence of hand numbness. Measures of diagnostic test accuracy and regression analysis were used to assess for any correlation between symptoms and radiographic findings.

Results: Referral of pain to the shoulder and neck stiffness showed small degrees of correlation with cervical degenerative joint disease, however, these correlations were not maintained when age was accounted for. Only age showed consistent statistical significance as a predictor for degree of disc degeneration (correlation coefficient (95% confidence interval): 0.06 (0.055, 0.066)); the presence of facet hypertrophy (odds ratio (95% confidence interval): 1.12 (1.09, 1.15)); or uncinate process hypertrophy (odds ratio (95% confidence interval): 1.15 (1.12, 1.18)). Neck stiffness demonstrated a small degree of diagnostic test accuracy for the degree of cervical disc degeneration (area under the curve (95%CI): 0.62 (0.56, 0.68)) and the presence of either facet (diagnostic OR (95%CI):1.69 (1.04, 2.76)) and uncinated process hypertrophy (LR+ (95%CI): 1.17 (1.00, 1.38)).

Conclusion: The results of this study indicate that clinical symptoms such as pain level, headaches, shoulder referral and hand radiculopathy or numbness are not reliably correlated with radiographic findings of degenerative joint disease in the cervical spine. A small increase in diagnostic accuracy between the presence of neck stiffness and all forms of cervical degenerative joint disease is shown, however, this increase is not at the level expected to change clinical practice.

Keywords: Degenerative joint disease, Osteoarthritis, Cervical spine, Neck pain, Neck stiffness, Sensitivity and specificity

* Correspondence: hazel.jenkins@mq.edu.au
Macquarie University, Sydney, Australia

Background

Neck pain is a widespread entity that affects a large majority of the population. The prevalence is greatest amongst middle-aged people, with approximately 66% of individuals experiencing neck pain and related symptoms at some stage in their lives [1,2]. Neck pain is also the second most frequent musculoskeletal complaint presenting to primary healthcare practitioners [3] and most people with neck pain do not experience a complete resolution of symptoms [4]. Although there is a large prevalence of neck pain, neck pain is difficult to diagnose [4] and therefore, to treat.

Among the many causes of neck pain, degenerative joint disease of the cervical spine is a common condition affecting the synovial joints [5] with a prevalence of 3.3 cases per 1000 people [6]. It is characterised by a series of degenerative changes comprising intradiscal tears with subsequent disc space loss, osteophytic growths and spur formation, ligamentous hypertrophy and capsular thickening [7]. Cervical spine degenerative joint disease occurs mostly in 4th and 5th decades and is associated with the natural aging process [8]. It also varies in presentation, with the most common complaints consisting of neck pain, activity related neck stiffness, headaches and upper limb referral [7].

Magnetic resonance imaging (MRI) remains the most advanced assessment tool to evaluate degenerative changes, however the costs and accessibility to this type of imaging requires clinicians to differentiate those patients that require this level of investigation. Plain film radiography is the most commonly used modality to diagnose degenerative joint disease [9], however the literature indicates that radiographic findings do not correlate well with pain and symptoms [10,11]. It also has been suggested that the use of plain film radiography based solely on the suspicion of detecting degenerative changes is not clinically justified [12,11].

Marchiori and Henderson [13] compared radiographic findings of spinal degeneration with severity and chronicity of cervical pain and any resulting lifestyle changes in 700 consecutive patients referred for a cervical radiographic examination. The authors concluded that increasing levels of spinal degeneration are related to increased chronicity of patient complaints. Gore et al. [14] in 1987 completed an investigation in 205 patients previously seen for a neck complaint. A follow up radiographic examination was conducted after a minimum of ten years to assess for subsequent spinal degeneration. The results concluded no significant relationship between the degree of spinal degeneration and patient symptoms at either initial presentation or at follow up. Heller et al. [11] examined the relation between symptoms and changes seen on radiograph in a hospital setting. Using the symptoms of pain in the arm or shoulder, shoulder blade, neck, and back of the head and stiffness in the neck, they concluded

that there were few and inconsistent relationships between symptoms and changes on radiograph. However, they did not examine whether hallmark symptoms could be predicting factors in diagnosing the severity or grade of cervical degenerative joint disease.

The aim of this study was to assess for correlation and the diagnostic test accuracy of hallmark symptoms in determining the presence, type and severity of cervical degenerative joint disease on radiograph.

Methods

Sample selection

The subjects included in this study were patients attending one of three Macquarie University Chiropractic Teaching Clinics who had cervical radiographs taken between April 2010 to June 2012. Of the 502 studies taken in this period, 180 were excluded, as they were: under 18 years of age, had incomplete or absent patient files or the cervical radiographic quality was too poor to interpret (non-diagnostic). This study complies with national research ethics guidelines and was approved by the Macquarie University Human Research Ethics Committee (HREC), approval number: 5201300294.

Data collection

Two members of the research team accessed the chiropractic clinic's radiographic report database to find all cervical spine radiographs taken within the selected time period. The radiographic reports were assessed and the following information was recorded: name, date of birth, gender and presence of degenerative joint disease (Yes/No) on cervical anteroposterior (AP) and lateral views. The AP and lateral radiographs reported to have signs of cervical degenerative joint disease were then accessed and graded using the Kellgren and Lawrence Osteoarthritis Severity Grading System [15-17] by the same two research members. The presence of facet hypertrophy and uncinate process hypertrophy was also recorded (Yes/No). The assessed radiographic reports were reported by chiropractic radiologists at the time of imaging. The two members of the research team assessing the radiographs for the grading of degenerative joint disease were both in their final year of chiropractic studies.

The names of the included patients were then provided to three other research team members, also in their final year of chiropractic studies, uninvolved with the radiographic data collection to preserve blinding. These researchers located the corresponding patient files in the clinics and extracted clinical data taken at the time of cervical radiographic referral, relating to the following: cervical pain levels (measured on the visual analogue scale (VAS)); the presence (Yes/No) as reported by the patient of: headaches, neck stiffness, pain referral to shoulders, radicular symptoms to the hands and numbness in the hands. Data pertaining to initial consultation, previous treatment or management plans was not recorded.

The recorded data was allocated to an independent group member, also in their final year of chiropractic studies, with no involvement in the radiographic or clinical data collection processes, to analyse and compare the results. Intra- and inter-observer reproducibility on the radiographic evaluations and extraction of clinical data was not performed, however, the radiographic evaluations were performed independently by two members of the research team. Results were compared and any discrepancies were discussed and arbitrated by the group supervisor, a chiropractic radiologist. Extraction of clinical data was from standardised files used in a chiropractic teaching institution. Files were excluded from analysis if they had incomplete or ambiguous data with respect to the symptoms being assessed.

Instruments

Kellgren and Lawrence osteoarthritis severity grade

Disc degeneration is a component of cervical degenerative joint disease. Kellgren developed certain criteria to classify and grade disc degeneration in the spine [15-17]. It uses the presence and severity of osteophytes, disc space narrowing and sclerosis to grade the level of degenerative disc disease present within a vertebral level on a grade of 1to 4 as outlined in Table 1. This assessment tool was selected based on its accuracy, reproducibility and recent validation for osteoarthritis in the cervical spine [18].

Presence of facet joint hypertrophy and uncinate process hypertrophy

These radiographic findings are also components of cervical degenerative joint disease [5]. Disc degeneration, facet joint hypertrophy and uncinate process hypertrophy may occur independently or in combination with each other. There is no known grading scale for facet joint and uncinate process hypertrophy, therefore the presence or absence of these findings was assessed (Yes/No).

Visual Analogue Scale (VAS)

The VAS is a subjective measurement of a person's pain intensity on a scale of 0 (no pain) to 10 (worst pain you have ever felt). This scale was used as it's a commonly implemented tool for patients presenting at the student

clinics. The VAS is also considered valid, reliable and appropriate for clinical use [19,20].

Presence of headaches, neck stiffness, referral to shoulder, radicular symptoms in hands and numbness in hands

These symptoms are common complaints associated with cervical degenerative joint disease which are well described in the literature [5]. The presence of these symptoms was recorded (Yes/No) as reported in the clinical files at the time of radiographic referral.

Data analysis

Linear or logistic regression analysis was used to assess for correlations between radiographic findings of cervical degenerative joint disease as the dependent variable and independent predictor variables. The independent predictor variables assessed were: gender, age, VAS, presence of neck stiffness, presence of headache, presence of shoulder referral and presence of hand radiculopathy or numbness.

Diagnostic accuracy testing was used to assess dichotomous data. Dichotomous data included the presence of facet hypertrophy and uncinate hypertrophy as dependent variables. These were tested for positive and negative correlations to the presence or absence of headache, neck stiffness, shoulder referral, hand radiculopathy and hand numbness as predictor variables. Sensitivity, specificity, positive predictive value (PPV), negative predictive value (NPV), positive likelihood ratio (LR+), negative likelihood ratio (LR-) and diagnostic odds ratios (OR) were calculated with 95% confidence intervals (95%CI).

ROC curves were used to assess for the diagnostic test accuracy of continuous data compared to dichotomous data. Comparisons were made between the grade of disc degeneration as a dependent variable and the presence of headache, shoulder pain, neck stiffness, hand radiculopathy or hand numbness as independent predictor variables. The area under the ROC curve with 95%CI was calculated to assess for statistical significance of the diagnostic test accuracy.

Results

322 subjects were included in the study. Of these, 162 (50.3%) subjects were male, the mean age was 40.5 (standard deviation 17.4) and 78 (24.2%) subjects had no radiographic signs of cervical degenerative joint disease.

Table 1 Kellgren-Lawrence grading scale [15]

Grade 0	No signs of degenerative disc disease
Grade 1	Minimal anterior osteophytes
Grade 2	Definite anterior osteophytosis with possible narrowing of the disc space and some sclerosis of vertebral plates
Grade 3	Moderate narrowing of the disc space with definite sclerosis of vertebral plates and osteophytes
Grade 4	Severe narrowing of the disc space with definite sclerosis of vertebral plates and multiple large osteophytes

Table 2 outlines the distribution of radiographic findings degenerative joint disease in the cervical spine.

Kellgren Lawrence grade of cervical disc degeneration

Linear regression analysis was conducted to examine the relationship between the Kellgren Lawrence grade of disc degeneration and the independent predictor variables. A significant trend could only be extrapolated for age as an independent variable. As demonstrated in Figure 1, the correlation coefficient (95%CI) of 0.06 (0.055, 0.066) shows a positive trend and variation around the regression line is acceptable as indicated by the R^2-value of 0.61. This indicates that for every 16.7 years a person ages, their grade of cervical disc degeneration is expected to increase by 1 on the Kellgren Lawrence grading scale.

Assessment of diagnostic accuracy between the Kellgren Lawrence grade of disc degeneration and specified symptomatologies was performed using ROC curves. The presence of neck stiffness and the presence of shoulder referral did show mild evidence of diagnostic accuracy in predicting disc degeneration as depicted in Figures 2 and 3. The area under the curve (95%CI) measured 0.62 (0.56, 0.68) and 0.60 (0.54, 0.67) respectively. Although these values were statistically significant the clinical significance is uncertain as these values do not represent high levels of diagnostic accuracy. The area under the curve (Area under curve (95%CI)) for headaches (0.43 (0.36, 0.50)), hand radiculopathy (0.57 (0.47, 0.67)) and hand numbness (0.57 (0.47, 0.68)) did not exhibit statistical significance. Therefore, the presence of headaches, hand radiculopathy and hand numbness did not predict the grade of disc degeneration on cervical radiograph.

Presence of cervical facet joint hypertrophy

Logistic regression analysis was conducted to examine the relationship between presence of facet joint hypertrophy and the independent predictor variables. Only age showed a significant relationship with an odds ratio (95%CI) of 1.12 (1.09, 1.15). Therefore, for every year increase in age the odds of having facet hypertrophy increase by 1.12.

Table 3 depicts the diagnostic accuracy outcomes for the presence of facet joint hypertrophy and the presence

of specified symptomatologies. The presence of neck stiffness was the only symptom to demonstrate statistically significant diagnostic accuracy with diagnostic OR (95% CI) of 1.69 (1.04, 2.76). Despite being statistically significant, however, this only represents a small increase in the odds of having facet hypertrophy on radiograph in the presence of neck stiffness. Hand radiculopathy and hand numbness both exhibited a high specificity for the presence of facet joint hypertrophy on radiograph at 0.89 (0.84, 0.93) and 0.90 (0.85, 0.94) respectively. Therefore, if there is no facet joint hypertrophy on radiograph then it is unlikely that the patient will have presented with hand radiculopathy or hand numbness.

Presence of cervical uncinate process hypertrophy

Logistic regression analysis was conducted to examine the relationship between presence of uncinate process hypertrophy and the independent predictor variables. Only age showed a significant relationship with an odds ratio (95% CI) of 1.15 (1.12, 1.18). Therefore, for every year increase in age the odds of having uncinate process hypertrophy increase by 1.15.

Table 4 depicts the diagnostic accuracy outcomes for the presence of uncinate process hypertrophy and the presence of specified symptomatologies. Neck stiffness demonstrated a small positive correlation with the presence of uncinate process hypertrophy with a sensitivity (95% CI) of 0.70 (0.61, 0.77) and LR+ (95% CI) of 1.17 (1.00, 1.38). Therefore, the presence of neck stiffness correlates with a mild increase in the odds of having uncinate process hypertrophy on radiograph. Hand radiculopathy and hand numbness both exhibited a high specificity for the presence of uncinate process hypertrophy on radiograph at 0.91 (0.85, 0.94) and 0.92 (0.87, 0.95) respectively. Therefore, if there is no uncinate process hypertrophy on radiograph then it is unlikely that the patient will have presented with hand radiculopathy or hand numbness.

Discussion

In this study, symptomatology was not correlated with the presence of cervical degenerative joint disease. The only independent predictor to show consistent significant

Table 2 Distribution of radiographic findings of cervical spine degenerative joint disease

Disc degeneration		Facet hypertrophy		Uncinate process hypertrophy	
Kellgren Lawrence grade	No. (%)	Presence (Y/N)	No. (%)	Presence (Y/N)	No. (%)
0	78 (24.2)	Y	118 (36.6)	Y	141 (43.8)
1	101 (31.4)	N	204 (63.4)	N	181 (56.2)
2	54 (16.8)				
3	45 (14)				
4	44 (13.7)				
Total	322 (100)	Total	322 (100)	Total	322 (100)

No.: Number of subjects exhibiting the finding; Y: Yes; N: No.

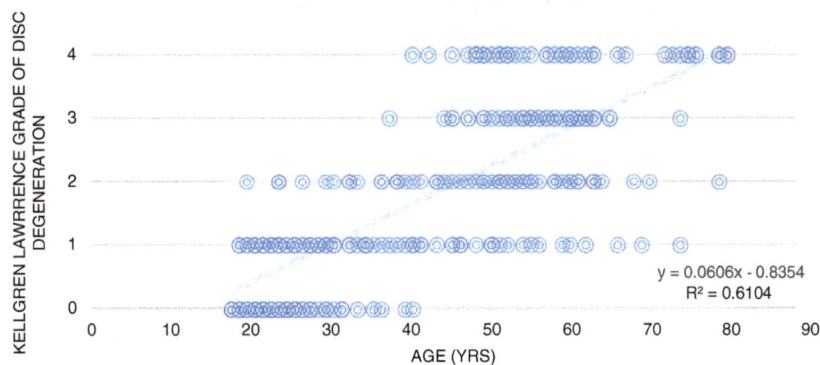

Figure 1 Correlation of disc degeneration vs age.

correlation with radiographic findings of degenerative joint disease was age. Cervical pain levels, measured by VAS, and the presence of headaches did not provide any increase in diagnostic accuracy for the presence of cervical degenerative joint disease. Hand radiculopathy and hand numbness did not show any correlations with grade of degenerative disc disease, however they did exhibit high specificity for the presence of facet joint or uncinate process hypertrophy. Although a correlation between radiographic findings and symptomatology is evident here, clinically this result does not aid the clinician in predicting the presence or absence of cervical degenerative joint disease from the presence or absence of these symptoms.

The presence of pain referring to the shoulder exhibited statistically significant but low diagnostic test accuracy with the grade of degenerative disc disease in the cervical spine. The area under the ROC curve, despite being statistically significant at 0.60 (95%CI: 0.54, 0.67), only represents a low level of accuracy in predicting radiographic findings of degenerative disc disease from the presence of shoulder referral. Similarly the accuracy of the presence of neck stiffness in predicting cervical disc degeneration also had an area under the ROC curve of 0.62 (95%CI: 0.55, 0.68), indicating a statistically significant result but of low diagnostic accuracy.

As a symptom, the presence of neck stiffness showed mild diagnostic test accuracy with all radiographic findings associated with degenerative joint disease of the cervical spine. The correlation of the presence of neck stiffness with radiographic evidence of cervical degenerative joint disease is plausible considering the combination of hypertrophic changes to the articular surfaces of

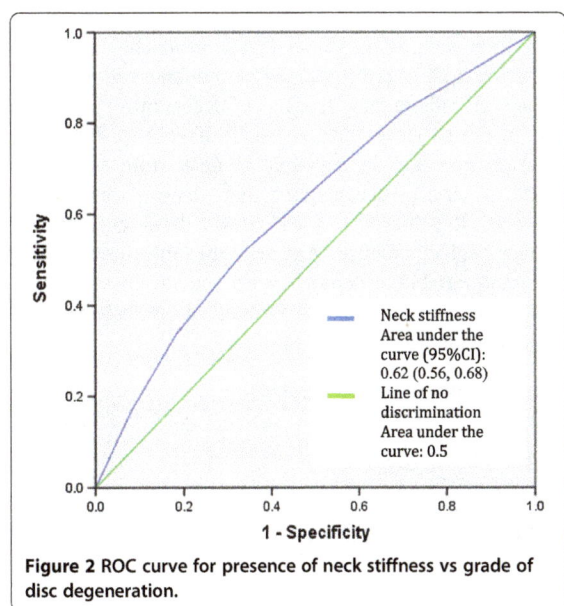

Figure 2 ROC curve for presence of neck stiffness vs grade of disc degeneration.

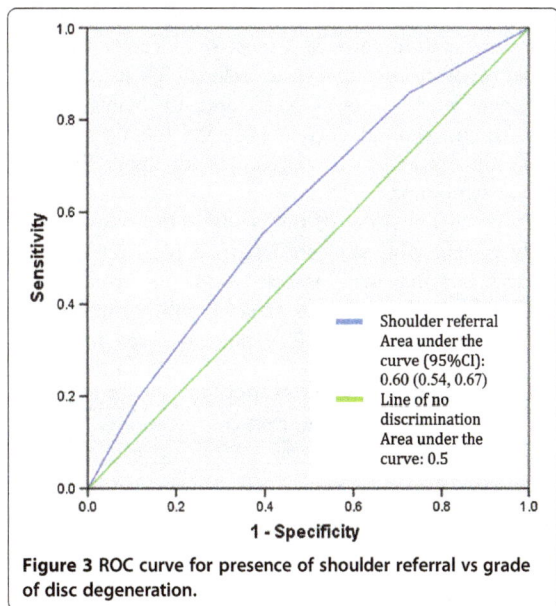

Figure 3 ROC curve for presence of shoulder referral vs grade of disc degeneration.

Table 3 Diagnostic accuracy of specified symptomatologies for facet joint hypertrophy

	Sensitivity (95%CI)	Specificity (95%CI)	PPV (95%CI)	NPV (95%CI)	LR+ (95%CI)	LR- (95%CI)
Headache	0.28 (0.21, 0.37)	0.65 (0.59, 0.71)	0.32 (0.24, 0.42)	0.61 (0.54, 0.67)	0.81 (0.57, 1.14)	1.1 (0.95, 1.28)
Neck stiffness	0.71 (0.63, 0.79)	0.4 (0.34, 0.47)	0.41 (0.34, 0.48)	0.71 (0.62, 0.78)	1.2 (1.02, 1.41)	0.71 (0.51, 0.98)
Shoulder referral	0.41 (0.32, 0.5)	0.64 (0.57, 0.7)	0.4 (0.31, 0.49)	0.64 (0.57, 0.71)	1.13 (0.85, 1.5)	0.93 (0.77, 1.11)
Hand Radiculopathy	0.14 (0.09, 0.21)	0.89 (0.84, 0.93)	0.42 (0.28, 0.58)	0.64 (0.58, 0.69)	1.26 (0.69, 2.3)	0.99 (0.89, 1.06)
Hand Numbness	0.1 (0.06, 0.17)	0.9 (0.85, 0.94)	0.36 (0.22, 0.53)	0.63 (0.58, 0.69)	0.99 (0.5, 1.94)	1.0 (0.93, 1.08)

the joints, osteophyte formation and resulting muscle tension that can cause neck stiffness [21]. However, the LR+ for both facet joint and uncinate process hypertrophy, despite exhibiting statistical significance, were at values associated with low levels of diagnostic accuracy that would not be expected to change clinical practice [22]. In addition, when regression analysis was performed, and age and gender were also accounted for, neck stiffness did not show statistically significant correlation with any form of cervical spine degenerative joint disease.

The results of this study agree with previous studies that the severity of cervical degeneration is not correlated with the degree of pain perceived [3,10,12,14]. This study adds to the body of evidence in this area by assessing the different radiographic findings associated with cervical degenerative joint disease individually and by grading the extent of degenerative disc disease using established grading criteria. Symptoms associated with cervical degenerative joint disease were also assessed individually for diagnostic accuracy. Although results were similar between disc degeneration, facet joint hypertrophy and uncinate process hypertrophy, some statistically significant differences were noted. The grade of disc degeneration correlated most significantly with the presence of neck stiffness or referral of pain to the shoulder, whereas, facet joint and uncinate process hypertrophy showed correlation with the presence of neck stiffness and high specificity with upper limb radicular symptoms.

The main limitation of this study is the retrospective study design. Only subjects who had been referred for cervical imaging were assessed and this would have skewed the sample towards subjects with symptomatology. In addition, clinical files were accessed to obtain data regarding presenting symptoms and, therefore, inter-practitioner inconsistencies when recording symptomatic data at the time of presentation could not be accounted for. Any files with missing data were excluded from the study to limit the associated bias. A prospective study would control for these limitations, however, the results of this study do not provide compelling evidence that a prospective study in this field would produce results that would lead to a change in clinical practice. Finally, this study only assessed for the presence of degeneration in any one of cervical discs, facet joints or uncovertebral joints. It did not account for presentations of multi-level or concomitant degenerative findings. These additional findings may help differentiate between levels of severity of cervical degeneration, however, a validated scale for this assessment could not be found in the current literature. Validation of a more precise scale to grade the severity of cervical degeneration may allow for further research into this area and a better understanding of any association between symptomatology and cervical degenerative joint disease.

Conclusion

In conclusion, the results of this study indicate that clinical symptoms such as pain level (VAS), headaches, shoulder referral and hand radiculopathy or numbness do not correlate with radiographic findings of degenerative joint disease in the cervical spine. A small increase in diagnostic accuracy between the presence of neck stiffness and all forms of cervical degenerative joint disease was shown. However, this increase is not at the level expected to change clinical practice. Age was the only independent predictor variable to demonstrate a statistically significant correlation with radiographic findings of cervical spine degenerative joint disease.

Table 4 Diagnostic accuracy of specified symptomatologies for uncinate process hypertrophy

	Sensitivity (95% CI)	Specificity (95% CI)	PPV (95% CI)	NPV (95% CI)	LR+ (95% CI)	LR- (95% CI)
Headache	0.3 (0.24, 0.39)	0.66 (0.59, 0.73)	0.42 (0.33, 0.51)	0.55 (0.48, 0.61)	0.91 (0.66, 1.26)	1.05 (0.9, 1.22)
Neck stiffness	0.7 (0.61, 0.77)	0.41 (0.34, 0.48)	0.48 (0.41, 0.55)	0.63 (0.54, 0.71)	1.17 (1.0, 1.38)	0.75 (0.55, 1.01)
Shoulder referral	0.44 (0.36, 0.52)	0.66 (0.59, 0.73)	0.5 (0.42, 0.59)	0.6 (0.53, 0.66)	1.23 (0.98, 1.7)	0.85 (0.71, 1.02)
Hand Radiculopathy	0.15 (0.1, 0.22)	0.91 (0.85, 0.94)	0.55 (0.4, 0.7)	0.58 (0.52, 0.63)	1.59 (0.87, 2.89)	0.94 (0.86, 1.02)
Hand Numbness	0.13 (0.08, 0.19)	0.92 (0.87, 0.95)	0.55 (0.38, 0.7)	0.57 (0.52, 0.63)	1.54 (0.81, 2.95)	0.95 (0.88, 1.03)

Consent

Written informed consent was obtained from the patient for the publication of this report and any accompanying images.

Abbreviations

AP: Anteroposterior; VAS: Visual analogue scale; PPV: Positive predictive value; NPV: Negative predictive value; LR+: Positive likelihood ratio; LR-: Negative likelihood ratio; OR: Odds ratio; 95%CI: 95% confidence intervals.

Competing interests

The authors declare that they have no competing interests.

Authors' contributions

IR was involved in the conception and design of the research, collection and interpretation of the data, and drafting and editing of the final manuscript. AP was involved in the conception and design of the research, data collection and drafting and editing of the final manuscript. LO was involved in design of the research, statistical analysis and interpretation of the data and drafting and editing of the final manuscript. AB was involved in design of the research, data collection and drafting and editing of the final manuscript. KK was involved in design of the research, data collection and editing of the final manuscript. JW was involved in design of the research, data collection and editing of the final manuscript. HJ was involved in conception, design and supervision of the research, statistical analysis and interpretation of the data and editing of the final manuscript. All authors read and approved the final manuscript.

References

1. Binder AI. Cervical spondylosis and neck pain. Br Med J. 2007;334:527–31.
2. Feder R, Hartvigsen J. Neck pain and disability due to neck pain: what is the relation? Eur Spine J. 2008;17:80–8.
3. Bovim G, Schrader H, Sand T. Neck pain in the general population. Spine (Phila Pa 1976). 1994;19(12):1307–9.
4. Abhishek A, Doherty M. Diagnosis and clinical presentation of osteoarthritis. Rheum Dis Clin North Am. 2013;39(1):45–66.
5. Haldeman S, Carroll K, Cassidy DJ, Schubert J, Nygren A. The bone and joint decade 2000–2010 task force on neck pain and its associated disorders: executive summary. Eur Spine J. 2008;17 Suppl 1:S5–7.
6. Cassidy JD, Cote P, Carrol L. The Saskatchewan health and back pain survey. The prevalence of neck pain and related disability in Saskatchewan adults. Spine (Phila Pa 1976). 1998;23(17):1860–6. discussion 1867.
7. Butler JS, Oner FC, Poynton AR, O'Byrne JM. Degenerative cervical spondylosis: a natural history, pathogenesis and current management strategies. Advances in Orthopedics. 2012;2012:916–87.
8. Lestini WF, Wiesel SW. The pathogenesis of cervical spondylosis. Clin Orthop Relat Res. 1989;239:69–93.
9. Ory PA. Radiography in the assessment of musculoskeletal conditions. Best Practice and Research Clinical Rheumatology. 2003;17(3):495–512.
10. Laplante BL, DePalma MJ. Spine osteoarthritis. Am Acad Physical Medicine and Rehabilitation. 2012;4(5 Suppl):S28–36.
11. Heller CA, Stanley P, Lewis-Jones B, Heller RF. Value of x ray examinations of the cervical spine. Br Med J (Clin Res Ed). 1983;287(6401):1276–8.
12. French SD, Walker BF, Cameron M, Pollard HP, Vitiello AL, Reggars JW, et al. Risk management for chiropractors and osteopaths: imaging guidelines for conditions commonly seen in practice. Aust Chir Osteo. 2003;11(2):41–8.
13. Marchiori DM, Henderson CNR. A cross-sectional study correlating degenerative findings to pain and disability. Spine (Phila Pa 1976). 1996;21(23):2747–51.
14. Gore DR, Sepie SB, Gardner GM, Murray PM. Neck pain: a long-term follow up of 205 patients. Spine (Phila Pa 1976). 1987;12(1):1–5.
15. Kellgren JH, Lawrence JS. Radiological assessment of osteo-arthrosis. Ann Rheum Dis. 1957;16:494–501.
16. Chapman JR, Dettori JR, Norvell DC. Spine Classifications and Severity Measures. New York: Thieme Verlag; 2009. p. 186–7.
17. Kellgren JH, Ball J. Atlas of standard radiographs: the epidemiology of chronic rheumatism, vol II. Oxford, England: Blackwell Scientific; 1963.
18. Ofiram E, Garvey TA, Schwender JD. Cervical degenerative index: a new quantitative radiographic scoring system for cervical spondylosis with interobserver and intraobserver reliability testing. J Orthop Traumatol. 2009;10(1):21–6.
19. Williamson A, Hoggart B. Pain: a review of three commonly used pain rating scales. J Clin Nurs. 2005;14:798–804.
20. Misailidou V, Paraskevi M, Beneka A, Karagiannidis A, Godolias G. Assessment of patients with neck pain: a review of definitions, selection criteria, and measurement tools. J Chiropr Med. 2010;9(2):49–59.
21. Hunter DJ. In the clinic: osteoarthritis. Ann Intern Med. 2007;147(3):ITC8-1–ITC8-16.
22. Fischer J, Bachmann L, Jaeschke R. A readers' guide to the interpretation of diagnostic test properties: clinical example of sepsis. Intensive Care Med. 2003;29:1043–51.

3

Attitudes toward drug prescription rights: a survey of Ontario chiropractors

Peter Charles Emary[1,2*] and Kent Jason Stuber[3]

Abstract

Background: Several published surveys have shown that chiropractors are generally split in their opinions regarding the right to prescribe drugs in chiropractic practice. Many of these studies have been limited by low response rates, leaving the generalizability of their findings open to question. The aim of the current study was to ascertain the general attitudes of chiropractors in Ontario, Canada toward the inclusion of drug prescription rights in their scope of practice. Relationships between these attitudes and the number of years in practice including differences in philosophical orientation were also explored.

Methods: A 14-item questionnaire was developed and invitations sent via e-mail to all eligible 2,677 chiropractors in active practice registered electronically with the College of Chiropractors of Ontario in February 2015. Data were collected and analyzed using descriptive and inferential statistics.

Results: 960 questionnaires were completed for a 36 % response rate. The majority of respondents agreed that chiropractors should be permitted to prescribe musculoskeletal medications such as over-the-counter and prescription-based analgesics, anti-inflammatories, and muscle relaxants. Over two-thirds also felt that with limited prescriptive authority chiropractors could help reduce patients' reliance on these types of drugs. Over three-quarters were opposed however to chiropractors having full prescribing rights. The majority indicated they recommend over-the-counter medications to acute and chronic patients to some extent in clinical practice. Nearly two-thirds perceived their knowledge of musculoskeletal medications as high or very high, while a similar proportion perceived their knowledge of drugs for non-musculoskeletal conditions to be low or very low. A majority of respondents felt that further education in pharmacology would be necessary for those in the profession wishing to prescribe medications. More recent graduates and those who espoused a broad scope of chiropractic practice were most in favour of limited prescribing rights for the profession.

Conclusions: A majority of responding Ontario chiropractors expressed interest in expanding their scopes of practice to include limited drug prescription. These results together with those of other recent surveys could indicate a shift in chiropractors' attitudes toward drug prescription rights within the profession. Further surveys and/or qualitative studies of chiropractors in other jurisdictions are still needed.

Keywords: Chiropractic, Attitudes, Knowledge, Drug prescription, Cross-sectional survey

* Correspondence: pcemary@hotmail.com
[1]Master of Science (MSc) Candidate, MSc Advanced Professional Practice (Clinical Sciences), Anglo-European College of Chiropractic, 13-15 Parkwood Road, Bournemouth, Dorset, BH5 2DF, UK
[2]Private Practice, 201C Preston Parkway, Cambridge, ON N3H 5E8, Canada
Full list of author information is available at the end of the article

Introduction

In some jurisdictions in the world chiropractors can gain licensure to prescribe medications from a limited formulary of over-the-counter (OTC) and/or prescription-based medications for common musculoskeletal conditions, such as non-steroidal anti-inflammatory drugs (NSAIDs), analgesics, and muscle relaxants [1, 2]. Some within the profession feel that such prescribing rights are necessary if chiropractors are to assume the role of 'primary spine care providers' within the healthcare system [3, 4]. Prescribing drugs in chiropractic nevertheless remains a contentious issue and continued incorporation of these rights into the scope of chiropractic practice has major implications for the profession.

To date several published surveys [5–9] have shown that chiropractors are generally split in their opinions regarding the right to prescribe drugs in chiropractic practice. This split in opinions is most pronounced in countries where chiropractors are not currently licensed to prescribe medications. Conversely, in jurisdictions where chiropractors are licensed to prescribe from a limited formulary, such as in Switzerland, the majority perceive this right as an advantage for the profession [1, 10]. Moreover, continuing education in pharmacology is viewed by Swiss chiropractors as a necessary component of this privilege [10].

Yet despite being divided over prescribing rights in general, there is evidence to suggest that many chiropractors often recommend OTC medications to patients in practice. For example, while just over half of respondent chiropractors from surveys in Australia [5] and Oklahoma, USA [6] were supportive of prescribing rights, between 66 % and 87 % indicated they recommend non-prescription analgesics and anti-inflammatories with variable frequency to their patients. This would suggest that chiropractors that are against prescribing rights for the profession may not be entirely averse to relevant pharmaceutical use by their patients in clinical practice. As such further investigation into the frequency of OTC drug recommendation by practising chiropractors would be informative.

Contention also exists over the scope of prescription-based drug use in chiropractic practice. In New Mexico, USA, for example, chiropractors can gain licensure to prescribe from a limited formulary of musculoskeletal medications [2]. However, chiropractors in this state have also made recent attempts to expand their current formulary to include additional prescription drugs as well as drugs to be administered by injection [11] in order for chiropractors to operate as 'primary care physicians' [12]. Concerning the issue of full prescribing rights however, evidence from the literature suggests that chiropractors are generally opposed [5, 6, 8]. In Canada, the current knowledge and attitudes of chiropractors toward full prescribing rights is unknown and research concerning limited prescribing rights is scarce.

Questions also remain as to why the chiropractic profession is split toward prescribing rights in the first place. Some evidence suggests that this division in attitudes may be reflective of differences in philosophical orientation, with so-called 'mixer' chiropractors being in favour and 'straight' chiropractors being opposed [8]. However further research is needed in order to validate these findings, particularly within the current environment of the chiropractic profession [13, 14]. Several of the aforementioned surveys [1, 5–9] have also been limited by low response rates, leaving the generalizability of their findings open to question. As such further surveys and/or qualitative research studies are warranted in order to clarify the general attitude of chiropractors toward drug prescription in chiropractic.

The aim of this study was therefore to ascertain the general attitude (s) of chiropractors from Ontario, Canada toward the inclusion of drug prescription rights in their scope of practice. In doing so, three main areas were investigated: (i) Ontario chiropractors' attitudes and opinions to drug prescription rights, (ii) the frequency of OTC drug recommendation by Ontario chiropractors, and (iii) Ontario chiropractors' current knowledge of drug prescription. This study also sought to determine if there was a relationship between Ontario chiropractors' attitudes toward drug prescription rights and (a) the number of years in chiropractic practice or employment, and (b) philosophical orientation/preferred style of practice.

Methods
Study design

A survey of all 2,900 chiropractors in active chiropractic practice registered through the 2014–2015 electronic directory of the College of Chiropractors of Ontario (CCO) [15] was carried out using an online, anonymous, 14-item self-administered questionnaire (see Additional file 1 for a copy of the survey instrument). Ontario chiropractors who were retired and/or who did not have an e-mail address listed with the CCO at the time of the survey were excluded. The current questionnaire was partially based on questionnaires previously used in assessing chiropractors' opinions toward drug prescription rights [5, 8].

All qualified participants in this study were contacted via e-mail messages, at one-week intervals, up to six times over the course of six weeks. The first e-mail was a pre-notification message containing an introduction to the survey and its purpose, as well as a link to a review article on the topic of prescribing rights in chiropractic [13]. The next four e-mail messages, which included up to three reminder notifications for non-responders, were distributed through SurveyMonkey® and included a cover letter, a link to the survey instrument, as well as opt-out instructions. A final e-mail reminder was sent to non-responders on the final day before the survey was closed.

Survey instrument
The questionnaire was divided into four sections. Section 1 consisted of four questions recorded on a 5-point Likert scale ranging from 'strongly agree' to 'strongly disagree' that focused on chiropractors' attitudes to drug prescription rights. Section 2 consisted of two questions regarding OTC drug recommendations in chiropractic practice. Responses to both questions were recorded on a 5-point scale ranging from 'never' to 'routinely.' Section 3 contained three questions asking about the chiropractors' current knowledge of drug prescription. Responses to the first two questions were recorded on a 5-point Likert scale ranging from 'very high' to 'very low.' Responses to the third question were recorded on a 3-point 'yes,' 'no,' or 'don't know' verbal scale. Section 4 asked demographic questions including: (i) age, (ii) gender, (iii) chiropractic college of graduation, (iv) number of years in chiropractic practice or employment, and (v) chiropractic philosophical orientation/scope of practice. For this last item, respondents were asked to choose between one of three categories, as defined by McDonald et al. [8], which best described their philosophical orientation / preferred scope of practice. The three categories included: 'broad scope' (i.e. the often described chiropractic "mixer"), 'middle scope,' and 'focused scope' (i.e. the often described "straight" chiropractors).

Pilot testing
An assessment of the questionnaire's face validity [16, 17] was undertaken through peer review and a pilot study. For the pilot study a random sample of 20 chiropractors registered with the Waterloo Regional Chiropractic Society, a diverse group of currently 39 chiropractors practising within the region of Waterloo, Ontario, Canada (and representative of the target population), was used. The names of each of the 39 registered chiropractors were entered into a computer-based random number generator and the first 20 listed after randomization were selected. Each pilot study participant was asked to complete the questionnaire online, using SurveyMonkey®, and to give feedback concerning its face validity (i.e. whether or not the questionnaire adequately assessed Ontario chiropractors' general attitudes to drug prescription rights), as well as general feedback regarding the time to complete the survey, individual item comprehension, and issues of ambiguity. There were 12 responses to the pilot study (60 % response rate) and feedback primarily consisted of comments relating to wording and clarity. All respondents affirmed the questionnaire's face validity. This feedback

was used to further revise the questionnaire, and the final survey instrument was created online and administered through SurveyMonkey®.

Data analysis
Responses to all questions were analyzed using descriptive statistics. Central tendencies were measured as means and standard deviations for continuous data, while medians were used for ordinal data [18]. Categorical data were presented as proportions. Inferential statistics were used to investigate any differences in opinion between chiropractors who: (i) had been in practice or employed for different amounts of time (i.e. 0 to 15 years, or greater than 15 years), and (ii) had differing views regarding chiropractic philosophy/scope of practice. It was hypothesized, a priori, that chiropractors with a higher number of years in practice and/or who preferred a focused (or 'straight') chiropractic scope of practice would hold more negative views toward drug prescription rights. Relationships between these two grouping variables and the various attitudinal response variables from section 1 of the questionnaire were explored using the chi-square test of independence for nominal/categorical data [18]. In order to evaluate differences between these groups, responses to the four Likert scale items in section 1, which provided ordinal data on chiropractors' attitudes to drug prescription rights, were collapsed and recoded as categorical data (e.g. 'strongly agree'/ 'agree,' 'neutral,' and 'disagree'/ 'strongly disagree'). Statistical significance was set at $p < 0.05$, and all data analysis was carried out using SPSS (Statistical Program for the Social Sciences, © IBM SPSS Statistics, Version 20).

Ethical considerations
Prior to data collection, ethics approval (E67/05/15) was obtained through the Anglo-European College of Chiropractic Research Ethics Sub-Committee. The Research Ethics Board Secretariat for Health Canada was also contacted and further ethics review in Canada was deemed not necessary due to the nature of the research being undertaken in this study. All data collected for this study was recorded anonymously and stored securely in a password protected electronic database.

Results
After removing duplicate and invalid e-mail addresses from the 2014–2015 CCO directory, the questionnaire was sent to 2,847 chiropractors in Ontario, representing more than two-thirds (68.0 %) of all chiropractors in active practice registered with the CCO at the time of the survey (February 2, 2015 to February 27, 2015). One hundred and seventy questionnaires were automatically returned as undeliverable due to change of recipient e-mail addresses ($n = 77$) or those previously having

opted out of receiving SurveyMonkey® surveys ($n = 93$). Of the remaining 2,677 questionnaires that were sent, completed questionnaires were received from 960 respondents (35.9 % response rate), representing the views of nearly one-quarter of the profession in Ontario at the time.

Table 1 provides demographic comparisons between the study sample and the general population of Ontario chiropractors. With respect to philosophical orientation, nearly one-third (31.7 %) of respondents classified themselves as practising within a 'broad scope' of chiropractic practice, over half (54.8 %) were 'middle scope,' and the remaining 13.4 % (128/952) of respondents identified themselves as 'focused scope' chiropractors.

Ontario chiropractors' attitudes to drug prescription rights obtained from section 1 of the questionnaire are summarized in Fig. 1. The majority of respondents were in favour of incorporating limited drug prescription rights within their scope of practice. Nearly two-thirds (65.0 %) were in agreement that chiropractors should be able to gain an expanded scope to allow for prescription of OTC medications for common musculoskeletal conditions (Fig. 1a). Similarly, the majority (61.7 %) agreed that chiropractors should be able to gain an expanded scope of practice to allow for the prescription of a limited number of prescription-based musculoskeletal medications (Fig. 1b). Respondents were not in favour of chiropractors having full prescribing rights, with a large majority (76.6 %) disagreeing that chiropractors should be able to gain an expanded scope to allow for the prescription of any and all medications, including controlled substances (Fig. 1c). Finally, a majority (68.3 %) of respondents agreed that if given limited prescriptive authority chiropractors could play a role in counselling patients against overuse and over-reliance on medications for musculoskeletal conditions (Fig. 1d).

Responses to section 2 of the questionnaire asking about the frequency of OTC drug recommendation are shown in Fig. 2. Overall, the majority of respondents indicated that they recommend OTC drugs to patients to some extent in clinical practice. Respondents also suggested OTC medications more frequently to acute patients (Fig. 2a) than chronic patients (Fig. 2b).

Responses to section 3 of the questionnaire exploring current knowledge of drug prescription are summarized in Fig. 3. Respondents were generally confident regarding their perceived knowledge towards prescribing musculoskeletal medications (Fig. 3a), but less so for drugs used in treating non-musculoskeletal conditions (Fig. 3b). A large majority (76.7 %) of respondents also felt that completion of a formal postgraduate certificate program in pharmacology/drug administration should be required for those in the profession wishing to prescribe medications (Fig. 3c).

Comparisons between Ontario chiropractors' attitudes to drug prescription rights and the number of years in practice are displayed in Table 2. A statistically significant greater proportion of respondents with less than 15 years' experience agreed that Ontario chiropractors should be able to prescribe OTC and prescription-based musculoskeletal medications compared to those with more than 15 years' experience. Respondents with more than 15 years' experience also disagreed significantly more so than those with less than 15 years' experience regarding the idea that chiropractors with limited prescriptive authority could counsel patients on musculoskeletal medication use. With respect to the issue of full prescribing rights, no statistically significant difference in opinion was found between chiropractors who had been in practice or employed for different amounts of time.

Table 1 Demographic comparison of study respondents versus all Ontario chiropractors in active practice at the time of the survey

Variable	Study respondents	All Ontario chiropractors[a]
	($n = 960$)	($n = 4,189$)
Mean (SD) age, years	44 (11)	44 (11)
Gender		
• Male, %	70 (670/951)	64 (2679/4187)
• Female, %	30 (281/951)	36 (1508/4187)
College of graduation		
• CMCC, %	72 (689/952)	73 (3033/4178)
• USA, %	26 (245/952)	26 (1100/4178)
• Outside USA, %	2 (15/952)	1 (35/4178)
• UQTR, %	0 (3/952)	0 (9/4178)
Mean (SD) years in practice	17 (11)	15 (12)

SD = standard deviation, *CMCC* = Canadian Memorial Chiropractic College, *USA* = United States of America, *UQTR* = Université de Québec à Trois Riviéres
[a]Values derived from demographic data provided by the College of Chiropractors of Ontario (as of December 5, 2014)

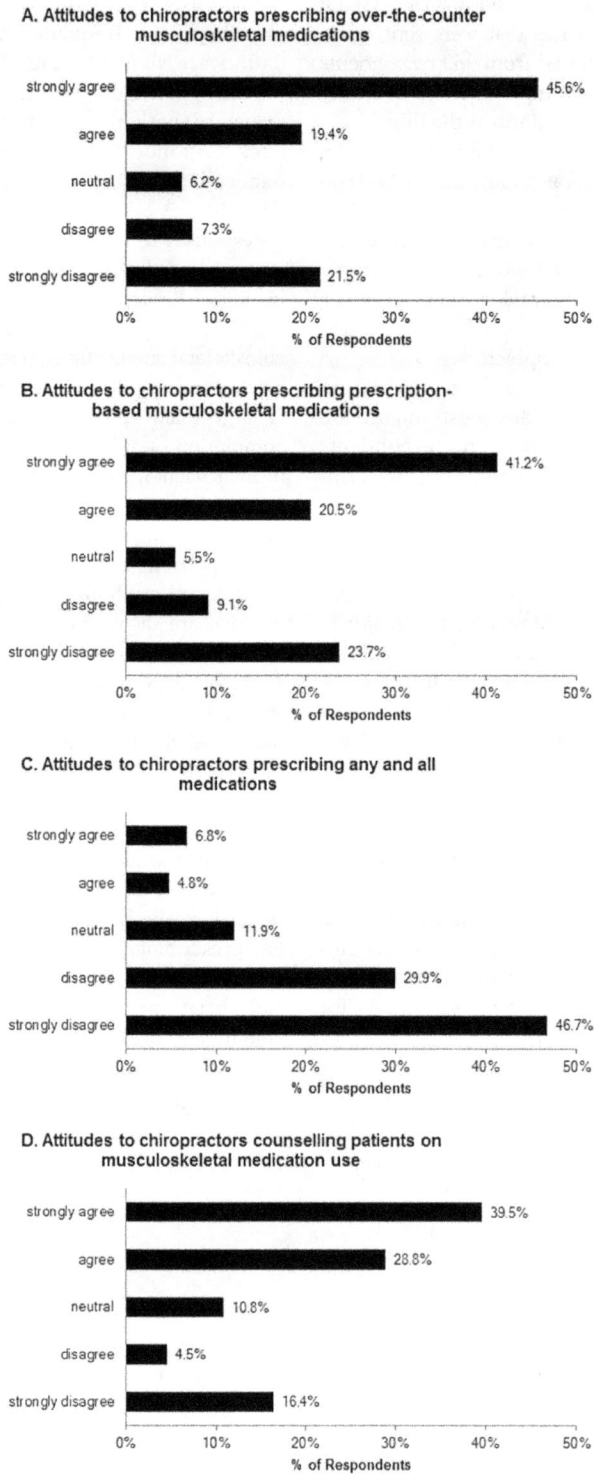

A. Attitudes to chiropractors prescribing over-the-counter musculoskeletal medications

- strongly agree — 45.6%
- agree — 19.4%
- neutral — 6.2%
- disagree — 7.3%
- strongly disagree — 21.5%

% of Respondents

B. Attitudes to chiropractors prescribing prescription-based musculoskeletal medications

- strongly agree — 41.2%
- agree — 20.5%
- neutral — 5.5%
- disagree — 9.1%
- strongly disagree — 23.7%

% of Respondents

C. Attitudes to chiropractors prescribing any and all medications

- strongly agree — 6.8%
- agree — 4.8%
- neutral — 11.9%
- disagree — 29.9%
- strongly disagree — 46.7%

% of Respondents

D. Attitudes to chiropractors counselling patients on musculoskeletal medication use

- strongly agree — 39.5%
- agree — 28.8%
- neutral — 10.8%
- disagree — 4.5%
- strongly disagree — 16.4%

% of Respondents

Fig. 1 (See legend on next page.)

(See figure on previous page.)
Fig. 1 Ontario chiropractors' attitudes to drug prescription rights. (**a**) Responses regarding attitudes to chiropractors prescribing over-the-counter musculoskeletal medications ($n = 958$), median value = 'agree.' (**b**) Responses regarding attitudes to chiropractors prescribing prescription-based musculoskeletal medications ($n = 952$), median value = 'agree.' (**c**) Responses regarding attitudes to chiropractors prescribing any and all medications ($n = 958$), median value = 'disagree.' (**d**) Responses regarding attitudes to chiropractors counselling patients on musculoskeletal medication use ($n = 955$), median value = 'agree'

Comparisons between Ontario chiropractors' attitudes to drug prescription rights and differences in philosophical orientation are displayed in Table 3. Among 'broad scope' respondents an overwhelming majority were in agreement that Ontario chiropractors should be able to gain an expanded scope to allow for prescription of OTC and prescription-based analgesics, NSAIDs, and muscle relaxants. Relatively few of the 'focused' group respondents held the same opinion. 'Middle scope' chiropractors were also in favour of limited prescribing rights, although to a lesser extent than their 'broad scope' colleagues supporting the idea of being able to prescribe OTC and prescription-based musculoskeletal medications. Similarly, a large majority of 'broad scope' and 'middle scope' respondents agreed that if given limited prescriptive authority, chiropractors could play a role in counselling patients against overuse and over-reliance on drugs commonly prescribed for musculoskeletal conditions. In contrast, less than one-quarter of 'focused scope' respondents supported this idea. Regarding full prescribing rights, nearly one-quarter of the 'broad scope' group agreed that Ontario chiropractors should be able to gain an expanded scope allowing for the prescription of any and all medications, including controlled substances, however the proportion of 'middle scope' and 'focused scope' chiropractors who similarly agreed was considerably lower.

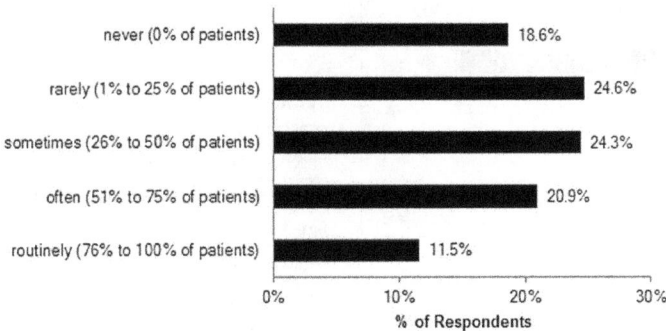

Fig. 2 Frequency of over-the-counter drug recommendation by Ontario chiropractors. (**a**) Responses regarding the frequency of over-the-counter drug recommendation to acute patients in clinical practice ($n = 955$), median value = 'sometimes.' (**b**) Responses regarding the frequency of over-the-counter drug recommendation to chronic patients in clinical practice ($n = 957$), median value = 'rarely'

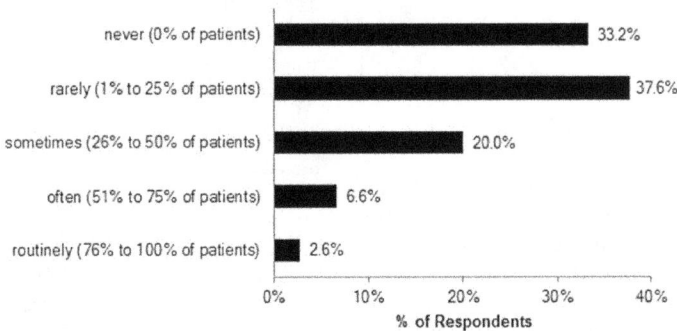

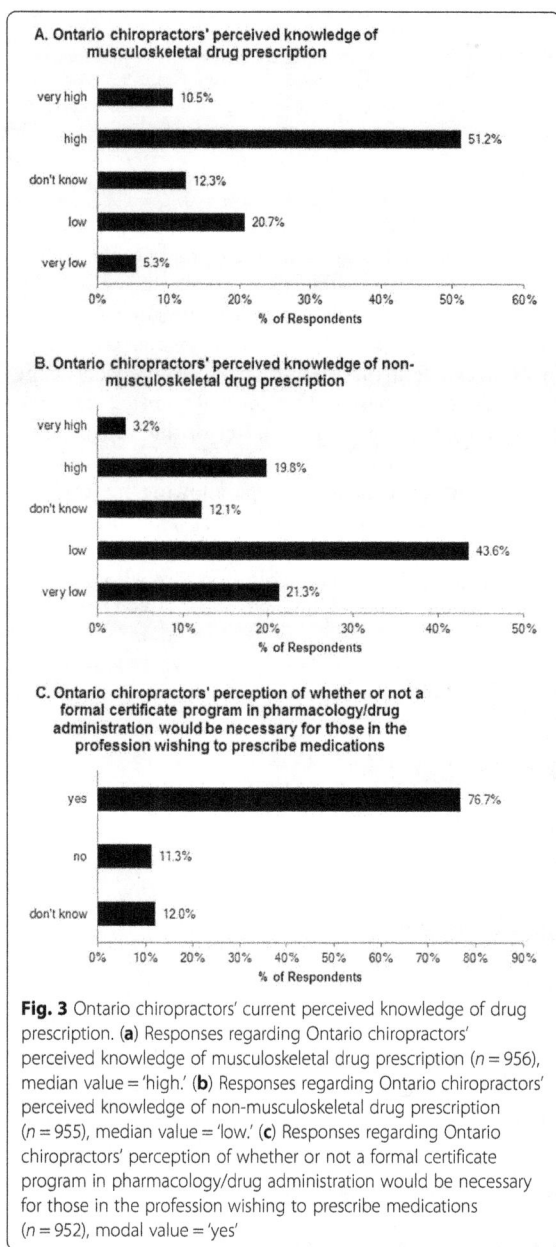

Fig. 3 Ontario chiropractors' current perceived knowledge of drug prescription. (**a**) Responses regarding Ontario chiropractors' perceived knowledge of musculoskeletal drug prescription ($n = 956$), median value = 'high.' (**b**) Responses regarding Ontario chiropractors' perceived knowledge of non-musculoskeletal drug prescription ($n = 955$), median value = 'low.' (**c**) Responses regarding Ontario chiropractors' perception of whether or not a formal certificate program in pharmacology/drug administration would be necessary for those in the profession wishing to prescribe medications ($n = 952$), modal value = 'yes'

Table 2 Comparison of Ontario chiropractors' attitudes to drug prescription rights based on the number of years in practice

Years in practice	Agree %	Neutral %	Disagree %
Attitudes to chiropractors prescribing OTC MSK medications[a]			
0 to 15 years	69.8 (369/529)	5.5 (29/529)	24.8 (131/529)
>15 years	59.3 (248/418)	6.9 (29/418)	33.7 (141/418)
Attitudes to chiropractors prescribing prescription-based MSK medications[b]			
0 to 15 years	65.8 (347/527)	4.9 (26/527)	29.2 (154/527)
>15 years	56.5 (234/414)	6.0 (25/414)	37.4 (155/414)
Attitudes to chiropractors prescribing any and all medications[c]			
0 to 15 years	12.5 (66/529)	11.7 (62/529)	75.8 (401/529)
>15 years	10.8 (45/418)	12.2 (51/418)	77.0 (322/418)
Attitudes to chiropractors counselling patients on MSK medication use[d]			
0 to 15 years	71.8 (379/528)	12.3 (65/528)	15.9 (84/528)
>15 years	64.2 (267/416)	8.9 (37/416)	26.9 (112/416)

OTC = over-the-counter, MSK = musculoskeletal
[a] $\chi^2_{2df} = 11.24$; $P = 0.004$
[b] $\chi^2_{2df} = 8.55$; $P = 0.014$
[c] $\chi^2_{2df} = 0.68$; $P = 0.714$
[d] $\chi^2_{2df} = 18.07$; $P < 0.001$

Table 3 Comparison of Ontario chiropractors' attitudes to drug prescription rights based on philosophical orientation

Philosophical orientation	Agree %	Neutral %	Disagree %
Attitudes to chiropractors prescribing OTC MSK medications[a]			
Broad scope	93.0 (281/302)	1.3 (4/302)	5.6 (17/302)
Middle scope	62.2 (324/521)	8.8 (46/521)	29.0 (151/521)
Focused scope	11.0 (14/127)	6.3 (8/127)	82.7 (105/127)
Attitudes to chiropractors prescribing prescription-based MSK medications[b]			
Broad scope	90.9 (271/298)	1.7 (5/298)	7.4 (22/298)
Middle scope	57.0 (296/519)	7.3 (38/519)	35.6 (185/519)
Focused scope	12.6 (16/127)	6.3 (8/127)	81.1 (103/127)
Attitudes to chiropractors prescribing any and all medications[c]			
Broad scope	23.9 (72/301)	17.3 (52/301)	58.8 (177/301)
Middle scope	6.1 (32/522)	10.7 (56/522)	83.1 (434/522)
Focused scope	5.5 (7/127)	3.9 (5/127)	90.6 (115/127)
Attitudes to chiropractors counselling patients on MSK medication use[d]			
Broad scope	90.0 (271/301)	4.3 (13/301)	5.6 (17/301)
Middle scope	66.2 (344/520)	14.2 (74/520)	19.6 (102/520)
Focused scope	23.8 (30/126)	11.9 (15/126)	64.3 (81/126)

OTC = over-the-counter, MSK = musculoskeletal
[a] $\chi^2_{4df} = 296.23$; $P < 0.001$
[b] $\chi^2_{4df} = 254.18$; $P < 0.001$
[c] $\chi^2_{4df} = 89.81$; $P < 0.001$
[d] $\chi^2_{4df} = 221.24$; $P < 0.001$

Discussion

The main finding of this study was that the majority of Ontario chiropractors who responded to this survey were in favour of incorporating limited drug prescription rights into their scope of practice. Nearly two-thirds agreed that chiropractors should be permitted to prescribe OTC and prescription-based analgesics, NSAIDs, and muscle relaxants. Almost 70 % also felt that with limited prescriptive authority chiropractors could help counsel patients against overuse and over-reliance on these types of medications. This level of support for chiropractic prescribing rights is in contrast to that of previously published research which has shown that the profession has generally been divided on this topic [13]. A majority (55.2 %) of respondents from a recent survey of North American chiropractic students [19] were also not in favour of expanding the chiropractic scope of practice to include drug prescription. The current study's findings are nevertheless in line with those of several recent unpublished surveys where between 55 % and nearly 80 % of respondents supported the idea of chiropractors prescribing musculoskeletal medications [20, 21] (B. Haig, Chief Executive Officer, Ontario Chiropractic Association; personal communication, 3 November 2014). These conflicting results in the literature reiterate the need for further investigation in order to clarify the general attitude of chiropractors internationally towards drug prescription in the profession.

In spite of this, evidence from two of the aforementioned surveys including that in the present study indicate that there may be a growing interest among Ontario chiropractors towards limited chiropractic prescribing rights. For instance, in surveys involving members of the Ontario Chiropractic Association from 2007 and 2011 (B. Haig, Chief Executive Officer, Ontario Chiropractic Association; personal communication, 3 November 2014), increasing majorities (55 % and 61 %) of respondents respectively were in favour of chiropractors prescribing anti-inflammatory and/or analgesic medications. An even greater majority favouring limited prescribing rights in the present study suggests that there may be a possible shift in chiropractors' attitudes toward drug prescription rights occurring within the profession in Ontario.

In Switzerland, where chiropractors already have limited prescribing rights, the profession is more united regarding drug prescription in chiropractic [1, 10] and is strongly integrated and accepted by the medical community [22]. As such Swiss chiropractors have cultural authority within the musculoskeletal domain. For instance, chiropractic is among one of five government-recognized medical professions in Switzerland (i.e. human medicine, chiropractic medicine, veterinary medicine, dentistry, and pharmacology), and chiropractic treatment is fully covered under the Swiss national health insurance program [22]. If chiropractors in other countries wish to gain drug prescription privileges however, there are numerous implications to consider. These would include, but are not limited to, the need for additional education and training for chiropractors in pharmacology and toxicology, necessary regulatory and legislative changes, consideration of legal and ethical issues, and increases to chiropractic malpractice/liability insurance coverage [13, 23].

Concerning the issue of pharmacology education, the current study found that Ontario chiropractors were quite confident regarding their perceived knowledge towards prescribing musculoskeletal medications. In fact, nearly two-thirds of respondents indicated that their current knowledge of these drugs was 'high' or 'very high.' Interestingly nearly equal numbers perceived their current knowledge of drugs for non-musculoskeletal conditions as 'low' or 'very low.' The first finding is surprising given that the basic chiropractic educational curriculum contains only 12 h of coursework in pharmacology [24]. A possible explanation is that over 72 % of respondents in the current study graduated from the Canadian Memorial Chiropractic College where students presently receive 30 h of training in pharmacology and toxicology [25]. Although this number of hours in pharmacology education is above the World Health Organization standards for chiropractic, students in other healthcare professions such as dentistry complete an average of almost 70 h [26] and chiropractic students in Switzerland take over 80 h in pharmacology at the University of Zürich (C.K. Peterson, personal communication, 18 January 2015). Regardless of how confident Ontario chiropractors might be regarding their perceived knowledge towards musculoskeletal medications, further undergraduate and/or post-graduate education and training would be necessary in order to competently prescribe these types of medications in clinical practice. In fact, this view was supported by a large majority of respondents in the current study as over three-quarters felt that completion of a formal postgraduate certificate program in pharmacology/drug administration should be required for those in the profession wishing to prescribe medications. Currently, chiropractors in New Mexico, USA must complete a two-year postgraduate Master of Science degree in 'Advanced Clinical Practice' [4, 27] before they can obtain a license to prescribe from the limited chiropractic formulary in that state [2]. This postgraduate program offers further training in pharmacology [27] and could serve as a model for the profession, particularly in other jurisdictions where chiropractic prescribing rights are being considered.

Despite evidence to suggest that chiropractors in Ontario and elsewhere are interested in gaining limited prescriptive privileges, a large majority of respondents in the current study did not favour the idea of chiropractors having full prescribing rights. More than three-quarters disagreed that chiropractors should be able to gain an expanded scope to allow for the prescription of any and all medications, including controlled substances. This finding is consistent with those of previous surveys of chiropractors from Australia [5], the United States [6], and North America [8] where respondents were generally opposed to chiropractors writing drug prescriptions for non-musculoskeletal conditions. This is also in accord-ance with the views of those in the medical profession whose members would likely oppose such an expansion to the chiropractic scope of practice as well [23]. On the other hand, if chiropractors would focus their scope to treating spine-related/musculoskeletal conditions there is evidence to suggest that medical doctors would support limited prescription privileges for the chiropractic profes-sion [22, 23, 28]. Some chiropractors in New Mexico, USA have nevertheless attempted to expand their existing formulary to beyond a limited number of medications, and this has been met by opposition from both the medical and chiropractic professions in that state [11].

Another finding of the current study was that a large number of Ontario chiropractors in this survey tend to recommend OTC drugs to their patients. For instance, when asked how often they suggested non-prescription analgesic and NSAID medications to acute and chronic patients in clinical practice, 81 % and 67 % of respon-dents indicated that they did so to some extent respect-ively. These non-prescription drug utilization rates are comparable to those of other published studies of prac-tising chiropractors [1, 5, 6, 10, 22], and are congruent with current evidence-based guidelines [29–31]. This nevertheless suggests that several chiropractors in Ontario are making treatment recommendations that are outside of their current legislative scope of practice [32]. Arguably however, this study's findings indicate the need to align the chiropractic scope of practice with current scientific evidence as well as individual practi-tioner behaviour. The findings of this study also suggest that many chiropractors support OTC drug use in clin-ical practice no matter what their personal stance is on prescribing rights for the profession. For at least some of these chiropractors this points to a disconnect between traditional chiropractic philosophy (i.e. non-drug, non-surgical health care) and once again, actual practice behaviour. Interestingly, the remaining respondents in the present study indicated that they would 'never' rec-ommend OTC analgesics and NSAIDs to their patients. It is unclear if these participant responses were based on individual chiropractic philosophical orientation, or simply that these clinicians felt that OTC drug recommen-dation was outside the scope of chiropractic practice.

When exploring possible reasons for why some chiro-practors have differing views toward drug prescription, an association was found in this study between respon-dents' opinions and the number of years in practice. For instance, chiropractors who had practised for 15 years or less were significantly more in favour of musculoskeletal drug prescription rights versus those with greater than 15 years' experience. This difference in opinion between the two groups could possibly reflect slightly differing views toward evidence-based practice. For example,

several clinical guidelines endorse the use of mild anal-gesics and/or anti-inflammatories in the management of various musculoskeletal conditions [29–31]. Yet some literature suggests that more experienced practitioners are less likely to view research evidence as valuable or necessary in their day-to-day clinical practice [33–35]. The current study did not directly inquire about respon-dents' attitudes to evidence-based practice, so it is unclear whether this characteristic actually influenced respondent opinions toward drug prescription in the survey. The dif-ferences may have once again been based more on respon-dents' philosophical orientation and/or attitudes toward current chiropractic scope of practice. Regardless, the majority of respondents from both groups (greater than 15 years versus 15 years or less in practice) still favoured the idea of limited prescribing rights for chiropractors despite their overall practice experience.

As for philosophical orientation, this study showed that there was a strong relationship between this variable and Ontario chiropractors' attitudes to drug prescription rights. For instance, almost all of the 'broad scope' respondents in the survey were in favour of Ontario chiropractors gaining prescriptive rights for treating musculoskeletal conditions, whereas very few of the 'focused scope' group felt the same way. These findings are consistent with those from the study by McDonald et al. [8] where more than three-quarters of broad scope respondents supported limited prescribing rights compared to less than one-fifth of focused scope chiro-practors who similarly agreed. The majority of 'middle scope' respondents in the current study also favoured musculoskeletal prescribing rights. The majority (53.5 %) of middle scope respondents in the McDonald et al. [8] survey supported limited chiropractic prescribing rights as well, but to a lesser extent than those in the current study. Where broad and middle scope chiropractors from the present study disagreed was regarding full prescribing rights; nearly one-quarter of respondents in the broad scope group agreed that chiropractors should be permit-ted to write prescriptions for any and all medications while virtually none in the middle scope group held a similar view. Akin to the situation in New Mexico, USA, however, this attitude of favouring full prescribing rights for chiropractors by some broad scope respondents is in contrast to the general view held by many others in the profession [5, 6, 8].

There may be a middle ground concerning chiroprac-tic prescribing rights where some level of agreement within the profession could be reached. For instance, evidence from the literature including results from the current study suggest that among chiropractors who hold favourable views toward drug prescription, pre-scription privileges limited to within a musculoskeletal scope of practice would be preferred [5, 6, 8]. A large majority of respondents in the current study also agreed that with limited prescriptive authority chiropractors could advise patients against overusing analgesic and anti-inflammatory medications. Evidence to support this notion can be found in Switzerland where chiropractors tend to prescribe medications significantly less so than asked for by their patients [10]. With the over-prescription of drugs such as opioids in countries like the United States [36], the ability of chiropractors to counsel patients on musculoskeletal drug use is something that all members of the profession should be interested in, regardless of philosophical orienta-tion. In fact, a large majority of broad and middle scope chiropractors in the current study supported this potential role for the profession. Focused scope re-spondents did not, however, as less than one-quarter similarly agreed. As such, these findings along with those of others [8] suggest that complete consensus on the topic of chiropractic prescribing rights will likely remain elusive for the profession given the philosoph-ical views traditionally held by this minority (13 % in the current study) group of chiropractors. However in light of the fact that physiotherapists are inter-ested in and are gaining limited drug prescription rights in some countries [37, 38], it is imperative that the remaining majority of the chiropractic profession continues this discussion. Further surveys and/or qualitative studies of chiropractors' opinions toward gaining prescription privileges in these and other jurisdictions would be timely. In Canada, the results of the current study may be taken to other provinces in order to complete a nationwide survey. If the same findings are confirmed elsewhere, it would argue for a national campaign to reform the chiropractic scope of practice acts across the country.

Limitations
This study has some limitations. First, the overall response to the survey was relatively low (36 %) thus raising the likelihood of non-response/exclusion bias in the results [18]. However, the number of responses ($n = 960$) obtained in this study was higher than those of other published surveys on chiropractic prescribing rights [1, 5–10], and when comparing demographic characteristics the sample appears to be representative of the general population of practising chiropractors in Ontario (see Table 1). Nevertheless, a 64 % non-response rate suggests that these survey results should be interpreted with caution as respondents' views to-ward drug prescription rights obtained may not be generalizable to those of all Ontario chiropractors.

A second limitation of this study is that it excluded re-tired chiropractors and those not on the electronic 2014–2015 directory of the CCO. As these groups

represented the minority (32 %) of all licensed chiro-practors in Ontario at the time of the survey, this was felt to be less of an issue. Nonetheless, there is a risk that retired chiropractors and/or those who did not have an e-mail address listed with the CCO may have held systematically different views toward drug prescription rights compared to chiropractors listed on the electronic CCO directory.

Thirdly, chiropractors' attitudes to drug prescription rights were measured in this study using a closed-answer format only. Although good for aggregating data from large study populations, the disadvantage to using this survey method is that it does not allow par-ticipants to expand upon responses or offer alternative viewpoints [17], and this would have prevented any 'richness' to the responses in the current study. On the other hand, open-answer questions take longer to complete which can dissuade participants from responding [17]. These questions can also be laborious (and expensive) to analyze qualitatively [17], particu-larly with large data sets, and was beyond the scope of the current study.

Conclusions
This study revealed that a majority of Ontario chiro-practors were in favour of incorporating limited drug prescription rights into their scope of practice, were generally confident regarding their knowledge of musculoskeletal medications, and tended to recom-mend OTC drugs such as mild analgesics and/or anti-inflammatories to patients to some extent in clinical practice. However, respondents did not favour the idea of chiropractors having full prescribing rights, were not confident in their knowledge of drugs for non-musculoskeletal conditions, and felt that further edu-cation and training in pharmacology should be neces-sary for those in the profession wishing to prescribe medications. Those who had been in practice for less than 15 years favoured musculoskeletal prescribing rights more so than chiropractors with more than 15 years' experience; however the overall majority in both groups still favoured limited prescribing rights for the profession. As for philosophical orientation, the majority of broad and middle scope respondents in this study also favoured limited chiropractic prescribing rights, whereas those in the focused scope group did not. Further surveys and/or qualitative studies of chi-ropractors in other jurisdictions are needed in order to validate these findings.

Additional file

Additional file 1: Survey instrument.

Abbreviations
CCO: College of Chiropractors of Ontario; CMCC: Canadian Memorial Chiropractic College; MSK: Musculoskeletal; NSAIDs: Non-steroidal anti-inflammatory drugs; OTC: Over-the-counter; SD: Standard deviation; SPSS: Statistical Program for the Social Sciences; UQTR: Université de Québec à Trois Riviéres; USA: United States of America.

Competing interests
The authors declare that they have no competing interests.

Authors' contributions
KJS conceived of the study and participated in its design. PCE was responsible for study design; data collection, analysis, and interpretation; and drafted the initial manuscript. Both authors reviewed the literature and also drafted, revised, and approved the final manuscript.

Acknowledgements
This study formed the main part of a Master of Science dissertation undertaken by PCE and supervised through the Anglo-European College of Chiropractic.

Author details
[1]Master of Science (MSc) Candidate, MSc Advanced Professional Practice (Clinical Sciences), Anglo-European College of Chiropractic, 13-15 Parkwood Road, Bournemouth, Dorset, BH5 2DF, UK. [2]Private Practice, 201C Preston Parkway, Cambridge, ON N3H 5E8, Canada. [3]Division of Graduate Education and Research, Canadian Memorial Chiropractic College, 6100 Leslie Street, Toronto, ON M2H 3J1, Canada.

References
1. Robert J. The multiple facets of the Swiss chiropractic profession. Eur J Chiropr. 2003;50:199–210.
2. New Mexico Regulation & Licensing Department. New Mexico administrative code: chiropractic advanced practice certification registry. [http://www.rld.state.nm.us/uploads/files/2010%20APC%20Formulary.pdf] [Accessed 9 October 2013].
3. Erwin MW, Korpela AP, Jones RC. Chiropractors as primary spine care providers: precedents and essential measures. J Can Chiropr Assoc. 2013;57:285–91.
4. Wisconsin Chiropractic Association. Filling the shortage of primary care health care providers in Wisconsin: the Primary Spine Care Physician, a new class of health care provider. [http://www.wichiro.org/wpwca/wp-content/uploads/2014/09/PSPC_white_paper.pdf] [Accessed 30 January 2015].
5. Jamison JR. Chiropractic in the Australian health care system: the chiropractors' comment on drug therapy. Chiropr J Aust. 1991;21:53–5.
6. Jacobson BH, Gemmell HA. A survey of chiropractors in Oklahoma. J Chiropr Educ. 1999;13:137–42.
7. Wilson FJH. A survey of chiropractors in the United Kingdom. Eur J Chiropr. 2003;50:185–98.
8. McDonald WP, Durkin KF, Pfefer M. How chiropractors think and practice: the survey of North American chiropractors. Semin Integr Med. 2004;2:92–8.
9. Pollentier A, Langworthy JM. The scope of chiropractic practice: a survey of chiropractors in the UK. Clin Chiropr. 2007;10:147–55.
10. Wangler M, Zaugg B, Faigaux E. Medication prescription: a pilot survey of Bernese doctors of chiropractic practicing in Switzerland. J Manipulative Physiol Ther. 2010;33:231–7.
11. International Chiropractors Association. ICA News – August 2013. [http://www.thechiropracticchoice.com/thechiropracticchoice.com/NEW-MEXICO-COURT-OF-APPEALS-SETS-ASIDE%20IMPROPERLY-ENACTED-CHIROPRACTIC-RULE.pdf] [Accessed 12 November 2013].
12. Lehman JJ, Suozzi PJ, Simmons GR, Jegtvig SK. Patient perceptions in New Mexico about doctors of chiropractic functioning as primary care providers with limited prescriptive authority. J Chiropr Med. 2011;10:12–7.
13. Emary PC, Stuber KJ. Chiropractors' attitudes toward drug prescription rights: a narrative review. Chiropr Man Therap. 2014;22:34.
14. The Chiropractic Report. The prescription drug debate. Should the chiropractic profession remain drug free? [https://www.chiropracticreport.com/index.php/past-issues/view_document/68-no-6-the-prescription-drug-debate] [Accessed 23 July 2014].
15. College of Chiropractors of Ontario. CCO publications: 2014–15 directory. [http://www.cco.on.ca/site_documents/87854-1_ChiroCollege_Directory.pdf] [Accessed 1 December 2014].
16. Boynton PM. Administering, analysing, and reporting your questionnaire: hands-on guide to questionnaire research. BMJ. 2004;328:1372–5.
17. Boynton PM, Greenhalgh T. Selecting, designing, and developing your questionnaire: hands-on guide to questionnaire research. BMJ. 2004;328:1312–5.
18. Haneline MT. Evidence-based chiropractic practice. Sudbury : Jones and Bartlett; 2007.
19. Gliedt JA, Hawk C, Anderson M, Ahmad K, Bunn D, Cambron J, et al. Chiropractic identity, role and future: a survey of North American chiropractic students. Chiropr Man Therap. 2015;23:4.
20. British Chiropractic Association. Limited prescribing rights. reading: British Chiropractic Association, In Touch. Newsletter. 2009;142:4–5.
21. Alabama State Chiropractic Association: 2010 Scope of Practice Survey. [http://www.mccoypress.net/subluxation/docs/ASCAscope.pdf] [Accessed 11 March 2015].
22. Humphreys BK, Peterson CK, Muehlemann D, Haueter P. Are Swiss chiropractors different than other chiropractors? Results of the job analysis survey 2009. J Manipulative Physiol Ther. 2010;33:519–35.
23. The College of Family Physicians of Canada. Position statement. Prescribing rights for health professionals. [http://www.cfpc.ca/uploadedFiles/Resources/Resource_Items/CFPC20Position20Statement20Prescribing20Rights20January202010.pdf] [Accessed 23 September 2013].
24. World Health Organization. WHO guidelines on basic training and safety in chiropractic. [http://apps.who.int/medicinedocs/documents/s14076e/s14076e.pdf] [Accessed 6 November 2013].
25. Canadian Memorial Chiropractic College. Academic calendar 2014–2015. [http://www.cmcc.ca/document.doc?id=1756] [Accessed 15 December 2014].
26. Gautam M, Shaw DH, Pate TD, Lambert HW. Pharmacology education in North American dental schools: the basic science survey series. J Dent Educ. 2013;77:1013–21.
27. National University of Health Sciences. Family Practice Residency. [http://www.nuhs.edu/academics/college-of-continuing-education/residency-programs/family-practice/] [Accessed 13 April 2015].
28. Jha NK. Letter to the Editor. J Can Chiropr Assoc. 2014;58:97–8.
29. Chou R, Huffman LH. Medications for acute and chronic low back pain: a review of the evidence for an American Pain Society/American College of Physicians Clinical Practice Guideline. Ann Intern Med. 2007;147:505–14.
30. Dagenais S, Tricco AC, Haldeman S. Synthesis of recommendations for the assessment and management of low back pain from recent clinical practice guidelines. Spine J. 2010;10:514–29.
31. Wong JJ, Côté P, Shearer HM, Carroll LJ, Yu H, Varatharajan S, et al. Clinical practice guidelines for the management of conditions related to traffic collisions: a systematic review by the OPTIMa Collaboration. Disabil Rehabil. 2015;37:471–89.
32. College of Chiropractors of Ontario. Standard of Practice S-001. Chiropractic scope of practice. [http://www.cco.on.ca/site_documents/S-001.pdf] [Accessed 19 June 2015].
33. Dysart AM, Tomlin GS. Factors related to evidence-based practice among U.S. occupational therapy clinicians. Am J Occup Ther. 2002;56:275–84.
34. Valdes K, von der Heyde R. Attitudes and opinions of evidence-based practice among hand therapists: a survey study. J Hand Ther. 2012;25:288–95.
35. Walker BF, Stomski NJ, Hebert JJ, French SD. A survey of Australian chiropractors' attitudes and beliefs about evidence-based practice and their use of research literature and clinical practice guidelines. Chiropr Man Therap. 2013;21:44.
36. Manchikanti L, Helm 2nd S, Fellows B, Janata JW, Pampati V, Grider JS, et al. Opioid epidemic in the United States. Pain Physician. 2012;15:ES9–38.

37. Chartered Society of Physiotherapy. Landmark decision gives UK physios a world first in prescribing rights. [http://www.csp.org.uk/news/2012/07/24/landmark-decision-gives-uk-physios-world-first-prescribing-rights#!] [Accessed 2 October 2013].
38. My Health Career. Prescribing rights for physiotherapists - by Tim Barnwell APA Sports Physiotherapist. [https://www.myhealthcareer.com.au/physiotherapy/prescribing-tim-barnwell] [Accessed 26 June 2015].

4

Short term treatment versus long term management of neck and back disability in older adults utilizing spinal manipulative therapy and supervised exercise: a parallel-group randomized clinical trial evaluating relative effectiveness and harms

Corrie Vihstadt[1], Michele Maiers[1*], Kristine Westrom[1], Gert Bronfort[2], Roni Evans[2], Jan Hartvigsen[3] and Craig Schulz[1]

Abstract

Background: Back and neck disability are frequent in older adults resulting in loss of function and independence. Exercise therapy and manual therapy, like spinal manipulative therapy (SMT), have evidence of short and intermediate term effectiveness for spinal disability in the general population and growing evidence in older adults. For older populations experiencing chronic spinal conditions, long term management may be more appropriate to maintain improvement and minimize the impact of future exacerbations. Research is limited comparing short courses of treatment to long term management of spinal disability.

The primary aim is to compare the relative effectiveness of 12 weeks versus 36 weeks of SMT and supervised rehabilitative exercise (SRE) in older adults with back and neck disability.

Methods/Design: Randomized, mixed-methods, comparative effectiveness trial conducted at a university-affiliated research clinic in the Minneapolis/St. Paul, Minnesota metropolitan area.

Participants: Independently ambulatory community dwelling adults ≥ 65 years of age with back and neck disability of minimum 12 weeks duration (n = 200).

Interventions: 12 weeks SMT + SRE or 36 weeks SMT + SRE.

Randomization: Blocked 1:1 allocation; computer generated scheme, concealed in sequentially numbered, opaque, sealed envelopes.

Blinding: Functional outcome examiners are blinded to treatment allocation; physical nature of the treatments prevents blinding of participants and providers to treatment assignment.

Primary endpoint: 36 weeks post-randomization.

(Continued on next page)

* Correspondence: mmaiers@nwhealth.edu
[1]Northwestern Health Sciences University, Wolfe-Harris Center for Clinical Studies, 2501 W 84th Street, Bloomington, MN 55431, USA
Full list of author information is available at the end of the article

(Continued from previous page)

Data collection: Self-report questionnaires administered at 2 baseline visits and 4, 12, 24, 36, 52, and 78 weeks post-randomization. Primary outcomes include back and neck disability, measured by the Oswestry Disability Index and Neck Disability Index. Secondary outcomes include pain, general health status, improvement, self-efficacy, kinesiophobia, satisfaction, and medication use. Functional outcome assessment occurs at baseline and week 37 for hand grip strength, short physical performance battery, and accelerometry. Individual qualitative interviews are conducted when treatment ends. Data on expectations, falls, side effects, and adverse events are systematically collected.

Primary analysis: Linear mixed-model method for repeated measures to test for between-group differences with baseline values as covariates.

Discussion: Treatments that address the management of spinal disability in older adults may have far reaching implications for patient outcomes, clinical guidelines, and healthcare policy.

Trial registry: www.ClinicalTrials.gov; Identifier: NCT01057706.

Keywords: Neck disability, Back disability, Spinal manipulative therapy, Exercise therapy, Older adults, Mixed-methods, Comparative effectiveness

Background

Musculoskeletal complaints such as back and neck pain are common in the general population but are particularly troublesome in older adults [1] and into extreme old age [2]. In a one to three month time period, approximately 20-35% of older adults report low back pain [3-6], 5-22% report neck pain [4-6], and 9-11% suffer concurrent low back and neck pain [5,6]. Chronic musculoskeletal pain and disability are often associated with increased dependence [1], decreased physical functioning [1,6,7], and other co-morbidities [6,8], which can inhibit vital social activities and quality of life [7], as well as contribute independently to mortality [9]. Healthcare expenditures for back and neck problems have increased with limited improvement in health status [10,11]. A Medicare claims analysis found back pain to be the second most costly chronic non-cancer pain condition; the adjusted cost attributed to back pain per affected member was $2888 annually [12]. With nearly 40 million older adults living in the US [13], this quickly growing age group [14] is projected to double by 2040 [13]. Subsequently, investigating conservative non-pharmacological treatments that temper the effects of back and neck problems is an important public health issue [12].

In the general population, exercise therapy has demonstrated effectiveness for back and neck pain and disability [15,16], particularly when tailored to the individual. Evidence suggests that older adults who exercise experience reduced risk of disability and functional decline [17]. Accordingly, regular exercise is recommended to maintain health and functional ability among older adults [18]. Importantly, Hayden et al. found exercise combined with conservative treatment such as manual therapy improved functional outcomes in the general population with chronic low back pain [15].

Approximately 11–17% of older Americans seek care from chiropractors annually [19,20]. While a majority of research has focused on short and intermediate term effectiveness of spinal manipulative therapy (SMT) in the general population [16,21], there is a limited, yet growing body of evidence suggesting effectiveness of SMT for back-related disability in older adults [22,23]. Considering that back and neck pain are often chronic in nature and part of a constellation of co-morbidities that impact functional ability [24], a long term management approach may be more appropriate to effectively address back and neck disability in older adults. Long term management may aid in maintaining the improvement in functional capacity achieved during a short course of treatment [25] and may minimize the impact of future exacerbations [26]. This theory is supported by a small study showing that nine months of continued treatment with SMT sustained participants' improvement in low back pain and disability compared to those receiving only one month of SMT [27]; however, the effectiveness of long term management of back and neck disability in older adults has yet to be investigated in a full scale trial [28].

Aims

The primary aim is to compare the effectiveness of 12 versus 36 weeks spinal manipulative therapy and supervised rehabilitative exercise (SMT + SRE) by assessing change in the Neck Disability Index (NDI) and Oswestry Disability Index (ODI) at 36 weeks.

Four secondary aims assess between-group differences in:

1) secondary patient-rated outcome measures at week 36 at 78, including disability at week 78
2) functional outcomes at week 37
3) patients' perceptions of treatment
4) cost effectiveness and cost utility at weeks 36, 52, and 78. This aim will be described and reported elsewhere.

Methods/Design

Ethical approval from Northwestern Health Sciences University's (NWHSU) institutional review board (IRB) was received in October 2009.

Design & setting

This randomized, observer-blinded, comparative effectiveness trial is being conducted at the Wolfe-Harris Center for Clinical Studies at NWHSU in Bloomington, Minnesota. Notice of privacy practices and written informed consent are secured from all subjects prior to participation.

Methodological changes to study protocol

The initial study protocol was a three-arm trial, which included a minimal-intervention comparison group of SRE alone for 36 weeks. Slower than projected enrollment and award reductions from the funding agency prompted changes to the study protocol 18 months after recruitment began. A modified study design was proposed by study investigators and approved by the steering committee, funding agency, IRB, and data and safety monitoring board (DSMB). The initial design, modified design, and rationales for each change are described in Table 1. The following three secondary aims were added to use the data collected from those already randomized to the SRE alone group:

A) assess within group change for all patient-rated outcomes at weeks 36 and 78

B) assess within group change for functional outcomes at week 37

C) describe participants' perceptions of treatment

The remainder of this manuscript describes the methodology for the modified trial.

Participants

This study will enroll 200 older adults who report functional disability in the back and neck regions. See Figure 1 for participant flow through the study.

Recruitment strategy

Participants from the Minneapolis/St. Paul metropolitan area are recruited through targeted mailing of brochures, church bulletins, movie theater advertisements, distributed flyers and posters, informational presentations, letters to physicians, and online strategies such as the NWHSU's website, Craigslist®, and Facebook®.

Inclusion/exclusion criteria

To be eligible, participants need to be 65 years of age or older with self-reported back and neck disability.
Inclusion criteria are:

- Back and neck disability of ≥ 12 weeks duration
- Back and neck disability, defined as
  ◦ 10% or higher on Neck Disability Index (NDI),

Table 1 Differences between the initial and modified trial designs and precipitating reasons for the change

Initial design	Modified design	Rationale
Three-arm trial (n = 300)	two-arm trial (n = 200)	Enrollment
• 36 weeks SMT + SRE (n = 88)	• 36 weeks SMT + SRE (n = 100)	Funding
• 12 weeks SMT + SRE (n = 124)	• 12 weeks SMT + SRE (n = 100)	
• 36 weeks SRE alone (n = 88)		
n = 300	n = 200 (for primary and secondary aims 1–4)	Enrollment
	n = 18 (for additional secondary aims A-C)	Funding
Randomization ratio 1:1.4:1	Final randomization ratio 1:1	Enrollment
		Funding
Pertinent inclusion/exclusion criteria:	Pertinent inclusion/exclusion criteria:	Enrollment
• NDI and ODI ≥ 15% each at both baseline evaluations	• NDI and ODI ≥ 10% each AND combined score of ≥ 25% at first baseline evaluation only	
Functional outcomes:	Functional outcomes:	Funding
• short physical performance battery		
• hand grip strength		
• accelerometry	• short physical performance battery	
• postural sway	• hand grip strength	
• range of motion	• accelerometry	
• static endurance		

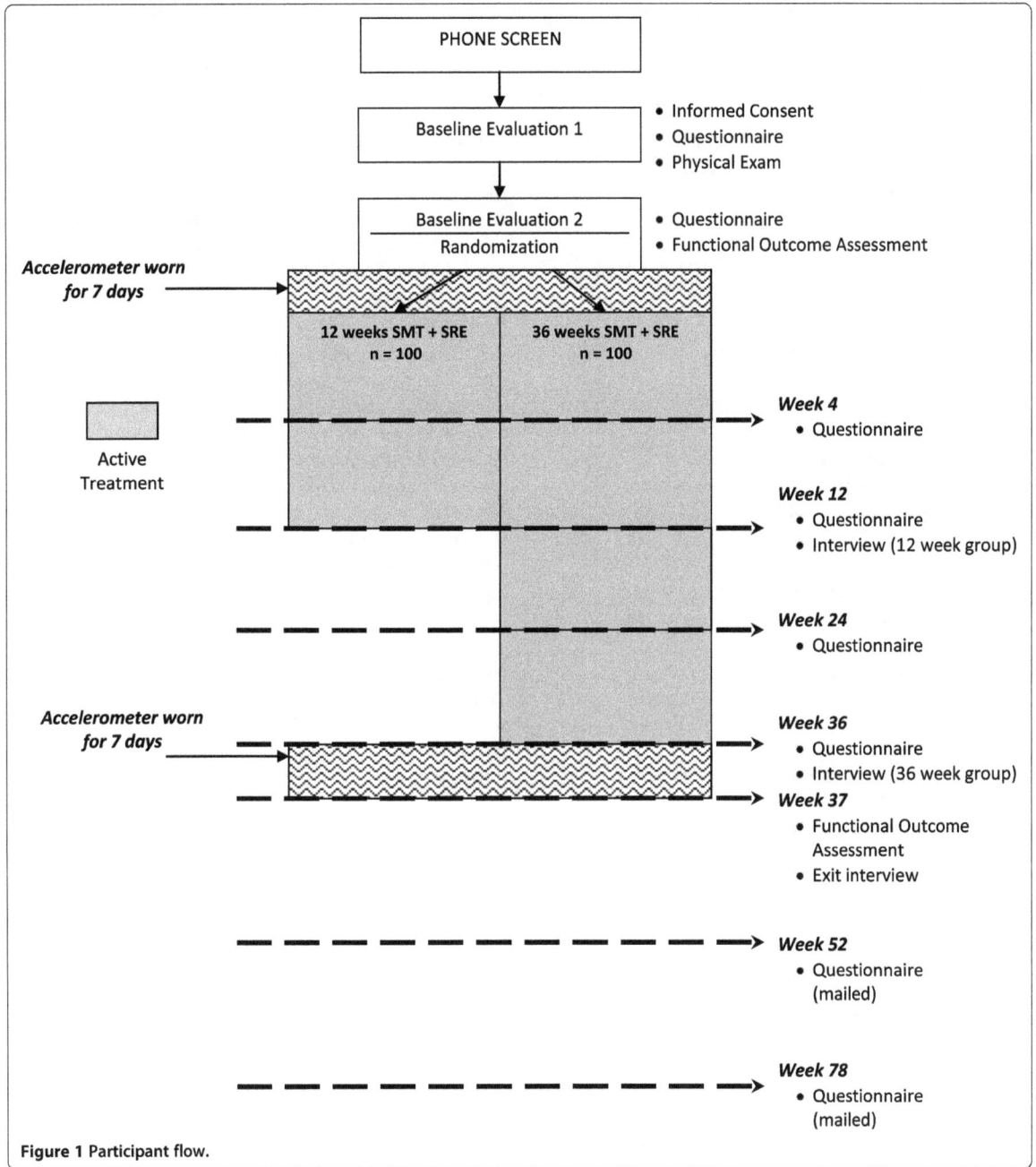

Figure 1 Participant flow.

∘ 10% or higher on Oswestry Disability Index (ODI), and
∘ A combined score (NDI + ODI) of at least 25%
- Stable pain medication plan 4 weeks prior to baseline
- Ability to read and speak English
- Community dwelling

- Ability to ambulate without the aid of a wheelchair or motorized scooter

Exclusion criteria are:

- Surgical spinal fusion [29]
- Multiple incidents of spinal surgery [29]

- Spinal surgery in the last 6 months
- Ongoing non-pharmacological treatment for a spinal condition
- Less than 25 on the Folstein Mini-Mental State Examination [30,31]
- Untreated or unstable clinical depression screened by the Geriatric Depression Scale [32-34]
- Current or pending financial compensation for a neck or back condition [35,36]
- Co-morbid conditions
  ◦ Ongoing substance abuse
  ◦ Body mass index ≥ 40
  ◦ Stage III or IV cancer diagnosis in the past 5 years or active cancer treatment
  ◦ Uncontrolled hypertension
  ◦ Advanced Parkinson's Disease
  ◦ Advanced multiple sclerosis
  ◦ Uncontrolled metabolic disease
  ◦ Diffuse idiopathic skeletal hyperostosis
- Contraindication to SMT
  ◦ Advanced spinal stenosis [37]
  ◦ Spinal fracture [37]
  ◦ Stroke or transient ischemic attack
  ◦ Inflammatory or destructive tissue changes of spine
  ◦ Bleeding disorder [38]
  ◦ Severe osteoporosis [38]
  ◦ Progressive neurological deficits or cauda equina syndrome [38]
- Contraindication to SRE
  ◦ Advanced cardiovascular or pulmonary disease [39]

Eligibility determination
Phone screen
Certified study personnel administer a computer-guided questionnaire to interested individuals by phone. Responses are directly entered into a computer program that determines general eligibility for the first baseline evaluation. Baseline evaluation consists of two visits, 7–21 days apart, which serve as a compliance check and provide a more accurate baseline estimate.

First baseline evaluation
The first baseline evaluation includes informed consent, cognitive function assessment, self-report questionnaire including demographic and outcome measures, and a history and examination by a licensed clinician. The physical examination focuses on the cervical and lumbar spine and assesses posture, gait, range of motion, orthopedic and neurologic tests. Unless recent imaging is available, cervical and lumbar plain radiographs and bone mineral density scans of the distal radius and ulna are taken to rule out exclusionary co-morbidities and contraindications (e.g., spinal stenosis, osteoporosis). Potential participants

that qualify at the first baseline evaluation are reviewed by a group of clinicians and investigators who reach consensus on eligibility (qualify, does not qualify, or referral if necessary).

Second baseline evaluation
A second baseline evaluation includes an informed consent (i.e., review of study activities), a self-report questionnaire, and functional outcome assessment. Consenting participants are then randomly allocated by staff masked to upcoming treatment assignment.

Randomization
Restricted randomization employs a 1:1 allocation ratio. The randomization scheme was generated by an independent statistician using randomly permuted block sizes created with a computerized random number generator. As participants become eligible for randomization, sequentially numbered, opaque, sealed envelopes containing treatment assignments are drawn and opened by study staff in the participant's presence. The randomization scheme and block sizes are concealed from all study staff including those who take part in eligibility determination, enrollment, and randomization.

Blinding
Functional outcome examiners are blinded to participant treatment assignment. The physical nature of the treatments prevents blinding of participants and providers to treatment assignment.

Interventions
Participants receive both SMT and SRE for either 12 weeks or 36 weeks. All are requested to abstain from seeking treatment for their back or neck outside the study. Treatment protocols are based on previous studies by the investigators [40] and study clinicians input. The approach to treatment is pragmatic in nature intended to reflect real-world, patient-centered practice and is tailored to participants' age, physical condition, and preferences [23]. Standardized forms are used to document treatment procedures, adverse events, and participant compliance; all forms are reviewed daily for completeness and protocol compliance. See Table 2 for descriptions of the interventions.

Spinal manipulative therapy (SMT)
SMT and mobilization are defined as the application of manual force to the spinal joints. Each SMT appointment is approximately 20 to 30 minutes and includes history, examination, and treatment. Appointments focus on complaints of the cervical and lumbar spine; however, other musculoskeletal complaints may be addressed if it impacts spine-related disability (e.g., hip complaint

Table 2 Descriptions of the interventions

Intervention	Type	Program design	Delivery method	Dose
SMT	High velocity, low amplitude manipulation (can be drop-table assisted) [41]	Individualized: spinal regions treated and type of therapy used is determined by the chiropractor [42,43]	Treatment delivered by licensed chiropractors with at least 5 years experience	20 to 30 minute visits
				Minimum: 1 visit/month
	Low velocity, low amplitude mobilization			Maximum: 2 visits/week
	Manual distraction, gentle soft tissue massage, hot or cold therapy, and active or passive muscle stretching to facilitate SMT			Individualized: Number of treatments determined by chiropractor & patient [40,44,45]
SRE	Aerobic warm up	Partially individualized: exercise selection, progression, and repetitions are determined by patient's abilities and tolerance	Supervised by exercise therapists*	45 to 60 minute sessions
	Stretching, strengthening, and balance exercises		One-on-one	Minimum: 1 session/month
	Advice to stay active; self-care tips for pain management [46,47]		Uses resistance bands, stability trainers, chairs	Home exercise encouraged between sessions

*Exercise therapists are under the supervision of treating chiropractors.

can be addressed if it impacts low back). Treatment areas are identified by palpatory spine tenderness [42], decreased vertebral motion, abnormal joint play, or abnormal end feel determined by passive motion tests [43]. Treatment procedures include high velocity low amplitude thrust, which can be drop-table assisted [41], and low velocity low amplitude mobilization. Manual distraction, gentle soft tissue massage, hot or cold therapy, and active or passive muscle stretching can be used to facilitate or as an adjunct to SMT.

Frequency of SMT treatment
The minimum frequency of SMT appointments is one per month with a maximum of two per week. The number and frequency of appointments are determined by the chiropractor and patient, guided by responses to a modified version of the Measure Yourself Medical Outcome Profile [44,45].

Supervised rehabilitative exercise (SRE)
Exercise therapy is defined as progressive stretching, strengthening, and balance exercises, which use resistance bands and stability trainers. SRE sessions are delivered by exercise therapists, under the supervision of chiropractors, in individual 45 to 60 minute sessions. There are 4 sessions spaced throughout the 12 week intervention and 10 sessions in the 36 week intervention. Exercises focus on increasing spinal mobility, strengthening supporting spinal musculature, and increasing overall stability and proprioception (see Table 3). All sessions include a 5 to 10 minute aerobic warm up on a treadmill or stationary bike. At the first session, participants are given information about their spine-related condition, self-care tips for pain management, and benefits of exercise for back and neck problems. Participants

review goals of the SRE program and set personal activity goals with their therapist. During the second session, strengthening exercises and body mechanics for activities of daily living are introduced. Exercises are introduced at an intensity commensurate to the participant's level of fitness and abilities based upon the therapist's assessment. Subsequent sessions review previous exercises and check for proper form. Ongoing encouragement to promote physical activity and movement to decrease fear avoidance is provided [46,47].

Participants are encouraged to perform the exercises at home between supervised sessions (see Table 3). To encourage compliance with home exercise, exercise logs, resistance bands, stability trainers, and exercise handouts are provided. The handouts feature pictures of older adults performing the exercise with simple written instructions.

Compliance
To be considered compliant in the 36 week group, participants must attend one SMT appointment per month for eight of the nine months and eight of ten SRE sessions. Compliance in the 12 week group is defined as attending one SMT appointment per month for all three months and three of four SRE sessions.

Rescue medication & reasons for withdrawal
For individuals experiencing acute exacerbation of pain, rescue medications are available by prescription from a study medical doctor following an evidence-based protocol. If a participant becomes involved with litigation for a neck- or back-related condition, demonstrates progressive neurological signs, or develops any co-morbidity that increases the risk of study participation (e.g., a new transient ischemic attack), they are withdrawn from

Table 3 Details of exercises in SRE program

Type (Freq) Exercise	Sets	Repetitions	Exercise description	Progressions
Stretching (performed daily at home)				
head retraction	1	5	Seated with head in neutral position, alternate retracting head back and returning to neutral.	
cat camel	1	5	Begin with the pelvis in a neutral position, alternate between arching the back in a "C" shape forward and backward.	1: Seated 2: Hands/knees
shoulder shrug	1	1	Seated with head and neck in neutral position, raise shoulders in a cephalic direction, and release.	
neck forward bend	1	1	Seated with head in neutral position, flex head forward to bring chin toward the chest.	
neck side bend	1	1	Seated with head in neutral position, keep shoulders stationary, tip head to side approximating ear to shoulder. Release & repeat on other side.	
hamstring stretch	1	1	Seated with one leg straight and one leg bent, flex at the waist while keeping leg straight. Repeat on other side.	
seated hip stretch	1	1	Seated, place one ankle on the opposite knee. Use the hand to add pressure on bent knee to externally rotate the hip. Repeat on other side.	
Balance (performed daily at home)				
knee lift	up to 2	up to 5	Stand next to a chair; bend one knee to lift the foot a few inches off the floor; slowly lower foot to floor. Repeat on other side.	1: Chair assisted 2: Stability trainer, chair assisted 3: Unassisted 4: Stability trainer, unassisted
stance/lunge	up to 2	up to 5	Stance: Stand with feet together, step forward so heel touches the opposite foot's toes. Return to the start position; repeat on other side.	1: Semi-tandem stance, chair assisted 2: Semi-tandem stance, unassisted 3: Stability trainer, semi-tandem stance, chair assisted 4: Stability trainer, semi-tandem stance, unassisted 5: Semi-tandem lunge, chair assisted 6: Stability trainer, semi-tandem lunge, chair assisted 7: Tandem stance, chair assisted* 8: Tandem stance, unassisted* 9: Stability trainer, tandem stance, chair assisted*
			Lunge: Begin with feet together, take an exaggerated step forward. Lower the knee of the back leg towards the ground and then rise to return to starting position with the feet together. Repeat on other side.	10: Stability trainer, tandem stance, unassisted*
Strengthening (performed every other day at home)				
bird dog	up to 2	up to 5	Begin on hands and knees, extend either one or two (contra lateral) extremities parallel to floor. Return to start position; repeat on other side.	1: Hands/knees leg only 2: Hands/knees, leg and arm combined 3: Stability trainer, hands/knees, leg and arm combined
push up	up to 2	up to 10	From a plank position, lower the body by bending the arms, keeping the back straight. Return to start position.	1: Wall 2: Kneeling 3: Full body

Table 3 Details of exercises in SRE program *(Continued)*

abdominal curl	up to 2	up to 10	Lie face up on floor with one knee bent and one leg straight; lift the shoulders off the ground and flex at the waist; release. After first set, switch bent knee.	1: Supine on floor, hands at side
				2: Supine on floor, arms on chest
				3: Supine on floor, hands behind head
				4: Supine on floor, hands overhead
				5: Stability
				trainer, hands at side
				6: Stability trainer, arms on chest
				7: Stability trainer, hands behind head
				8: Stability trainer hands overhead
resisted head retraction	up to 2	up to 10	Seated with head in neutral position facing a closed door. A resistance band is looped around the head/forehead with end secured by a firmly closed door. Alternate head retraction and release.	1: Yellow Theraband®
				2: Red Theraband®
				3: Green Theraband®
chair squat	up to 2	up to 10	Stand in front of a chair, bend knees and hips to lower body to a seated position; return to standing.	1: Two handed assist
				2: Arms at sides
				3: Arms crossed
				4: Arms out front
				5: Stability trainer, arms at sides
				6: Stability trainer, arms crossed
				7: Stability trainer, arms out front

*Only one set is required to progress.
Sets and repetitions listed are for each side, if appropriate. Progressions are introduced when the participant can complete the maximum number of sets and repetitions with proper form. Neutral position of the head implies a relaxed posture, the ears aligned with the shoulders. Neutral pelvis cues the patient to position themselves with a slight, not exaggerated, lordosis in the lumbar spine.

treatment by the steering committee. Participants with medical conditions that warrant additional follow up and treatment are referred.

Data collection

Outcome measures are collected through self-report questionnaires, interviews, and blinded functional assessments (see Table 4 for data collection schedule). Patient flow characteristics (i.e., number evaluated, disqualified, etc.) are monitored according to the Consolidated Standards of Reporting Trials (CONSORT) guidelines for standardized reporting of clinical trials [48].

Primary outcome measures
Self-report questionnaires
Back and neck disability The Oswestry Disability Index [50,64] (ODI) version 2.0 (section 4, item 6, has been modified to read "I am in bed most of the time.") and the Neck Disability Index [49] (NDI) are valid and reliable outcome measures for back- and neck-related disability. The NDI was derived from the ODI; therefore, both instruments have similar measurement properties, which may aid in the comparison of results. Each outcome measure has 10 sections, each section with six

possible responses that reflect increasing disability (0 = no disability, 5 = maximal disability).

Secondary outcome measures
Self-report questionnaires
Pain Patients with spinal conditions consider pain to be one of the most important outcome measures [65]. Participants are asked to rate their typical level of neck, mid back, arm, low back, and leg pain during the past week on an 11-box scale (0 = no pain, 10 = worst pain possible); one response for each area [51].

General Health The EuroQol EQ-5D [52] is used to determine the participant's general health state. It is a multi-attribute utility scale that measures five dimensions (mobility, self-care, usual activities, pain/discomfort, anxiety/depression) with three response levels (no problem, moderate problem, severe problem). It also includes a visual analog scale, the EuroQol thermometer, which measures overall health status.

Improvement Improvement in both back and neck problems after starting treatment in the study is measured using a single nine-point ordinal scale (1 = no symptoms/

Table 4 Data collection schedule

	BEV1	BEV2	W4	W12	W24	W36	W37	W52	W78
Demographics	X								
Clinical characteristics/physical examination	X								
Self-report outcome measures									
Disability: NDI [49] and ODI [50]	X	X	X	X	X	X		X	X
Pain: 11-box scale [51]	X	X	X	X	X	X		X	X
General health: EuroQol EQ-5D [52]	X	X	X	X	X	X		X	X
Improvement [40,53,54]			X	X	X	X		X	X
Pain Self-Efficacy Questionnaire [55]	X	X	X	X	X	X		X	X
Tampa Scale for Kinesiophobia [56,57]	X	X	X	X	X	X		X	X
Satisfaction [40,53,54]			X	X	X	X		X	X
Medication use [40,53]	X	X	X	X	X	X		X	X
Expectations [40,53]		X		X	X	X	X		
Falls [58]		X		X	X	X		X	X
*Side effects [40,59]			X	X	X	X			
Home exercise frequency			X	X	X	X		X	X
Self-reported influence	X	X	X	X	X	X		X	X
Functional outcome measures									
Hand grip strength [60]		X					X		
Short physical performance battery (SPPB) [61,62]		X					X		
Accelerometry (7 days) [63]		X				X			
Qualitative data collection									
Interviews					X 12wk	X 36wk			

BEV = Baseline evaluation; W = weeks post-randomization; 12wk = 12 week treatment group only; 36wk = 36 week treatment group only.
*Also collected at treatment visits during intervention phase: BL2-W12 for 12wk group; BL2-W36 for 36wk group.

100% improvement, 9 = as bad as it could be/100% worse) [40,53,54].

Self-efficacy The Pain Self-Efficacy Questionnaire is a valid and reliable [55] 10-item scale used to assess the participant's confidence level (0 = not at all confident, 6 = completely confident) when performing physical and social activities in the presence of chronic pain.

Kinesiophobia The Tampa Scale of Kinesiophobia [56,57] measures fear of movement and (re)injury; it has been shown to be valid and reliable in chronic pain conditions [66] including back pain [67]. It is a 17-item tool that is scored using a four-point Likert scale (1 = strongly disagree, 4 = strongly agree).

Satisfaction Participants will rate how satisfied they are with the care they have received in the study on a seven-point scale (1 = completely satisfied/couldn't be better, 7 = completely dissatisfied, couldn't be worse) [40,53,54].

Medication Use Participants report frequency of use for over-the-counter and prescription medications for their back or neck problem during the past week; this is measured using an eight-point scale (0 = have not taken any, 7 = every day). Participants then identify the medications used during the past week [40,53].

Improvement, satisfaction, and medication use outcome measures have not been tested for validity or reliability.

Functional outcome measures
Functional outcome assessments take approximately 30 minutes and occur at baseline and week 37.

Functional ability
Hand Grip Strength Hand grip strength, a surrogate of overall functional ability and mortality [68-70], measures the grip strength exerted in a maximum effort using a hand-held hydraulic dynamometer (JAMAR Hand Dynamometer, Therapeutic Equipment Corporation, Clifton, NH) [71,72]. The procedure and scoring rubric are from Mathiowetz et al. [60]. This test was modified by alternating hands between each measurement; further, it is considered invalid if the participant cannot perform 3 or more contractions or if there is more than a 20 kg difference between any two measurements.

Short Physical Performance Battery (SPPB) The SPPB is shown to predict future disability in healthy community dwelling older adults over the age of 70 [62]. Adapted from the National Institute on Aging, it is comprised of three tests: gait speed, standing balance, and chair rising [61]. Each component of the SPPB is scored on a five-point scale (0 = inability to perform, 4 = highest level of performance); these are summed to produce a composite score. The protocols and scoring rubrics are based on the method developed by Guralnik et al. [62]. Modifications of the SPPB include reordering of the tests and performing tests on a force plate. Specifically, gait speed is performed first with the shoes on, while the two remaining components are completed in stocking feet on the force plate. The force plate records ground reaction forces during the standing balance and chair stand tests (Bertec Force Plate, Model #4060-NC, Bertec, Inc, Columbus, OH) using Motion Monitor data acquisition software (Innovative Sports Training, Inc, Chicago, IL) to define the participant's center-of-pressure.

Physical activity
Accelerometry A valid and reliable measure for physical activity is an accelerometer [63], which measures activity in three planes including the intensity and duration of movement. The GT3X accelerometer (Actigraph, Inc, Pensacola, FL) is worn for 7 consecutive days at 2 time points: prior to both the first treatment visit and week 37. The GT3X is light (19 grams), small (4.6 x 3.3 x 2.5 cm), and worn at the hip.

Qualitative interviews
One-on-one interviews are conducted upon completion of treatment [73]. The interview format is semi-structured; trained interviewers follow a standardized protocol for conducting interviews [74] beginning with open-ended questions followed by probing questions to elicit underlying reasons and additional details:

- When you have discomfort or pain in your neck or back, how does it affect you? *(Probes: Can you tell me more about that? In what ways does it affect your life?)*
- Do you expect your neck and back problems will improve, stay the same, or get worse in the future? *(Probes: In what way?)*
- In general, when seeking care for your neck and back problems, what types of things make a treatment worthwhile to you? *(Probes: Overall, what do you look for in a treatment? What makes a treatment worth investing your time, energy, or money in?)*
- In your opinion, what was the most beneficial/helpful part of being in this study? *(Probes: Why is that? Was there anything you liked about the study?)*

- What was the least beneficial/helpful part of being in this study? *(Probes: Why is that? Was there anything you didn't like about the study?)*

Interviews are kept confidential to allow the participants to speak freely and audio-recorded if the participant consents [73]. Recorded interviews are transcribed for analysis; a portion of the transcriptions are cross-checked with the audio for quality assurance purposes.

Additional outcome measures
Falls
Data on falls is collected through a modified outcome measurement tool [58]. Participants are asked if they have fallen and landed on the floor or ground or have fallen and hit an object like a table or chair during the past four weeks. If they respond 'yes,' they are asked how many times they have fallen during the past four weeks (1, 2–3, 4–5, or 6 or more) and injuries sustained (broke or fractured bone, hit or injured my head, sprain or strain, bruise or bleeding, some other kind of injury, and no injuries).

Side effects
Participants report side effects by indicating 'yes' or 'no' to the following list of known contraindications and potential side effects of SMT and SRE:

- Increase in neck or back pain
- A different type of pain than usually experienced
- Dizziness or nausea[*]
- Increase in numbness or tingling in the arms/hands[*]
- Increase in numbness or tingling in the legs/feet[*]
- Numbness in the saddle area[*]
- Change in bowel or bladder habits[*]
- Increase in difficulty in lifting one or both feet while walking[*]
- Other

*Triggers a clinical evaluation by a study doctor to further assess the participant's condition.

For each side effect indicated, the participant rates the bothersomeness of the symptom on an ordinal 11-point scale (0 = not at all bothersome, 10 = extremely bothersome) [40,59].

Home exercise
Participants report how frequently they performed the study exercises in the past week; this is measured on an eight-point scale (0 = have not done any, 7 = every day).

These three additional outcome measures have not been tested for validity or reliability.

Adverse events and unanticipated problems

Expected and unexpected adverse events and unantici-pated problems (AE/UP) are captured when possible. Active surveillance of harms [75] occurs at every treat-ment visit through standardized treatment forms (see *Side Effects*). Passive surveillance of harms [75] occurs at all time points. AE/UPs are categorized by investiga-tors using a standardized form with categories congruent with U.S. Department of Health and Human Services [76]. Reportable AE/UPs are forwarded within 3 business days to the DSMB and funding agency and to the IRB within 10 business days. All AE/UPs are reported unblinded to the DSMB annually and to the IRB upon request.

Potential confounding variables

Variables that may influence outcomes, such as depres-sion, level of physical activity outside the study setting, ex-pectations to treatment, and other health care utilization, are measured and will be taken into account during the statistical analysis, if appropriate.

Depression

The Geriatric Depression Scale (short form) is adminis-tered at baseline to screen for depression in older, pos-sibly cognitively impaired populations [32-34].

Physical activity

Participants rate the amount of physical activity outside the study setting in their daily routine at baseline (none, very light, light, moderate, heavy, very heavy).

Expectations

Participants are asked just prior to randomization how they expect to respond to both treatment groups (much worse, worse, no change, better, or much better) [40,53,77]. Participants are also asked how much they expect their back or neck problem to change 3 months from now using a nine-point scale (1 = no symptoms/100% improvement, 9 = as bad as it could be/100% worse) at baseline and at weeks 12, 24, and 36. At week 52, participants are asked how they expect their back and neck problem to be six months from now.

Healthcare utilization

This is captured in self-report questionnaires by asking if participants have seen any non-study health providers for their back and neck problem in the last month. Treatment received from non-study providers is also captured in the standardized treatment forms.

Data analysis
Statistical methods

Data analyses will be conducted using SAS for Windows (Release 9.1 or higher). Descriptive statistics will be cal-culated to describe patient baseline characteristics in each treatment group and to assess comparability and generalizability. Baseline values of self-report outcome variables will be obtained by averaging the two baseline visits. Demographic and clinical variables determined by the investigators to impact outcomes or those that have a correlation of 0.5 or greater will be considered as other possible covariates [78]. Intention-to-treat analysis will be used; patients with one or more follow up measures will be included in the analysis. Normality assumptions will be evaluated through normal probability plots and data transformed, if necessary.

Sample size

Sample size is based on detecting a minimally important between group difference of 10% [79] in the ODI at week 36, with a variance of 0.20 [80,81]. Using baseline values as covariates in a two-arm design, 85 subjects per group allows a power of 0.90 to be achieved at an alpha level of 0.025. Assuming a 15% dropout or loss to follow up rate, 100 patients are required per group, for a total of 200 subjects.

Primary and secondary analyses

Primary analysis will use a linear mixed-model method for repeated data to test for between-group differences in neck and back disability separately at week 36, with baseline variables that may influence outcomes as covar-iates [82,83]. Secondary analysis of disability will include testing for between-group differences at weeks 4, 12, 24, 52, and 78, as well as within-group change at all time points. Longitudinal analysis will be performed through the short (weeks 4, 12, 24 and 36) and long term (weeks 4, 12, 24, 36, 52 and 78).

Secondary outcome measures, including pain, general health, improvement, self-efficacy, kinesiophobia, satisfac-tion, medication use, and functional outcome measures will be similarly calculated for within- and between-group differences. This study is not powered to detect change in the secondary outcome measures.

Content analysis of qualitative interviews will use both inductive and deductive approaches [84] to identify themes that occur in response to questions asked [85]. When coding is complete, frequency of themes will be quantified and representative quotations will be identified [85,86].

Confirmatory analyses

Additional confirmatory analysis will calculate the area under the curve for each variable, taking into account the increasing time intervals between assessments [87]. If the area under the curve analysis differs in result from the repeated measures, it suggests that the cumulative experience over time is different.

Discussion

This is one of the first full-scale randomized clinical trials to compare short term treatment and long term management using SMT and exercise to treat spine-related disability in older adults. It builds on previous research by the investigative team showing improvement with three months of SMT and exercise in similar populations, which regressed to baseline values in long term follow up without further intervention [88]. As back and neck pain in older adults are often chronic and among several co-morbidities [6,8], we theorized that long term management may result in sustained improvement compared to short term treatment. Identifying the most favorable duration of treatment is a pragmatic question common to patients, clinicians, policy makers, and third-party payers alike [25,89]. This is especially important to address in an older population, whose long term functional ability is essential to maintaining vitality and independence.

In addition to effectiveness, this trial systematically evaluates harms associated with SMT and SRE. There is a need to improve the reporting of harms in general [75], and in particular, those associated with exercise programs [90] and SMT [26,91] where evidence is limited [92,93]. Importantly, for older adults, the harms may be different from those experienced in general population due to the age-related changes and the natural history of other diseases [90]. This may cause concern for patients or practitioners, and the current lack of evidence highlights the importance of collecting this data [23,89]. For these reasons, this trial developed and implemented standardized, prospective data collection strategies to systematically report harms associated with SMT and SRE. Improved reporting of harms, in addition to effectiveness, will provide more balanced information on risks and benefits of these treatments, which then can be translated into clinical practice.

The qualitative component of this study explores older adults' experiences with back and neck problems, a condition which has been widely acknowledged as a complex phenomenon [94]. A patient's individual experience with back and neck problems is difficult to fully appreciate with quantitative data collection alone. Using a mixed-method approach allows this study to better understand the impact of study treatments through complementary approaches to data collection, facilitating a more robust interpretation and understanding of spine-related disability in older adults. Additionally, these results may enlighten the design and implementation of spine care treatment for older adults in both future research studies and clinical practice.

The Patient-Centered Outcomes Research Institute (PCORI) has called for "comparative clinical effectiveness research that will give patients and those who care for them the ability to make better-informed health decisions" [95]. Pragmatic study designs reflect real world practice, using input from stakeholders such as clinicians to answer practical questions [96]. This trial was designed with that goal in mind. Study clinicians were engaged in developing parameters for the study treatments to help investigators determine protocols for frequency of visits and specific therapies used in the treatment encounter. Further, care was individualized to patients according to their age, physical condition, and preferences. To that end, the interventions in this study are designed to be more reflective of clinical practice and increase the generalizability of results when the study is complete. Subsequently, clinically useful findings from this study may guide health care decisions and policy regarding conservative non-pharmacological management of spinal disability in older adults.

Trial status and timeline

Recruitment began in January 2010 and was completed in May 2013; participants received treatment through December 2013. Data collection will continue through 2014 which will be followed by data cleaning, analysis, and reporting in 2015.

Abbreviations

AE/UP: Adverse events and unanticipated problems; CONSORT: Consolidated Standards of Reporting Trials; DSMB: Data and safety monitoring board; HRSA: Health Resources and Services Administration; IRB: Institutional Review Board; NDI: Neck Disability Index; NWHSU: Northwestern Health Sciences University; ODI: Oswestry Disability Index; SMT: Spinal manipulative therapy; SPPB: Short Physical Performance Battery; SRE: Supervised rehabilitative exercise.

Competing interests

The authors declare that they have no competing interests.

Authors' contributions

MM, JH, RE, GB, KW, and CS are investigators for this trial; MM, as the principle investigator, has overall responsibility for the conduct of the trial. MM, JH, RE, GB, KW participated in the initial trial concept. MM, JH, RE, GB, KW, and CS contributed to protocol development, implementation and redesign. CV is a research fellow and a project manager for the trial. CV prepared the first draft of the manuscript and organized revisions under the mentorship of MM. All authors read, provided feedback, and approved the final manuscript.

Acknowledgements

The trial was funded by the U.S. Department of Health and Human Services Health Resources and Services Administration (HRSA), Bureau of Health Professions (BHPr), Division of Medicine and Dentistry (DMD), grant number R18HP15127. The content and conclusions of this manuscript are those of the authors and should not be construed as the official position or policy of, nor should any endorsements be inferred by the U.S. government, HHS, HRSA, BHPr, or the DMD.
The authors wish to thank the research clinicians and staff participating in the trial and study collaborators for their input during the design and implementation of this trial. Low technology exercise equipment for this study was kindly donated by Performance Health/Hygenics Corporation.

Author details

[1]Northwestern Health Sciences University, Wolfe-Harris Center for Clinical Studies, 2501 W 84th Street, Bloomington, MN 55431, USA. [2]University of Minnesota, Center for Spirituality and Healing, Mayo Memorial Building C592,

420 Delaware Street SE, Minneapolis, MN 55455, USA. [3]Institute of Sports Science and Clinical Biomechanics, University of Southern Denmark, Campusvej 55, Odense, M DK-5230, Denmark.

References

1. Thomas E, Peat G, Harris L, Wilkie R, Croft PR: The prevalence of pain and pain interference in a general population of older adults: cross-sectional findings from the North Staffordshire Osteoarthritis Project (NorStOP). Pain 2004, 110:361–368.
2. Hartvigsen J, Christensen K: Pain in the back and neck are with us until the end: a nationwide interview-based survey of Danish 100-year-olds. Spine 2008, 33:909–913.
3. Macfarlane GJ, Beasley M, Jones EA, Prescott GJ, Docking R, Keeley P, McBeth J, Jones GT: The prevalence and management of low back pain across adulthood: results from a population-based cross-sectional study (the MUSICIAN study). Pain 2012, 153:27–32.
4. Schopflocher D, Taenzer P, Jovey R: The prevalence of chronic pain in Canada. Pain Res Manag 2011, 16:445–450.
5. Strine TW, Hootman JM: US national prevalence and correlates of low back and neck pain among adults. Arthritis Rheum 2007, 57:656–665.
6. Hartvigsen J, Frederiksen H, Christensen K: Back pain remains a common symptom in old age. A population-based study of 4486 Danish twins aged 70–102. Eur Spine J 2003, 12:528–534.
7. Gill TM, Desai MM, Gahbauer EA, Holford TR, Williams CS: Restricted activity among community-living older persons: incidence, precipitants, and health care utilization. Ann Intern Med 2001, 135:313–321.
8. Magni G, Marchetti M, Moreschi C, Merskey H, Luchini SR: Chronic musculoskeletal pain and depressive symptoms in the National Health and Nutrition Examination. I. Epidemiologic follow-up study. Pain 1993, 53:163–168.
9. Nuesch E, Dieppe P, Reichenbach S, Williams S, Iff S, Juni P: All cause and disease specific mortality in patients with knee or hip osteoarthritis: population based cohort study. BMJ 2011, 342:d1165.
10. Martin BI, Deyo RA, Mirza SK, Turner JA, Comstock BA, Hollingworth W, Sullivan SD: Expenditures and health status among adults with back and neck problems. JAMA 2008, 299:656–664.
11. Weiner DK, Kim YS, Bonino P, Wang T: Low back pain in older adults: are we utilizing healthcare resources wisely? Pain Med 2006, 7:143–150.
12. Pasquale MK, Dufour R, Schaaf D, Reiners AT, Mardekian J, Joshi AV, Patel NC: Pain conditions ranked by healthcare costs for members of a national health plan. Pain Pract 2013, 14:117–131.
13. US Census Bureau: US Census Bureau Pop Projections. 2009. [https://www.census.gov/population/projections/data/national/2009.html] Last accessed: 07/08/2014.
14. Administration on Aging, U.S.Department of Health and Human Services: A Profile of Older Americans. 2009. [http://www.aoa.gov/aoaroot/aging_statistics/profile/2009/docs/2009profile_508.pdf] Last accessed: 07/08/2014.
15. Hayden JA, van Tulder MW, Tomlinson G: Systematic review: strategies for using exercise therapy to improve outcomes in chronic low back pain. Ann Intern Med 2005, 142:776–785.
16. Kay TM, Gross A, Goldsmith CH, Rutherford S, Voth S, Hoving JL, Bronfort G, Santaguida PL: Exercises for mechanical neck disorders. Cochrane Database Syst Rev 2012, 8:CD004250.
17. Paterson DH, Warburton DE: Physical activity and functional limitations in older adults: a systematic review related to Canada's Physical Activity Guidelines. Int J Behav Nutr Phys Act 2010, 7:38.
18. How much physical activity do older adults need? http://www.cdc.gov/physicalactivity/everyone/guidelines/olderadults.html Last accessed 5-31-2013.
19. Foster DF, Phillips RS, Hamel MB, Eisenberg DM: Alternative medicine use in older Americans. J Am Geriatr Soc 2000, 48:1560–1565.
20. Cheung CK, Wyman JF, Halcon LL: Use of complementary and alternative therapies in community-dwelling older adults. J Altern Complement Med 2007, 13:997–1006.
21. Gross A, Miller J, D'Sylva J, Burnie SJ, Goldsmith CH, Graham N, Haines T, Bronfort G, Hoving JL: Manipulation or mobilisation for neck pain. Cochrane Database Syst Rev 2010, CD004249.

22. Cecchi F, Molino-Lova R, Chiti M, Pasquini G, Paperini A, Conti AA, Macchi C: Spinal manipulation compared with back school and with individually delivered physiotherapy for the treatment of chronic low back pain: a randomized trial with one-year follow-up. Clin Rehabil 2010, 24:26–36.
23. Hondras MA, Long CR, Cao Y, Rowell RM, Meeker WC: A randomized controlled trial comparing 2 types of spinal manipulation and minimal conservative medical care for adults 55 years and older with subacute or chronic low back pain. J Manipulative Physiol Ther 2009, 32:330–343.
24. Manchikanti L, Singh V, Datta S, Cohen SP, Hirsch JA: Comprehensive review of epidemiology, scope, and impact of spinal pain. Pain Physician 2009, 12:E35–E70.
25. Descarreaux M, Blouin JS, Drolet M, Papadimitriou S, Teasdale N: Efficacy of preventive spinal manipulation for chronic low-back pain and related disabilities: a preliminary study. J Manipulative Physiol Ther 2004, 27:509–514.
26. Taylor DN: A theoretical basis for maintenance spinal manipulative therapy for the chiropractic profession. J Chiropr Humanit 2011, 18:74–85.
27. Senna MK, Machaly SA: Does maintained spinal manipulation therapy for chronic nonspecific low back pain result in better long-term outcome? Spine 2011, 36:1427–1437.
28. Hawk C, Cambron JA, Pfefer MT: Pilot study of the effect of a limited and extended course of chiropractic care on balance, chronic pain, and dizziness in older adults. J Manipulative Physiol Ther 2009, 32:438–447.
29. La Rocca H: Failed lumbar surgery: principles of management. In The Lumbar Spine. Edited by Weinstein JN, Weisel SW, International Society for the Study of the Lumbar Spine. Philadelphia, PA: W.B. Saunders; 1990:872–881.
30. Folstein MF, Folstein SE, McHugh PR: "Mini-mental state". A practical method for grading the cognitive state of patients for the clinician. J Psychiatr Res 1975, 12:189–198.
31. O'Bryant SE, Humphreys JD, Smith GE, Ivnik RJ, Graff-Radford NR, Petersen RC, Lucas JA: Detecting dementia with the mini-mental state examination in highly educated individuals. Arch Neurol 2008, 65:963–967.
32. Sheikh JI, Yesavage JA: Geriatric Depression Scale (GDS): recent evidence and development of a shorter version. Clin Gerontol 1986, 5:165–173.
33. Yesavage JA: Geriatric Depression Scale. Psychopharmacol Bull 1988, 24:709–711.
34. Yesavage JA, Brink TL, Rose TL, Lum O, Huang V, Adey M, Leirer VO: Development and validation of a geriatric depression screening scale: a preliminary report. J Psychiatr Res 1982, 17:37–49.
35. Rasmussen C, Leboeuf-Yde C, Hestbaek L, Manniche C: Poor outcome in patients with spine-related leg or arm pain who are involved in compensation claims: a prospective study of patients in the secondary care sector. Scand J Rheumatol 2008, 37:462–468.
36. Deyo RA: Early diagnostic evaluation of low back pain. J Gen Intern Med 1986, 1:328–338.
37. Spitzer WO: Scientific approach to the assessment and management of activity-related spinal disorders. A monograph for clinicians. Report of the Quebec Task Force on Spinal Disorders. Spine 1987, 12:S1–S59.
38. Eck JC, Circolone NJ: The use of spinal manipulation in the treatment of low back pain: a review of goals, patient selection, techniques, and risks. J Orthop Sci 2000, 5:411–417.
39. American Geriatrics Society Panel on Exercise and Osteoarthritis: Exercise prescription for older adults with osteoarthritis pain: Consensus practice recommendations. JAGS 2001, 49:808–823.
40. Maiers M, Hartvigsen J, Schulz C, Schulz K, Evans R, Bronfort G: Chiropractic and exercise for seniors with low back pain or neck pain: the design of two randomized clinical trials. BMC Musculoskelet Disord 2007, 8:94.
41. Bergmann TF, Peterson DH: Chiropractic Technique: Principles and Procedures. St. Louis: Mosby; 2011.
42. Hubka MJ, Phelan SP: Interexaminer reliability of palpation for cervical spine tenderness. J Manipulative Physiol Ther 1994, 17:591–595.
43. Seffinger MA, Najm WI, Mishra SI, Adams A, Dickerson VM, Murphy LS, Reinsch S: Reliability of spinal palpation for diagnosis of back and neck pain: a systematic review of the literature. Spine 2004, 29:E413–E425.
44. Paterson C: Measuring outcomes in primary care: a patient generated measure, MYMOP, compared with the SF-36 health survey. BMJ 1996, 312:1016–1020.

45. Paterson C, Britten N: In pursuit of patient-centred outcomes: a qualitative evaluation of the 'Measure Yourself Medical Outcome Profile'. *J Health Serv Res Policy* 2000, 5:27–36.

46. Engers A, Jellema P, Wensing M, van der Windt D, Grol R, van Tulder M: Individual patient education for low back pain; a systematic review. In *Low Back Pain in General Practice. Should Treatment be aimed at Psychosocial Factors?* Edited by Jellema P. Amsterdam, The Netherlands: Febodruk BV; 2005:123–156.

47. Burton AK, Waddell G, Tillotson KM, Summerton N: Information and advice to patients with back pain can have a positive effect. A randomized controlled trial of a novel educational booklet in primary care. *Spine* 1999, 24:2484–2491.

48. Schulz KF, Altman DG, Moher D: CONSORT 2010 statement: updated guidelines for reporting parallel group randomised trials. *BMJ* 2010, 340:c332.

49. Vernon H, Mior S: The Neck Disability Index: a study of reliability and validity. *J Manipulative Physiol Ther* 1991, 14:409–415.

50. Fairbank JC, Pynsent PB: The Oswestry Disability Index. *Spine* 2000, 25:2940–2953.

51. Jensen MP, Karoly P, Braver S: The measurement of clinical pain intensity: a comparison of six methods. *Pain* 1986, 27:117–126.

52. The EuroQol Group: EuroQol – a new facility for the measurement of health-related quality of life. *Health Policy* 1990, 16:199–206.

53. Bronfort G, Evans R, Nelson B, Aker P, Goldsmith C, Vernon H: A randomized clinical trial of exercise and spinal manipulation for patients with chronic neck pain. *Spine* 2001, 26:788–799.

54. Schulz CA, Hondras MA, Evans RL, Gudavalli MR, Long CR, Owens EF, Wilder DG, Bronfort G: Chiropractic and self-care for back-related leg pain: design of a randomized clinical trial. *Chiropr Man Therap* 2011, 19:8.

55. Nicholas MK: The pain self-efficacy questionnaire: Taking pain into account. *Eur J Pain* 2006, 11:153–163.

56. The Tampa scale. http://www.worksafe.vic.gov.au/__data/assets/pdf_file/0020/10964/tampa_scale_kinesiophobia.pdf *Last accessed* 5-31-2013.

57. Kori SH, Miller RP, Todd D: Kinesiophobia: A new view of chronic pain behavior. *Pain Management* 1990, 3:35–43.

58. Knudtson MD, Klein BE, Klein R: Biomarkers of aging and falling: the Beaver Dam eye study. *Arch Gerontol Geriatr* 2009, 49:22–26.

59. Westrom KK, Maiers MJ, Evans RL, Bronfort G: Individualized chiropractic and integrative care for low back pain: the design of a randomized clinical trial using a mixed-methods approach. *Trials* 2010, 11:24.

60. Mathiowetz V, Weber K, Volland G, Kashman N: Reliability and validity of grip and pinch strength evaluations. *J Hand Surg [Am]* 1984, 9:222–226.

61. Guralnik JM, Simonsick EM, Ferrucci L, Glynn RJ, Berkman LF, Blazer DG, Scherr PA, Wallace RB: A short physical performance battery assessing lower extremity function: association with self-reported disability and prediction of mortality and nursing home admission. *J Gerontol* 1994, 49:M85–M94.

62. Guralnik JM, Ferrucci L, Simonsick EM, Salive ME, Wallace RB: Lower-extremity function in persons over the age of 70 years as a predictor of subsequent disability. *N Engl J Med* 1995, 332:556–561.

63. Brage S, Brage N, Wedderkopp N, Froberg K: Reliability and validity of the computer science and applications accelerometer in a mechanical setting. *Meas Phys Educ Exerc Sci* 2003, 7:101–119.

64. Roland M, Fairbank J: The Roland-Morris Disability Questionnaire and the Oswestry Disability Questionnaire. *Spine* 2000, 25:3115–3124.

65. Evans RL, Maiers MJ, Bronfort G: What do patients think? Results of a mixed methods pilot study assessing sciatica patients' interpretations of satisfaction and improvement. *J Manipulative Physiol Ther* 2003, 26:502–509.

66. French DJ, France CR, Vigneau F, French JA, Evans RT: Fear of movement/(re)injury in chronic pain: a psychometric assessment of the original English version of the Tampa scale for kinesiophobia (TSK). *Pain* 2007, 127:42–51.

67. Vlaeyen JW, Kole-Snijders AM, Boeren RG, van Eek H: Fear of movement/(re)injury in chronic low back pain and its relation to behavioral performance. *Pain* 1995, 62:363–372.

68. Giampaoli S, Ferrucci L, Cecchi F, Lo NC, Poce A, Dima F, Santaquilani A, Vescio MF, Menotti A: Hand-grip strength predicts incident disability in non-disabled older men. *Age Ageing* 1999, 28:283–288.

69. Rantanen T, Volpato S, Ferrucci L, Heikkinen E, Fried LP, Guralnik JM: Handgrip strength and cause-specific and total mortality in older

disabled women: exploring the mechanism. *J Am Geriatr Soc* 2003, 51:636–641.

70. Taekema DG, Gussekloo J, Maier AB, Westendorp RG, de Craen AJ: Handgrip strength as a predictor of functional, psychological and social health. A prospective population-based study among the oldest old. *Age Ageing* 2010, 39:331–337.

71. Richards L, Palmiter-Thomas P: Grip strength measurement: a critical review of tools, methods, and clinical utility. *Crit Rev Phys Rehabil Med* 1996, 8:87–109.

72. Schmidt RT, Toews JV: Grip strength as measured by the Jamar dynamometer. *Arch Phys Med Rehabil* 1970, 51:321–327.

73. Britten N: Qualitative interviews in medical research. In *Qualitative Research in Health Care.* Edited by Mays N, Pope C. London: BMJ Publishing Group; 1996:28–35.

74. Newman I, Benz CR: *Qualitative-Quantitative Research Methodology: Exploring the Interactive Continuum.* Carbondale, IL: Southern Illinois University Press; 1998.

75. Ioannidis JP, Evans SJ, Gotzsche PC, O'Neill RT, Altman DG, Schulz K, Moher D: Better reporting of harms in randomized trials: an extension of the CONSORT statement. *Ann Intern Med* 2004, 141:781–788.

76. Guidance on reviewing and reporting unanticipated problems involving risks to subjects or others and adverse events. http://www.hhs.gov/ohrp/policy/advevntguid.html *Last accessed* 7-16-2014.

77. Evans R, Bronfort G, Nelson B, Goldsmith CH: Two-year follow-up of a randomized clinical trial of spinal manipulation and two types of exercise for patients with chronic neck pain. *Spine* 2002, 27:2383–2389.

78. Pocock SJ, Assmann SE, Enos LE, Kasten LE: Subgroup analysis, covariate adjustment and baseline comparisons in clinical trial reporting: current practice and problems. *Stat Med* 2002, 21:2917–2930.

79. Ostelo RW, Deyo RA, Stratford P, Waddell G, Croft P, Von Korff M, Bouter LM, de Vet HC: Interpreting change scores for pain and functional status in low back pain: towards international consensus regarding minimal important change. *Spine* 2008, 33:90–94.

80. Triano JJ, McGregor M, Hondras MA, Brennan PC: Manipulative therapy versus education programs in chronic low back pain. *Spine* 1995, 20:948–955.

81. Davidson M, Keating JL: A comparison of five low back disability questionnaires: reliability and responsiveness. *Phys Ther* 2002, 82:8–24.

82. Littell RC, Milliken GA, Stroup WW, Wolfinger RD: *SAS System for Mixed Models.* Cary, NC: SAS Publications; 1996.

83. Vonesh EF, Chinchilli VM: *Linear and Nonlinear Models for the Analysis of Repeated Measurements.* New York: Marcel Dekker, Inc.; 1997.

84. Lincoln YS, Guba EG: *Naturalistic Inquiry.* Beverly Hills, CA: Sage Publications, Inc.; 1985.

85. Bauer M: Classical Content Analysis: A Review. In *Qualitative Researching with Text, Image and Sound: A Practical Handbook for Social Research.* Edited by Bauer M, Gaskell G. London, UK: Sage Publications, Inc; 2000:131–151.

86. Tashakkori A, Teddlie C: *Mixed Methodology: Combining Qualitative and Quantitative Approaches.* Thousand Oaks, CA: Sage; 1998.

87. Matthews JN, Altman DG, Campbell MJ, Royston P: Analysis of serial measurements in medical research. *BMJ* 1990, 300:230–235.

88. Maiers M, Bronfort G, Evans R, Hartvigsen J, Svendsen K, Bracha Y, Schulz C, Schulz K, Grimm R: Spinal manipulative therapy and exercise for seniors with chronic neck pain. *Spine J* 2013, doi:10.1016/j.spinee.2013.10.035. [Epub ahead of print].

89. Hawk C, Schneider M, Dougherty P, Gleberzon BJ, Killinger LZ: Best practices recommendations for chiropractic care for older adults: results of a consensus process. *J Manipulative Physiol Ther* 2010, 33:464–473.

90. Liu CJ, Latham N: Adverse events reported in progressive resistance strength training trials in older adults: 2 sides of a coin. *Arch Phys Med Rehabil* 2010, 91:1471–1473.

91. Ernst E: Adverse effects of spinal manipulation: a systematic review. *J R Soc Med* 2007, 100:330–338.

92. Walker BF, Losco B, Clarke BR, Hebert J, French S, Stomski NJ: Outcomes of usual chiropractic, harm & efficacy, the ouch study: study protocol for a randomized controlled trial. *Trials* 2011, 12:235.

93. Dougherty PE, Hawk C, Weiner DK, Gleberzon B, Andrew K, Killinger L: The role of chiropractic care in older adults. *Chiropr Man Therap* 2012, 20:3.

94. Sweet WH: Pain–old and new methods of study and treatment. *Acta Neurochir Suppl* 1995, 64:83–87.

95. Patient-Centered Outcomes Research Institute: National Priorities and Research Agenda. www.pcori.org/research-we-support/priorities-agenda *Last accessed* 7-16-2014.
96. Selby JV, Beal AC, Frank L: The Patient-Centered Outcomes Research Institute (PCORI) national priorities for research and initial research agenda. *JAMA* 2012, **307:**1583–1584.

Evaluation of a modified clinical prediction rule for use with spinal manipulative therapy in patients with chronic low back pain: a randomized clinical trial

Paul E Dougherty[1,2,3*], Jurgis Karuza[2,4,5], Dorian Savino[1] and Paul Katz[6,7]

Abstract

Background: Spinal Manipulative Therapy (SMT) and Active Exercise Therapy (AET) have both demonstrated efficacy in the treatment of Chronic Lower Back Pain (CLBP). A Clinical Prediction Rule (CPR) for responsiveness to SMT has been validated in a heterogeneous lower back pain population; however there is a need to evaluate this CPR specifically for patients with CLBP, which is a significant source of disability.

Methods: We conducted a randomized controlled trial (RCT) in Veteran Affairs and civilian outpatient clinics evaluating a modification of the original CPR (mCPR) in CLBP, eliminating acute low back pain and altering the specific types of SMT to improve generalizability. We enrolled and followed 181 patients with CLBP from 2007 to 2010. Patients were randomized by status on the mCPR to undergo either SMT or AET twice a week for four weeks. Providers and statisticians were blinded as to mCPR status. We collected outcome measures at 5, 12 and 24-weeks post baseline. We tested our study hypotheses by a general linear model repeated measures procedure following a univariate analysis of covariance approach. Outcome measures included, Visual Analogue Scale, Bodily pain subscale of SF-36 and the Oswestry Disability Index, Patient Satisfaction and Patient Expectation.

Results: Of the 89 AET patients, 69 (78%) completed the study and of the 92 SMT patients, 76 (83%) completed the study. As hypothesized, we found main effects of time where the SMT and AET groups showed significant improvements in pain and disability from baseline. There were no differences in treatment outcomes between groups in response to the treatment, given the lack of significant treatment x time interactions. The mCPR x treatment x time interactions were not significant. The differences in outcomes between treatment groups were the same for positive and negative on the mCPR groups, thus our second hypothesis was not supported.

Conclusions: We found no evidence that a modification of the original CPR can be used to discriminate CLBP patients that would benefit more from SMT. Further studies are needed to further clarify the patient characteristics that moderate treatment responsiveness to specific interventions for CLBP.

Trial registration: ISRCTN30511490

Keywords: Clinical prediction rule, Chronic lower back pain, Spinal manipulative therapy, Active exercise therapy, Randomized controlled trial

* Correspondence: paul.dougherty@va.gov
[1]Canandaigua Veterans Affairs Medical Center, Canandaigua, NY, USA
[2]New York Chiropractic College, Seneca Falls, NY, USA
Full list of author information is available at the end of the article

Background

Chronic lower back pain (CLBP) is a significant public health problem in both Veterans and the general population [1,2]. Chronic Lower Back Pain is not only a problem in the US, the recent global burden of disease reports that it is one of the most common causes of years lived with disability [2]. Chronic lower back pain is secondary only to respiratory conditions in reasons for visiting primary care [3]. Despite over 200 treatments for CLBP, the costs of treating CLBP have risen 65% in the last 10 years with no appreciable improvement in patient outcomes [4,5].

One contributory factor is inappropriate management due to poor understanding of prognostic factors [6,7]. This is particularly relevant for primary care providers who must make decisions on management strategies for this very common problem [8]. Spinal Manipulative Therapy (SMT) and Active Exercise Therapy (AET) are two commonly utilized, evidence based, interventions for CLBP [9] however neither has shown superiority [10]. It has been hypothesized that identification of specific characteristics predicting clinical responsiveness to these interventions would improve the outcomes through appropriate management [11].

The desire to identify these specific patient characteristics has led to the development of clinical prediction rules (CPR). A CPR is a clinical tool that quantifies individual contributions that various components of the history as well as the physical examination results make towards the diagnosis, prognosis, or likely response to treatment in an individual patient [12]. The CPR for SMT (CPR SMT) was first reported in 2002 [12] and then a validation study was published in 2004 [13]. This CPR predicted responsiveness in patients with lower back pain (LBP) to SMT [13]. Although this is the most studied of the CPRs, it still has not achieved the level of validation to be recommended for general clinical practice [14]. Furthermore, the previous validation studies of CPR SMT included acute, sub-acute and chronic conditions, and so their generalizability specifically to CLBP is unclear. A recent systematic review stated that there "is a lack of good quality RCTs validating the effects of a clinical prediction rule for low back pain" [15].

The current study evaluates the generalizability of the CPR for SMT to a CLBP population. The current study modified the original CPR for SMT for use with a CLBP population therefore creating a modified CPR for SMT (mCPR) that applies four of the five originally proposed components of the CPR for SMT.

Study hypotheses

Based on previous data, our first hypothesis is that patients in both SMT and AET groups would demonstrate statistically and clinically significant improvements in disability and pain from baseline [9,10]. Our second hypothesis predicts that the mCPR moderates the comparative effectiveness of treatment in the SMT group but not the AET treatment group. Based on the data from Childs et al. [13], we hypothesized that the mCPR modifies the comparative effectiveness of (i.e., the differences between) the two treatment groups. We expect the comparative effectiveness between the two treatment arms for the positive on the mCPR group would be different from the comparative effectiveness between the two treatment arms for the negative on the mCPR group.

Methods

Trial design

The study was a prospective RCT using a stratified permutated block design conducted between 2007 and 2010. Chronic lower back pain patients were recruited and evaluated for their status on a mCPR for responsiveness to SMT. Patients were then randomized to receive either SMT or AET twice a week for four weeks. The protocol received Institutional Review Board approval through the Syracuse/Canandaigua Veterans' Affairs (VA) Medical Centers (MIRB#00367) and through the New York Chiropractic College (NYCC) (IRB#07-01). Trial Registration: ISRCTN30511490- http://www.controlled-trials.com/ISRCTN30511490/.

Participants

Our patients were 181 adults who met the following inclusions criteria. Inclusion: LBP for ≥12 weeks prior to enrollment, pain upon deep palpation of the lumbar erector spinae, LBP from L1 to sacroiliac joint inclusive, live within 50 miles of Rochester, NY, have a baseline >30 mm on the Visual Analogue Scale (VAS) [16] and >20% on the Oswestry Disability Index (ODI) [17]. Patients had to be willing to undergo no new or different treatment during the study intervention and follow up period, although they were allowed to continue any medications.

Exclusion: Radiographic or clinical evidence of cauda equina syndrome, spinal neoplasia or metastatic disease, destructive joint pathology such as rheumatoid arthritis, bowel/bladder dysfunction associated with the LBP, peripheral neuropathy or progressive lumbosacral radiculopathy, progressive myelopathy or neurogenic claudication and spinal surgery within the past six months. Patients were excluded if they had undergone a course of SMT or supervised AET within the six months prior to enrollment into the study and if they could not perform an exercise program based on a New York Heart Association Classification of grade III or IV [18].

To attempt to reduce any variability of the assessment of the mCPR physical examination elements, all study patients were screened by the same clinician, the VA patients were screened in a VA setting and the non-VA patients were screened at a local hospital clinic. Based on the response to the Fear Avoidance Belief Questionnaire (FABQ), subjective symptoms and the physical exam findings, patients were categorized in terms of whether they were positive or negative on the modified clinical prediction rule [13]. Patients within each group were then randomized into either the SMT or AET treatments.

Study settings
This multisite RCT was conducted in Rochester, NY at the VA Outpatient chiropractic and physical therapy clinics and two civilian outpatient chiropractic clinics and two civilian outpatient physical therapy clinics. The SMT interventions were carried out by licensed chiropractors (DC) and the AET interventions were carried out by licensed physical therapists (PT) at both the VA and in the private locations. Prior to initiation of the study the providers (DC and PT) met to discuss evaluation and treatment parameters and a video was made as a resource for all providers to refer to if they had questions.

Interventions
Spinal Manipulative Therapy, as defined in this study, included high velocity low amplitude spinal manipulation and/or flexion distraction therapy or mobilization, and advise on heat/ice all of which are commonly performed by manual therapists [19-21]. The practitioner was allowed to give the patient one of two stretches to do at home, either "cat/camel stretch" or "knee to chest stretch." While this definition differed from the original CPR validation study, it was felt that this allowed for greater generalizability of the SMT arm of the study to those who perform manual therapy.

Active Exercise Therapy included directional preference exercises, lumbar stabilization, general flexibility, and specific training exercises [22-24]. The therapists were given freedom to choose the active care exercise that they felt was best suited to the patient's needs, but could only utilize those exercises that were included in the protocol and no specific limit was given on the number of exercises that could be prescribed. No passive stretching or modalities such as electric stimulation or ultrasound were allowed. Both treatment were performed twice a week for four weeks [25].

Outcomes
The study evaluated improvement in pain using the VAS [16] and the SF-36 pain subscale [26] and disability using the ODI [17] in CLBP patients. The treatment outcomes are described in Table 1. All outcome measures have previously been validated in a CLBP population. Outcome measures were collected at baseline, 5, 12 and 24-weeks

post baseline. A face valid open-ended Patient Expectation scale was administered prior to and after randomization to detect potential patient bias associated with the assigned treatment intervention. This scale asked patients to "Circle below on the scale from 0 to 10 how confident you are that the treatment you will be receiving will be successful at reducing your low-back pain." Responses were measured on an 11 point scale anchored by "Not Confident" and "Confident". As an adjunct to the outcomes, we examined the patients' satisfaction at the end of the treatment at the last data collection point, the 24-week follow up visit, by administering a Patient Satisfaction survey [27]. We computed a mean patient treatment satisfaction score for each subject by averaging the ten patient satisfaction questions. Four of the items were reversed scored and were recoded so that the higher the score indicated the more satisfied the subject. The scale was reliable, (Cronbach's alpha = .85). We performed a 2×2 analysis of variance on the treatment satisfaction score with the mCPR and treatment arm as the two between subject factors.

Randomization
Randomization to treatments was through a random number producing algorithm. The same screening clinician performed the history and physical exam for all study participants. The screening clinician was blinded to the results of the FABQ, and thus did not assign the status on the rule. The study coordinator administered the baseline questionnaires including: VAS, ODI, SF-36, FABQ and the Patient Expectation scale. The de-identified results of the FABQ and the subjective and objective components of the mCPR were faxed to the evaluator who combined the data and determined the status on the mCPR. Once the status was determined the evaluator utilized the random number algorithm to assign the intervention. The assignment of treatment intervention was then faxed to the study coordinator who scheduled the first visit with the appropriate provider. The screening clinician, the statistician and the treating clinician were all blinded to the status on the mCPR. The patient data on the mCPR was revealed upon completion of the study. At the first treatment visit, the patient was given the second Patient Expectation scale. Patients were recruited through radio ads, posters, and physician recruitment.

Modified clinical prediction rule
The original study validating the CPR for SMT included acute, sub-acute and chronic lower back pain patients; however the median duration of pain for participants was 27 days [13]. Therefore, most of the patients in the original validation were classified as having acute and

Table 1 Summary of outcome measures

Variable	Definition
VAS: Visual Analogue Scale	A patient completed analogue measure that evaluates pain intensity on a 100 mm long horizontal line.
ODI Oswestry Disability Index	The back pain specific, self-rating scale to measure the degree of functional impairment that a subject is experiencing in a number of activities of daily living.
Patient Satisfaction	A self-developed questionnaire based on Cherkin's satisfaction questionnaire.
Patient Expectation	The recovery expectations measured using a time-based, specific single-item tool produced a strong prediction of outcome.
SF-36: Short Form-36 item health survey	A set of generic, coherent, and easily administered physical and mental quality-of-life measures.

sub-acute lower back pain. Given that much of the morbidity associated with back pain is in chronic lower back pain patients, we felt that it was necessary to assess a modification of the rule in an exclusively CLBP population. The original mCPR criteria included: pain <16 days, pain proximal to the knee, internal hip rotation of greater than 35 degrees, hypomobility of one or greater lumbar segments and FABQ work subscale score of less than 19 [12]. The original rule was modified to exclude the criteria concerning pain <16 days, this allowed for only CLBP patients to be included. In order for a patient to be considered positive on the mCPR, they had to have at least three of the four criteria positive from the original rule.

Power analysis

Paralleling Child et al's study [13], we based sample size calculation on our primary outcome disability measure, the ODI. Based on the work of Ostelo et al. [28] a minimally clinically significant outcome for the ODI is 10 points. Our power analysis was based on detecting a difference that size or larger when comparing the effectiveness between the two treatment arms in both the positive on the mCPR group and negative on the mCPR group at each time of measurement which would be necessary in the test of our second hypothesis. We required 112 patients in a balanced design, or 28 patients in each group assuming an α level of 0.05, two tailed test, and a power (1-beta) of .80. Our power analysis for our secondary outcomes, the VAS, and SF-36 pain sub score, required the same or fewer patients to detect the same clinically meaningful differences. Since we treated them as secondary outcomes, we did not perform an alpha correction for the power analysis. Because of difficulties in recruiting patients who were negative on the mCPR and given our randomization strategy we were forced to recruit additional patients who were positive on the mCPR until we reached the minimum number of patients who were negative on the mCPR. Rather than exclude them from the analyses, and thus possibly create a bias, we kept the additional

patients who were positive mCRP, which resulted in an excess of patients in the positive mCPR cells.

Statistical analyses

We tested our study hypotheses a repeated measures analysis of variance strategy using Statistical Package for the Social Sciences (SPSS) version 21. The patients' status on the mCPR (negative, positive) and the treatment group the patients were randomized to (SMT, AET) defined the between subject factors. The time of measurement (baseline, 5, 12 and 24-weeks post baseline) defined the within subject repeated measures factor. To control for age and length of pain significant differences and the fact that this was a multi-site study, we included them as covariates in the analyses.

We articulated our hypothesis in terms of main effects and interactions, as defined by our study design, and we employed traditional analyses of covariance tests of significance to test our derived hypothesis. We tested our hypothesis 1, which predicts significant clinical improvement in patients' outcomes in both SMT and AET, by testing the main effect of time. We would expect a significant main effect of time, which would reflect a significant improvement in outcomes from baseline in both treatment groups. We also tested for mean differences between treatment groups in response to treatment over time, which is tested by the treatment × time interaction, to see whether the pattern of improvement was similar in the two treatment groups.

We tested our hypothesis 2, which predicts that the mCPR modifies the comparative effectiveness of (i.e., the differences between) the two treatment groups, i.e., the comparative effectiveness between the treatment arms for the positive on the mCPR group is different from the comparative effectiveness between the treatment arms for the negative on the mCPR group by examining the mCPR × treatment × time of measurement interaction.

We report the effect sizes using partial eta^2. Partial eta^2 is an effect size measurement for analysis of variance with more than one independent variable and conceptually is the proportion of variance in the dependent variable explained by an effect while controlling for other effects.

We used an intention to treat approach that included all enrolled patients who met inclusion criteria regardless of whether they completed the study. Ten patients dropped out. There was no significant difference in the dropout rate across the study groups. We used multiple imputation to handle missing data. We conducted the multiple imputation using SPSS missing values module (version 21) with five imputation runs using an iterative Markov chain Monte Carlo (MCMC) method with a linear regression model and assuming data missing at random.

We included the outcome measures at baseline and followups, subject expectations for treatment effectiveness, and the subject characteristics, with categorical variables dummy coded, as the variables in the multiple imputation.

Results

A total 953 patients were phone screened of which 390 patients were physically screened. A total of 181 CLBP patients were enrolled; 89 were randomized into AET of these 69 (78%) completed the study and 92 to SMT of these 76 (83%) completed the study. (See Figure 1 for details).

Patient characteristics

As seen in Table 2, the sample was predominately white, male, overweight, and with a mean age ranging from 53 to 61 years. Most attended college or graduated from college. While patients who were recruited from and treated in VA clinics accounted for slightly less than half the patients, the percentage of VA patients across groups was not significantly different. Slightly more than one third of the patients self-reported arthritis on their clinical history, and about one third of the patients self-reported a depression diagnosis. We did not find any significant differences between patients who were positive on the mCPR and patients negative on the mCPR with the exception of age and self-report of pain duration. We included these patient characteristics as covariates in the analysis.

Also seen in Table 2, nearly all patients previously sought allopathic medicine treatment for the CLBP and a majority had previously sought chiropractic treatment in all groups.

We next examined patient expectations of the treatment's effectiveness prior to and after randomization to assure that patients who may have had preconceived biases toward one treatment or another would be detected, as this would have the potential to affect treatment responsiveness [29]. We performed a 4 × 2 analyses of variance with the study group as the between

subject factor, and the time of the expectation rating (prior to randomization and post randomization before the start of treatment) as the within subject factor. We present the group × time interaction in Table 3. Patients became slightly more positive in their expectations for the treatment's effectiveness after randomization to their treatment arm compared to their expectations prior to randomization (main effect of time, p = .02). This increase was similar across the four study groups, as indicated by the absence of a significant study group × time interaction (p = .43). This finding indicates that patients did not seem to lower their expectations once they knew which treatment they would be receiving.

Given that this was a multisite study, before combining the data, we tested for the presence of site differences. We ran preliminary analyses that included site of treatment as a between subject factor. We found no significant site of treatment main effects or interactive effects of site of treatment with treatment group, mCPR, or time of measurement on the outcome measures.

With the absence of site of treatment effects, we pooled data across treatment sites. Even so, we included site as a covariate in our analysis.

We performed separate analyses on our three outcome measures, i.e., VAS, ODI, and the SF-36 pain subscales. We present the means and standard deviations for the outcome measures at each point in time in Table 4.

Test of hypothesis 1

We found a significant time of measurement effect for VAS (p = .05, partial eta^2 = .02), ODI (p = .001, partial eta^2 = .04), and the SF-36 pain subscale (p = .003, partial eta^2 = .03). We found no significant treatment arm × time interactions (p > .50). The SMT and AET groups both exhibited similar improvements in pain and disability outcomes after treatment. To help interpret the significant main effect of time, we then tested the within-patients linear, quadratic, and cubic contrasts with analysis of variance for each of the three outcome measures. We only found significant linear contrasts for the VAS (p = .03), SF-36 pain subscale (p = .002) and ODI (p = .001) with pain and disability dropping from the baseline to the post treatment follow ups (see Figure 2). The pattern of results support hypothesis 1.

Test of hypothesis 2

We did not find significant mCPR × treatment × time of measurement interactions on the three outcome measures, VAS (p = .70), ODI (p = .76), and SF-36 pain subscale (p = .93). This is contrary to the expected pattern of results and so does not support hypothesis 2. We found no differences in the changes in treatment outcomes between SMT and AET in the positive on the mCPR group and no differences in the changes in

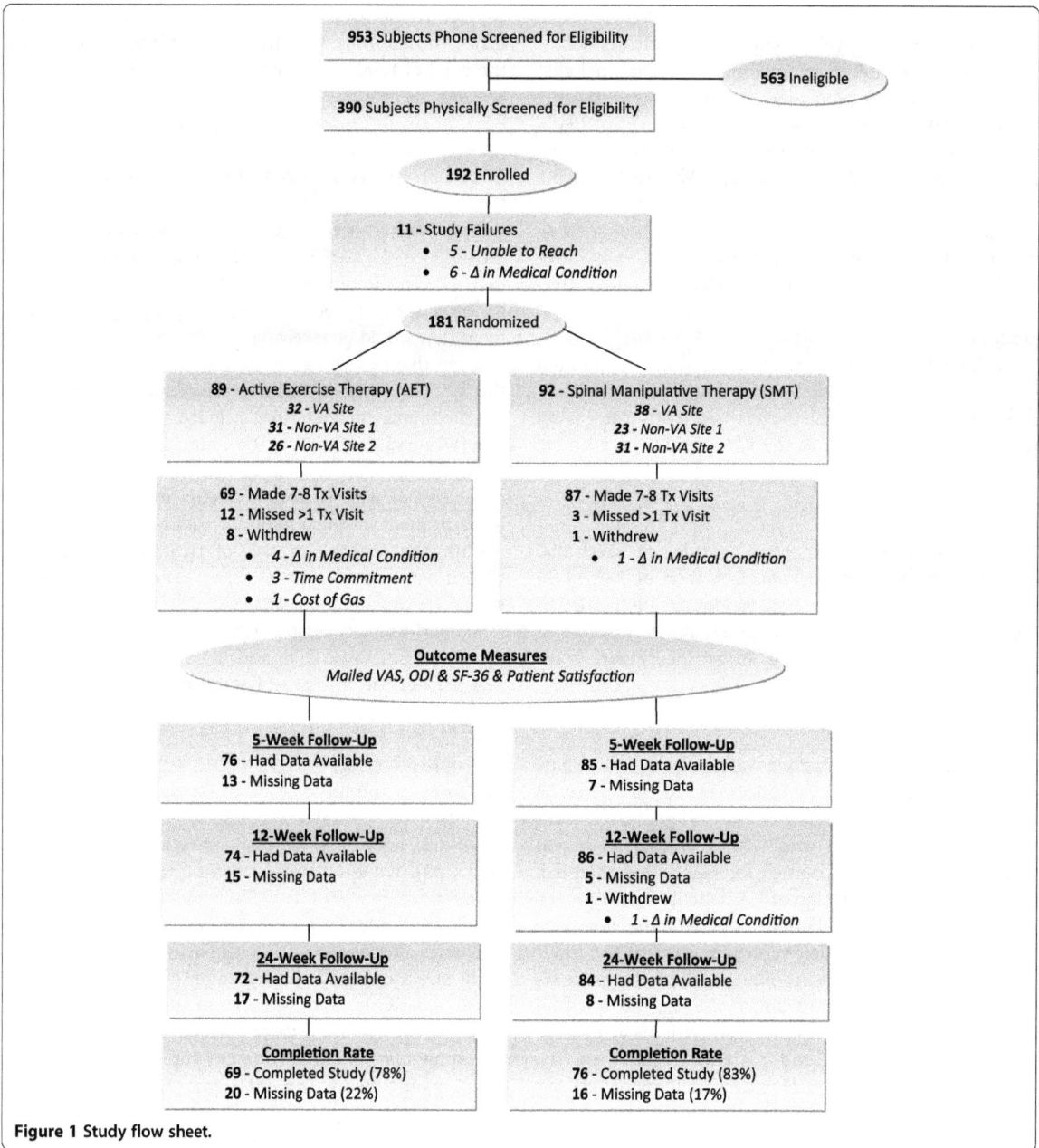

Figure 1 Study flow sheet.

treatment outcomes between SMT and AET in the negative on the mCPR group. We present the adjusted cell means and confidence intervals within the negative on the mCPR and positive on the mCPR groups for each of the follow up time points in Table 5.

Patient satisfaction

We found a significant mCPR x treatment arm interaction (p = .02, partial eta^2 = .03) on the patients' satisfaction

scores. As seen in Table 6, the positive on the mCPR group was equally satisfied with the AET and SMT. In contrast, the negative on the mCPR group was more satisfied with the AET than the SMT.

Harms

Adverse event (AE) and serious adverse event (SAE) data were tracked for each of the treatment groups, AET and SMT. Adverse event data was collected at each

Table 2 Patient demographics

Variable	Study group			
	SMT Negative mCPR N = 32 (St. Dev.)	SMT Positive mCPR N = 60 (St. Dev.)	AET Negative mCPR N = 28 (St. Dev.)	AET Positive mCPR N = 61 (St. Dev.)
Mean Age[a]	61.16 (16.24)	54.12 (16.04)	60.00 (15.00)	53.43 (18.18)
Mean Height (inches)	67.62 (4.14)	67.55 (4.08)	67.29 (3.36)	68.23 (5.82)
Mean Weight (pounds)	206.09 (39.36)	206.22 (49.34)	201.75 (34.07)	192.25 (44.31)
Mean BMI	31.84 (6.75)	31.71 (6.87)	31.34 (4.95)	29.34 (7.36)
Mean Pain Duration (mos)[b]	261.31 (237.90)	140.78 (196.29)	186.62 (188.63)	138.37 (152.13)
Arthritis	56%	40%	39%	38%
Osteoporosis	0%	2%	0%	0%
Depression	37%	45%	25%	28%
Female	25%	38%	24%	36%
White	91%	87%	82%	84%
African American	6%	8%	14%	11%
Hispanic	0%	5%	0%	5%
VA Patients	47%	37%	59%	30%
Education				
Some High School or Less	0%	5%	11%	8%
High School Graduate	41%	20%	18%	21%
Some College	31%	32%	43%	27%
College Graduate	8%	21%	26%	44%
Previous Treatment History				
Allopathic Medicine	87%	75%	93%	77%
Physical Therapy	41%	40%	52%	34%
Chiropractic	62%	55%	67%	52%
Surgery	16%	10%	26%	8%
Injection	12%	13%	26%	19%

[a]difference between positive and negative mCPR groups, p < .01.
[b]difference between positive and negative mCPR groups, p < .01.

treatment visit and patients also received phone calls during the 5, 12, and 24-week post baseline follow up period. For purpose of this protocol, an AE was defined as any undesirable medical event with new onset or significant exacerbation during the course of the study, regardless of whether or not it was considered to be related to study treatment. Each clinician rated each AE as to severity (a clinical judgment): mild, moderate or severe. An SAE was defined as any AE occurring during the study or within 30 days of conclusion of study participation resulting in any one of the following outcomes: death, life threatening persistent or significant disability/incapacity, hospitalization (when the result of an AE occurring during the study; note, hospitalization for an elective procedure or for treatment of a pre-existing condition not worsened during the study was not considered an SAE; admission to the ER for 23 hours or less was not considered a hospitalization), congenital anomaly, important medical event (i.e. an event that in the opinion of the investigator may jeopardize the participant and may require medical or surgical intervention to prevent one of the outcomes listed above). The Data Safety and Management Board (DSMB) met four times during the study (at 25%, 50%, 75%, and final enrollment), the DSMB evaluated the reported AEs and SAEs and found no issues with the reporting of these events and no trends that would require alteration of the study methods. A total of 243 AEs were reported over the course of the study with 54.7% in the AET group and 45.3% in the SMT group. Of the 133 AEs reported in the AET group, the DSMB judged 16 as definitely or probably associated with the intervention. Of the 110 AEs reported in the SMT group, the DSMB judged 14 as definitely or probably associated

Table 3 Patient expectation

	Patient expectation	
	Mean[a]	(±95% CI)
Negative on mCPR SMT (n = 32)		
Pre randomization	5.78	(5.09, 6.47)
Post randomization	6.03	(5.27, 6.79)
Negative on mCPR AET (n = 28)		
Pre randomization	6.14	(5.41, 6.88)
Post randomization	6.79	(5.97, 7.60)
Positive on mCPR SMT (n = 60)		
Pre randomization	6.62	(6.11, 7.12)
Post randomization	7.07	(6.51, 7.62)
Positive on mCPR AET (n = 61)		
Pre randomization	6.46	(5.95, 6.96)
Post randomization	6.47	(5.91, 7.04)

[a]patient expectation for treatment score. The higher the number the more confident the patient was with the treatment. Responses measured on a 11 point scale anchored by 0, not at all confident and 10, very confident.

with the intervention. The majority of AEs that were reported consisted of musculoskeletal soreness and resolved within the study period. During the study period there were 10 SAEs reported after the start of the treatments (5 in the AET group and 5 in the SMT group), the DSMB judged that none of the SAEs were associated with the study intervention.

Discussion
Interpretation
Recent literature has highlighted the lack of definitive data to emerge from RCTs evaluating CLBP, with no treatment producing consistently superior outcomes [29-32]. In keeping with this previous literature and supporting our first hypothesis, we found clinically and statistically significant improvements in outcomes from baseline to follow up in the groups receiving SMT and AET, which are both recognized as evidence based interventions for CLBP [10,31].

After an initial promising start in developing treatment based classification in lower back pain, two recent reviews did not identify any studies validating the use of a treatment based classification in CLBP [33,34]. The lack of data on specific patient factors that would moderate the treatment of CLBP is what makes the current study important. Our second hypothesis was that the status on the mCPR would moderate the effectiveness of SMT. If the mCPR moderated the effectiveness of SMT, then we would have expected a significant treatment × mCPR × time interaction. We did not find significant treatment × mCPR × time interaction and so we cannot support our second hypothesis.

Table 4 Intention to treat analysis

mCPR status treatment group time of measurement	Outcome measures		
	VAS[a] (St. Dev.)	ODI[b] (St. Dev.)	SF-36 Pain[c] (St. Dev.)
Negative on mCPR			
SMT (n = 32)			
Baseline	58.44 (15.46)	35.13 (8.55)	5.56 (1.20)
5-weeks	37.51 (28.89)	29.01 (14.66)	6.98 (1.66)
12-weeks	43.29 (24.62)	32.14 (15.77)	6.41 (1.92)
24-weeks	47.61 (25.66)	30.17 (15.69)	6.60 (2.06)
AET (n = 28)			
Baseline	65.36 (16.78)	37.04 (12.57)	5.35 (1.21)
5-weeks	36.50 (33.77)	30.15 (17.71)	6.56 (2.33)
12-weeks	42.00 (33.57)	32.91 (20.82)	6.54 (2.72)
24-weeks	52.54 (27.24)	32.71 (18.64)	6.44 (2.47)
Positive on mCPR			
SMT (n = 60)			
Baseline	61.25 (13.74)	33.62 (9.60)	5.78 (1.22)
5-weeks	34.86 (31.18)	26.71 (15.06)	7.10 (2.22)
12-weeks	40.43 (27.53)	29.64 (18.30)	6.57 (2.55)
24-weeks	38.47 (26.99)	23.16 (15.74)	7.51 (2.71)
AET (n = 61)			
Baseline	55.38 (16.64)	31.44 (10.05)	6.00 (1.52)
5-weeks	26.60 (33.48)	23.73 (17.14)	7.49 (2.57)
12-weeks	36.30 (29.64)	25.94 (19.90)	7.05 (2.98)
24-weeks	42.11 (31.77)	23.52 (18.98)	7.75 (3.08)

[a]the higher the number the higher the reported pain on a 100 point scale.
[b]the higher the number the more disability reported due to pain on a 100 point scale.
[c]the higher the number the *less* self-reported pain on the computed SF-36 pain subscale.

Our study results can be compared to the findings of Hancock et al. [35], that found the CPR performed no better than chance in identifying responsiveness to SMT among patients with acute lower back pain. Together the two studies (Hancock and our study) that attempted to apply the CPR to specific populations (Hancock et al. in acute lower back pain and ours in chronic lower back pain) suggest that the CPR, as it is able to be applied, does not seem to moderate the responsiveness to SMT of lower back pain patients, and thus suggesting a limited use of mCPR in clinical judgments of treatment selection for CLBP patients. We are aware of the fallacy of "proving" the null hypothesis of no effect, and so call for additional research to determine the effectiveness of the CPR as a clinical tool in predicting treatment responsiveness in lower back pain patients. Of particular note is the need for additional research to examine the role of other psychosocial factors in the prognosis of CLBP patients [36-39].

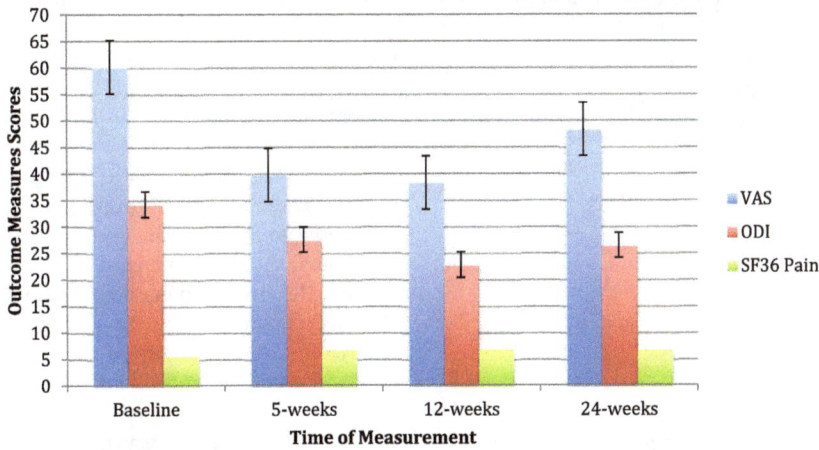

Figure 2 Adjusted Outcome Measures. VAS, ODI, and SF-36 Pain Subscale scores, adjusted for age, duration of pain, and treatment site, and 95% confidence intervals at baseline, post treatment 5, 12 and 24-weeks followup. Linear decrease significant for VAS (p = .03), ODI (p = .001) and SF-36 Pain Subscale (p = .002). The larger the score the more pain as measured by the VAS and disability as measured by the ODI. The larger the score the *less* pain as measured by the SF-36 Pain Subscale.

Limitations

Our study is limited by factors that may need to be addressed in future trials. The first limitation is that we modified a rule that was developed to be utilized in general population of LBP patients. The original rule defined a patient as positive on the rule, if the patient scored positive on four or more of the five criteria, one of which was pain <16 days (acute pain). Since all the patients had CLBP they could not meet the mCPR criteria of pain <16 days (i.e., acute pain). Using the original rule would have been overly restrictive by drastically limiting the universe of positive mCPR patients, who would have had to score positive on all the remaining four rule criteria.

We recognize that our study is limited to two different broadly defined interventions and that this limits the extent to which one can make definitive statements about the individual treatment nuances of each. We purposefully allowed for a more broadly defined SMT treatment, in order to capture more realistically the treatments of clinicians performing manual therapy. Allowing for a more encompassing definition has been seen in other studies, both of these studies allowed the SMT groups to utilize treatments outside of high velocity low amplitude SMT [40,41]. We however, realize that this comes at a price of clouding the impact of specific types of SMT, thus limiting the direct correlation

Table 5 Adjusted difference scores between SMT and AET groups

Time of measurement	Outcome measures		
	VAS[a] (±95% CI)	ODI[b] (±95% CI)	SF-36 pain[c] (±95% CI)
5-week Follow Up			
Negative on mCPR between	7.16 (−20.32, 34.62)	0.75 (−8.84, 10.23)	0.21 (−1.99, 2.42)
Positive on mCPR between	0.81 (−31.21, 32.83)	0.37 (−9.92, 10.66)	−0.03 (−2.84, 2.77)
12-week Follow Up			
Negative on mCPR between	5.36 (−68.25, 78.96)	2.58 (−10.18, 15,34)	−0.66 (−2.30, 0.98)
Positive on mCPR between	2.48 (−11.32, 16.27)	1.93 (−17.08, 20.94)	−0.50 (−2.48, 1.48)
24-week Follow Up			
Negative on mCPR between	−4.26 (−34.82, 26,29)	0.03 (−20.65, 20.70)	0.16 (−1.85, 2.17)
Positive on mCPR between	−8.50 (−48.75, 31.75)	−2.28 (−29.18, 24.62)	0.11 (−2.05, 2.26)

[a]A positive difference score indicates SMT group reported more pain in comparison to the AET group. A negative difference score indicates the AET group reported more pain in comparison to the SMT group. The larger the absolute value, the greater the difference.

[b]t A positive difference score indicates SMT group reported more disability in comparison to the AET group. A negative difference score indicates the AET group reported more disability in comparison to the SMT group. The larger the absolute value, the greater the difference.

[c]A positive difference score indicates SMT group reported less pain in comparison to the AET group. A negative difference score indicates the AET group reported less pain in comparison to the SMT group. The larger the absolute value, the greater the difference.

Table 6 Treatment satisfaction as a function of mCPR and treatment group

mCPR status	Treatment group	
	SMT	AET
	Mean[a] (±95% CI)	Mean (±95% CI)
Negative on mCPR	3.65[a] (3.42, 3.89) st dev = .76	4.14 (3.88, 4.04) st dev = .55
	n = 26	n = 21
Positive on mCPR	3.97 (3.80, 4.13) st dev = .58	3.96 (3.80, 4.13) st dev = .54
	n = 52	n = 49

[a]responses measured on five point Likert Scales anchored by 1 and 5. The higher the number the more satisfaction.

to the original CPR. Further studies may be used to address which specific aspects of the SMT (manipulative thrust or distraction) were the most effective. Another limitation is that the SMT group did allow for the recommendation of a simple stretching exercise (Cat/camel stretch); although allowing this did increase the generalizability of the study as a whole, it limits that ability to evaluate SMT alone. We also recognize the limitations due to the subjective nature of some of the assessment tools utilized in this study including the use of "deep palpation of erector spinae" and the use of "hypomobility of one or greater segments." These assessment tools have not demonstrated reliability or validity; however they are commonly utilized measures in clinical practice. We acknowledge that the use of these criteria could introduce certain selection bias in the inclusion criteria and the designation of status on the prediction rule; however the study utilized previously reported criteria [12]. To attempt to maintain reliability however, we did use a single screening clinician to perform all baseline screening examinations. Future study should work to identify reliable and valid criteria for identification of pain and hypomobility.

Generalizability

The current trial utilized easily administered tools (spinal mobility, hip motion, symptom characteristics and a simple questionnaire) to attempt to characterize those patients who would respond to one type of treatment over another. In addition, the interventions were designed to be easily generalizable to the typical practice of a manual therapist (PT, DC or Osteopath). This study was designed to apply a modification of a previously defined CPR and see if it was applicable to a different population and a more generalizable treatment method. This study should not be construed to discount the original CPR.

Conclusion

While patients benefited from both SMT and AET, the mCPR did not moderate the effectiveness of SMT, as we hypothesized. Future studies are needed to better understand the specific and non-specific nature of interventions for CLBP [42-45] and also to aid the general practitioner in his/her decision on what intervention may be most appropriate. Further studies are warranted to evaluate the underlying physiological and psychological mechanisms in CLBP in order to better address these underlying abnormalities with the most effective treatment. The results of these studies may help to inform development of a new CPR that would be applicable to CLBP. There is also a need for further studies to evaluate the role of predictive factors for responsiveness for conservative interventions that will be sensitive to the role of non-specific effects of both SMT and AET.

Abbreviations
AE: Adverse Event; AET: Active Exercise Therapy; CLBP: Chronic Lower Back Pain; CPR: Clinical Prediction Rule; CONSORT: Consolidated Standards of Reporting Trials; DC: Doctor of Chiropractic; DSMB: Data and Safety Monitoring Board; FABQ: Fear Avoidance Belief Questionnaire; HRSA: Health Resources and Services Administration; IRB: Institutional Review Board; LBP: Lower Back Pain; MCMC: Markov chain Monte Carlo; mCPR: Modified Clinical Prediction Rule; NYCC: New York Chiropractic College; ODI: Oswestry Disability Index; PT: Physical Therapist; RCT: Randomized Controlled Trial; SAE: Serious Adverse Event; SF-36: Short Form-36 Item Health Survey; SMT: Spinal Manipulative Therapy; SPSS: Statistical Package for the Social Sciences; VA: Veteran's Affairs; VAS: Visual Analogue Scale.

Competing interests
The authors declare that they have no competing interests.

Authors' contributions
All authors contributed to the research design and administration. JK performed the data analysis and PED performed the initial drafting of the manuscript. PED supervised the research and edited the final manuscript. All authors read and approved the final manuscript.

Acknowledgements
The authors would also like to acknowledge the practitioners who provided the clinical intervention for the study: Jim Codarro, PT, Jonathon Egan, DC, MPH, Brian Justice, DC, Andrew Opett, PT, DPT, OCS, CKTP, Scott Spinner, DC, Marcia Miller Spoto, PT, DC, OCS, John Ventura, DC, and Brian Westlake, PT, DPT, MPSPT, Cert. MDT.

Funding
This study was funded by a Department of Health and Human Services, Health Resources and Service Administration (HRSA) Chiropractic Demonstration grant. AWARD NO.: R18HP07641-03-03, GRANT NO.: R18HP07641.

Author details
[1]Canandaigua Veterans Affairs Medical Center, Canandaigua, NY, USA. [2]New York Chiropractic College, Seneca Falls, NY, USA. [3]University of Rochester School of Medicine and Dentistry, Rochester, NY, USA. [4]University of Rochester, Rochester, NY, USA. [5]State University of New York College at Buffalo, Buffalo, NY, USA. [6]University of Toronto, Toronto, ON, Canada. [7]Medical Affairs, Baycrest Geriatric Centre, Toronto, Canada.

References

1. Gironda RJ, Clark ME, Massengale JP, Walker RL: Pain among veterans of operations enduring freedom and Iraqi Freedom. *Pain Med* 2006, 7:339–343.

2. Vos T, Flaxman AD, Naghavi M, Lozano R, Michaud C, Ezzati M, Shibuya K, Salomon JA, Abdalla S, Aboyans V, Abraham J, Ackerman I, Aggarwal R, Ahn SY, Ali MK, Alvarado M, Anderson HR, Anderson LM, Andrews KG, Atkinson C, Baddour LM, Bahalim AN, Barker-Collo S, Barrero LH, Bartels DH, Basanez MG, Baxter A, Bell ML, Benjamin EJ, Bennett D, *et al*: Years lived with disability (YLDs) for 1160 sequelae of 289 diseases and injuries 1990–2010: a systematic analysis for the Global Burden of Disease Study 2010. *Lancet* 2012, 380:2163–2196.

3. Deyo RA, Weinstein JN: Low back pain. *N Engl J Med* 2001, 344:363–370.

4. Martin BI, Deyo RA, Mirza SK, Turner JA, Comstock BA, Hollingworth W, Sullivan SD: Expenditures and health status among adults with back and neck problems. *JAMA* 2008, 299:656–664.

5. Haldeman S, Dagenais S: A supermarket approach to the evidence-informed management of chronic low back pain. *Spine J* 2008, 8:1–7.

6. Fairbank J, Gwilym SE, France JC, Daffner SD, Dettori J, Hermsmeyer J, Andersson G: The role of classification of chronic low back pain. *Spine (Phila Pa 1976)* 2011, 36:S19–S42.

7. Apkarian AV, Baliki MN, Geha PY: Towards a theory of chronic pain. *Prog Neurobiol* 2009, 87:81–97.

8. Grotle M, Foster NE, Dunn KM, Croft P: Are prognostic indicators for poor outcome different for acute and chronic low back pain consulters in primary care? *Pain* 2010, 151:790–797.

9. Chou R, Qaseem A, Snow V, Casey D, Cross JT Jr, Shekelle P, Owens DK: Diagnosis and treatment of low back pain: a joint clinical practice guideline from the American College of Physicians and the American Pain Society. *Ann Intern Med* 2007, 147:478–491.

10. Chou R, Huffman LH: Nonpharmacologic therapies for acute and chronic low back pain: a review of the evidence for an American Pain Society/American College of Physicians clinical practice guideline. *Ann Intern Med* 2007, 147:492–504.

11. Hebert J, Koppenhaver S, Fritz J, Parent E: Clinical prediction for success of interventions for managing low back pain. *Clin Sports Med* 2008, 27:463–479.

12. Flynn T, Fritz J, Whitman J, Wainner R, Magel J, Rendeiro D, Butler B, Garber M, Allison S: A clinical prediction rule for classifying patients with low back pain who demonstrate short-term improvement with spinal manipulation. *Spine (Phila Pa 1976)* 2002, 27:2835–2843.

13. Childs JD, Fritz JM, Flynn TW, Irrgang JJ, Johnson KK, Majkowski GR, Delitto A: A clinical prediction rule to identify patients with low back pain most likely to benefit from spinal manipulation: a validation study. *Ann Intern Med* 2004, 141:920–928.

14. Haskins R, Rivett DA, Osmotherly PG: Clinical prediction rules in the physiotherapy management of low back pain: a systematic review. *Man Ther* 2012, 17:9–21.

15. Patel S, Friede T, Froud R, Evans DW, Underwood M: Systematic review of randomized controlled trials of clinical prediction rules for physical therapy in low back pain. *Spine (Phila Pa 1976)* 2013, 38:762–769.

16. Ohnmeiss DD: Million visual analog scale. In *Compendium of Outcome Instruments for Assessment and Research of Spinal Disorders*. Edited by Gatchel RJ. La Grange, Illinois: North American Spine Society; 2001:42–63.

17. Fairbank JC, Couper J, Davies JB, O'Brien JP: The Oswestry low back pain disability questionnaire. *Physiotherapy* 1980, 66:271–273.

18. Sharma S, Firoozi S, McKenna WJ: Value of exercise testing in assessing clinical state and prognosis in hypertrophic cardiomyopathy. *Cardiol Rev* 2001, 9:70–76.

19. Cherkin DC, Deyo RA, Battie M, Street J, Barlow W: A comparison of physical therapy, chiropractic manipulation, and provision of an educational booklet for the treatment of patients with low back pain. *N Engl J Med* 1998, 339:1021–1029.

20. Bronfort G, Goldsmith CH, Nelson CF, Boline PD, Anderson AV: Trunk exercise combined with spinal manipulative or NSAID therapy for chronic low back pain: a randomized, observer-blinded clinical trial. *J Manipulative Physiol Ther* 1996, 19:570–582.

21. Christensen MG, Kollasch MW, Ward R, Webb KR, Day AA, zumBrunnen J: *Job Analysis of Chiropractic: a project report, survey anlaysis, and summary of the practice of chiropractic within the United States*. Greeley: National Board of Chiropractic Examiners; 2005.

22. O'Sullivan PB, Phyty GD, Twomey LT, Allison GT: Evaluation of specific stabilizing exercise in the treatment of chronic low back pain with radiologic diagnosis of spondylolysis or spondylolisthesis. *Spine (Phila Pa 1976)* 1997, 22:2959–2967.

23. Hides JA, Jull GA, Richardson CA: Long-term effects of specific stabilizing exercises for first-episode low back pain. *Spine (Phila Pa 1976)* 2001, 26:E243–E248.

24. Wilke HJ, Wolf S, Claes LE, Arand M, Wiesend A: Stability increase of the lumbar spine with different muscle groups. A biomechanical in vitro study. *Spine (Phila Pa 1976)* 1995, 20:192–198.

25. Haas M, Groupp E, Kraemer DF: Dose–response for chiropractic care of chronic low back pain. *Spine J* 2004, 4:574–583.

26. McHorney CA, Ware JE Jr, Raczek AE: The MOS 36-Item Short-Form Health Survey (SF-36): II. Psychometric and clinical tests of validity in measuring physical and mental health constructs. *Med Care* 1993, 31:247–263.

27. Hertzman-Miller RP, Morgenstern H, Hurwitz EL, Yu F, Adams AH, Harber P, Kominski GF: Comparing the satisfaction of low back pain patients randomized to receive medical or chiropractic care: results from the UCLA low-back pain study. *Am J Public Health* 2002, 92:1628–1633.

28. Ostelo RW, Deyo RA, Stratford P, Waddell G, Croft P, Von KM, Bouter LM, de Vet HC: Interpreting change scores for pain and functional status in low back pain: towards international consensus regarding minimal important change. *Spine (Phila Pa 1976)* 2008, 33:90–94.

29. Iles RA, Davidson M, Taylor NF, O'Halloran P: Systematic review of the ability of recovery expectations to predict outcomes in non-chronic non-specific low back pain. *J Occup Rehabil* 2009, 19:25–40.

30. Hurwitz EL: Commentary: exercise and spinal manipulative therapy for chronic low back pain: time to call for a moratorium on future randomized trials? *Spine J* 2011, 11:599–600.

31. Rubinstein SM, Van MM, Assendelft WJ, De Boer MR, Van Tulder MW: Spinal manipulative therapy for chronic low-back pain: an update of a Cochrane review. *Spine (Phila Pa 1976)* 2011, 36:E825–E846.

32. Gore M, Tai KS, Sadosky A, Leslie D, Stacey BR: Clinical comorbidities, treatment patterns, and direct medical costs of patients with osteoarthritis in usual care: a retrospective claims database analysis. *J Med Econ* 2011, 14:497–507.

33. Kent P, Mjosund HL, Petersen DH: Does targeting manual therapy and/or exercise improve patient outcomes in nonspecific low back pain? A systematic review. *BMC Med* 2010, 8:22.

34. Hebert JJ, Koppenhaver SL, Walker BF: Subgrouping patients with low back pain: a treatment-based approach to classification. *Sports Health* 2011, 3:534–542.

35. Hancock MJ, Maher CG, Latimer J, Herbert RD, McAuley JH: Independent evaluation of a clinical prediction rule for spinal manipulative therapy: a randomised controlled trial. *Eur Spine J* 2008, 17:936–943.

36. Ramond A, Bouton C, Richard I, Roquelaure Y, Baufreton C, Legrand E, Huez JF: Psychosocial risk factors for chronic low back pain in primary care–a systematic review. *Fam Pract* 2011, 28:12–21.

37. Kongsted A, Johannesen E, Leboeuf-Yde C: Feasibility of the STarT back screening tool in chiropractic clinics: a cross-sectional study of patients with low back pain. *Chiropr Man Therap* 2011, 19:10.

38. Hill JC, Whitehurst DG, Lewis M, Bryan S, Dunn KM, Foster NE, Konstantinou K, Main CJ, Mason E, Somerville S, Sowden G, Vohora K, Hay EM: Comparison of stratified primary care management for low back pain with current best practice (STarT Back): a randomised controlled trial. *Lancet* 2011, 378:1560–1571.

39. Grotle M, Vollestad NK, Brox JI: Clinical course and impact of fear-avoidance beliefs in low back pain: prospective cohort study of acute and chronic low back pain: II. *Spine (Phila Pa 1976)* 2006, 31:1038–1046.

40. Haas M, Vavrek D, Peterson D, Polissar N, Neradilek MB: Dose–response and efficacy of spinal manipulation for care of chronic low back pain: a randomized controlled trial. *Spine J* 2014, 14:1106–1116.

41. Bronfort G, Maiers MJ, Evans RL, Schulz CA, Bracha Y, Svendsen KH, Grimm RH Jr, Owens EF Jr, Garvey TA, Transfeldt EE: Supervised exercise, spinal manipulation, and home exercise for chronic low back pain: a randomized clinical trial. *Spine J* 2011, 11:585–598.

42. Steiger F, Wirth B, de Bruin ED, Mannion AF: Is a positive clinical outcome after exercise therapy for chronic non-specific low back pain contingent upon a corresponding improvement in the targeted aspect(s) of performance? A systematic review. *Eur Spine J* 2012, 21:575–598.

43. Machado LA, Kamper SJ, Herbert RD, Maher CG, McAuley JH: **Analgesic effects of treatments for non-specific low back pain: a meta-analysis of placebo-controlled randomized trials.** *Rheumatology (Oxford)* 2009, **48:**520–527.

44. Fregni F, Imamura M, Chien HF, Lew HL, Boggio P, Kaptchuk TJ, Riberto M, Hsing WT, Battistella LR, Furlan A: **Challenges and recommendations for placebo controls in randomized trials in physical and rehabilitation medicine: a report of the international placebo symposium working group.** *Am J Phys Med Rehabil* 2010, **89:**160–172.

45. Dougherty P, Karuza J, Dunn A, Savino D, Katz P: **Spinal manipulative therapy for chronic lower back pain in older veteran's: a prospective, randomized, placebo-controlled trial.** *Geriatric Orthopaedic Surgery and Rehabilitation* in press.

Indicating spinal joint mobilisations or manipulations in patients with neck or low-back pain: protocol of an inter-examiner reliability study among manual therapists

Emiel van Trijffel[1,2*], Robert Lindeboom[1], Patrick MM Bossuyt[1], Maarten A Schmitt[2], Cees Lucas[1], Bart W Koes[3] and Rob AB Oostendorp[4,5]

Abstract

Background: Manual spinal joint mobilisations and manipulations are widely used treatments in patients with neck and low-back pain. Inter-examiner reliability of passive intervertebral motion assessment of the cervical and lumbar spine, perceived as important for indicating these interventions, is poor within a univariable approach. The diagnostic process as a whole in daily practice in manual therapy has a multivariable character, however, in which the use and interpretation of passive intervertebral motion assessment depend on earlier results from the diagnostic process. To date, the inter-examiner reliability among manual therapists of a multivariable diagnostic decision-making process in patients with neck or low-back pain is unknown.

Methods: This study will be conducted as a repeated-measures design in which 14 pairs of manual therapists independently examine a consecutive series of a planned total of 165 patients with neck or low-back pain presenting in primary care physiotherapy. Primary outcome measure is therapists' decision about whether or not manual spinal joint mobilisations or manipulations, or both, are indicated in each patient, alone or as part of a multimodal treatment. Therapists will largely be free to conduct the full diagnostic process based on their formulated examination objectives. For each pair of therapists, 2×2 tables will be constructed and reliability for the dichotomous decision will be expressed using Cohen's kappa. In addition, observed agreement, prevalence of positive decisions, prevalence index, bias index, and specific agreement in positive and negative decisions will be calculated. Univariable logistic regression analysis of concordant decisions will be performed to explore which demographic, professional, or clinical factors contributed to reliability.

Discussion: This study will provide an estimate of the inter-examiner reliability among manual therapists of indicating spinal joint mobilisations or manipulations in patients with neck or low-back pain based on a multivariable diagnostic reasoning and decision-making process, as opposed to reliability of individual tests. As such, it is proposed as an initial step toward the development of an alternative approach to current classification systems and prediction rules for identifying those patients with spinal disorders that may show a better response to manual therapy which can be incorporated in randomised clinical trials. Potential methodological limitations of this study are discussed.

Keywords: Manual therapy, Motion assessment, Diagnostics, Decision-making, Reliability, Clinical reasoning, Neck pain, Back pain

* Correspondence: e.vantrijffel@somt.nl
[1]Department of Clinical Epidemiology, Biostatistics & Bioinformatics, Academic Medical Centre, University of Amsterdam, Amsterdam, the Netherlands
[2]Institute for Master Education in Musculoskeletal Therapy, Amersfoort, the Netherlands
Full list of author information is available at the end of the article

Background

Neck and low-back pain are common and costly disorders in adult general populations [1-6]. Manual spinal joint mobilisations and manipulations are widely used treatments in patients with these complaints [7,8]. Although the underlying mechanisms of these treatments are far from understood, spinal joint mobilisations and manipulations are effective as well as cost-effective in patients with non-specific neck and low-back pain although no more effective than other treatment modalities [9-14].

Traditionally, manual therapy has a strong focus on the diagnostics, treatment, and evaluation of spinal joint function by emphasising the use of passive physiological and accessory movements [15-17]. Passive intervertebral motion (PIVM) assessment is used to judge the quantity and quality of functions of spinal motion segments and is assumed to play an important role in diagnostically classifying patients and selecting treatment [18]. Dutch, New Zealand, and USA manual therapists indeed believe that passive spinal mobility testing is important for deciding on manual mobilisation or manipulation as a treatment option [19,20]. Moreover, a recent international, multidisciplinary survey showed that PIVM assessment is the most commonly used impairment outcome measure in patients with neck pain [21].

In order to yield accurate and uniform decisions about treatment options for patients, test results need to be reliable [22]. Reliability is a component of reproducibility along with agreement and reflects the extent to which test results can diagnostically discriminate between patients despite measurement errors [23,24]. Agreement, on the other hand, concerns the possibility of examiners to obtain the same test results on different measurement occasions [25]. Systematic reviews have consistently shown poor inter-examiner reliability for spinal physical tests, and for PIVM assessment in particular [26-30]. However, the large majority of studies investigating the reliability of physical tests and PIVM assessment can be regarded as test research following a single-test or univariable approach, thus neglecting the multivariable character of the diagnostic process as opposed to diagnostic research [31].

Physiotherapists conduct a diagnostic process by collecting data through interview and physical examination and by generating hypotheses as to why a problem exists in order to reach a decision about appropriate patient management [32,33]. During this diagnostic process, manual therapists indeed seem to apply, amongst others, a hypothetico-deductive way of clinical reasoning [34,35]. PIVM assessment is usually conducted after history-taking, questionnaires, and other physical tests and is indicated after interpreting earlier clinical information and formulating specific hypotheses about spinal joint dysfunction [35]. Moreover, Canadian manual therapists reported to decide on manual mobilisation or manipulation based on their whole clinical assessment and clinical reasoning in a patient [36]. It is therefore reasonable to assume that the diagnostic process in manual therapy has a multivariable character.

Over the last three decades, many systems have been developed for classifying patients with spinal disorders, in particular for those with low-back pain [37]. A systematic review found 28 systems for classifying chronic low-back pain alone and it was concluded that there was insufficient evidence to support or recommend any particular system for use in clinical description, determining prognosis, or predicting response to treatment [38]. Some systems were tested for their inter-examiner reliability, but evidence was either conflicting or moderate to strong for poor reliability [27]. On the other hand, using clusters of tests for diagnosing sacroiliac joint dysfunction yielded acceptable reliability [39-41]. However, the majority of these systems either lack evidence for their reliability, only use certain parts of the clinical examination (e.g. only physical tests), are prescriptive in their application, do not include PIVM assessment, are not related to manual therapy interventions, or do not direct towards treatment decisions. Some systems [42,43] were developed as treatment-based classification algorithms for subgrouping patients with low-back pain and were strongly based on factors derived from several clinical prediction rules [44-47]. However, these rules lack validation, and methodological and statistical issues regarding their development have been raised [48]. In contrast to the field of classification systems for low-back pain, the development and number of systems for classifying neck pain patients lie far behind. Besides a treatment-based classification system for physiotherapy interventions [49], clinical prediction rules have been derived to identify factors that predict response to spinal manipulation in patients with neck pain but with identical problems as in the rules for low-back pain as mentioned above [50-55]. In a systematic review, Gemmell and Miller [56] found poor inter-examiner reliability of multitest regimens using only physical tests for identifying manipulable spinal lesions in chiropractic. Including pain scores and medical history next to manual examination of spinal motion segments resulted in high accuracy in identifying neck pain patients [57]. To summarise, however, the value of the diagnostic process as a whole to classify patients with neck or low-back pain in order to decide whether or not spinal mobilisations or manipulations are indicated remains unclear.

This is the protocol of a study that aims to determine the inter-examiner reliability among Dutch manual therapists of indicating spinal joint mobilisations or manipulations in patients with neck or low-back pain based on a multivariable, hypothesis-based diagnostic reasoning and decision-making process. Secondly, using univariable logistic regression analysis of concordant decisions about indications, we will explore which demographic, professional, and clinical factors can explain variation in reliability of therapists' decisions with specific attention to the contribution of PIVM assessment.

Methods

Design

This study will be conducted as a repeated-measures design in which pairs of manual therapists independently examine a consecutive series of patients with neck or low-back pain presenting in primary care physiotherapy in the Netherlands. Primary outcome measure is therapists' decision about whether or not spinal manual therapy (SMT) is indicated in each patient, alone or as part of a multimodal treatment. SMT is defined here as either spinal joint mobilisations or manipulations, or both. Therapists will largely be free to conduct the full diagnostic process as they are routinely used to.

Participants

Consecutive patients aged 18 years or older presenting with a primary complaint of neck or low-back pain, either referred to primary care physiotherapy by their general practitioner or medical specialist, or by self-referral, will be eligible for participation in the study. Neck pain is defined as pain in the region between the superior nuchal line, the external occipital protuberance, the spines of the scapula, the superior border of the clavicula, and the suprasternal notch, with or without radiation to the head, trunk, or upper limbs [58]. Patients will not be eligible when headache or dizziness is their dominant complaint. Low-back pain is defined as pain or discomfort localised below the costal margin and above the inferior gluteal folds, with or without radiation to the lower limbs [59]. All patients who are assumed to have non-specific or (non-serious) specific neck or low-back pain with a potential indication for SMT will be included. Patients who are not able to speak or read Dutch fluently will be ineligible. Patients will receive verbal and written information on all aspects of the study and will be asked to provide written consent at their inclusion. The Central Committee for Research involving Human Subjects (CCMO, the Hague, the Netherlands) decided that a full evaluation of the study protocol by a medical ethical committee was not required because patients will undergo a diagnostic process similar to routine daily practice.

Examiners

Examiners will be manual therapists working at least 20 hours a week in their private practices in the Netherlands and registered by the Dutch Association for Manual Therapy or the Royal Dutch Society for Physical Therapy. From a database of those graduated from the Institute for Master Education in Musculoskeletal Therapy (SOMT: Stichting Opleidingen Musculoskeletale Therapie, Amersfoort, the Netherlands), 14 pairs of manual therapists will be invited to participate. Each pair works together in the same practice and practices will be selected based on their ability to logistically organise the study. We aim to include therapists who vary in years of clinical experience in manual therapy. Therapists will attend an information session followed by a two-hour training session in which procedures for digitally registering data are explained and practised. They will not receive additional training in history-taking, physical examination procedures, or using questionnaires. Pairs of therapists will be strictly requested not to discuss their experiences during the study with each other until their last patient has been included. Gender, age, years of clinical experience in manual therapy, highest diploma, practice setting, weekly amount of work related to spinal disorders (hours), teaching experience (yes/no), and participation in research (yes/no) will be recorded as professional characteristics from the participating therapists.

In each practice, a third colleague will function as a research assistant to coordinate the inclusion and flow of patients. Research assistants will be instructed with respect to applying the inclusion criteria, the order of assigning patients to therapists, and assuring blinding procedures.

Procedures

From eligible patients, demographic (gender, age, marital status, working status) and clinical (type of complaints (neck or low-back pain), duration of complaints (days), radiation (yes/no), traumatic origin (yes/no), comorbidity (yes/no)) data will be recorded as baseline data by the local research assistant. In addition, baseline pain and disability will be determined using the Numeric Pain Rating Scale (NPRS 0–10, higher scores indicate higher pain intensity), and the Quebec Back Pain Disability Scale (QBPDS 0–100, higher scores indicate higher disability) for low-back pain patients and the Neck Disability Index Dutch Language Version (NDI-DLV 0–50, higher scores indicate higher pain and disability) for neck pain patients, respectively. The NPRS is a reliable and valid scale to measure pain intensity in adults [60]. The Dutch version of the QBPDS is a reliable and valid instrument for measuring disability in low-back pain patients [61] and the Dutch version of the NDI is recommended for measuring pain and disability in patients with neck pain [62].

All baseline data will be available to each therapist before he or she starts the diagnostic process. The first therapist of each pair will be the treating therapist to whom the patient was assigned to, so the order in which both therapists act as the first examiner will vary according to the practice's planning. The first therapist will screen all consecutive patients with neck or low-back pain for the presence of red flags [63]. In accordance with guidelines in the Netherlands [64], patients suspected of having serious (spinal or non-spinal) pathology will not enter the study which will be recorded. Patients will then undergo a full history-taking by the first therapist. The therapist will record his or her findings as well as proposed hypotheses about patient's health status by formulating explicit objectives for further examination. The therapist will then choose the diagnostic procedures (e.g. observation, physical tests, performance tests, questionnaires) that he or she plans to perform in the patient. After performing each procedure, its outcome will be recorded. If PIVM assessment is indicated, therapists will use three-dimensional coupled movements in flexion and extension directions for each individual motion segment [65]. Movements will be judged on mobility (hypermobile-normal-hypomobile), resistance perceived by the therapist during the movement (increased resistance or stiffness yes/no), resistance perceived by the therapist at the end of the movement (end-feel) (increased resistance or stiffness at the end of the movement yes/no), and pain provocation (yes/no). Therapists will perform a maximum of three repetitions for each movement per direction per spinal motion segment to afford the best stiffness discriminability [66].

The therapist will then be asked to record whether he or she has made any changes to the original examination objectives as well as to specify these changes, and a diagnostic conclusion in terms of specific or non-specific neck or low-back pain is given. Finally, the therapist will make the decision about whether or not SMT is indicated in the patient and, when indicated, it will also be stated whether mobilisations or manipulations, or both, are indicated, and to which spinal motion segments these techniques would be targeted. In addition, the therapist will rate his or her level of certainty of the primary decision about the indication on a bipolar seven-point scale ranging from −3 (completely uncertain) to 3 (completely certain). It will also be recorded which other interventions he or she believes would further be indicated in the patient. However, at this point, no actual treatment will be provided.

After the first therapist has performed the full examination, he or she will leave the examination room and the patient will be given a 10 minute break. After checking whether all data have been registered, the research assistant then guides the second therapist into the room and makes sure that there is no visual or verbal contact between the two therapists. The second therapist will then conduct the full diagnostic process, excluding the screening for red flags, whilst being unaware of the outcomes of the first examination. Patients will be requested not to mention any outcomes or conclusions from the first examination. Both therapists will record all their findings and data into a fit-for-purpose software program. The research assistant will check whether all data have been entered by both therapists.

Statistical analysis

Demographic and clinical baseline characteristics of patients will be summarised using descriptive statistics. Absolute and relative frequencies are used to describe categorical data. Ordinal data relating to patients' pain and disability will be described with their median and interquartile range. Normally distributed numerical data will be summarised by their mean and standard deviation. In case of non-normality, median and interquartile range are presented. Examination objectives as formulated by therapists will be classified by one researcher (EvT) according to the framework of the World Health Organization's *International Classification of Functioning, Disability and Health* (ICF) [67] to describe patients' functioning in terms of impairments of neuromusculoskeletal and movement-related functions, activity limitations and participation restrictions, and personal and environmental factors. Diagnostic procedures will be listed and described with their frequencies, and also outcomes of PIVM assessment, changes to the original examination objectives, diagnostic conclusions, and examiners' level of certainty of their decision about the treatment indication will be summarised. Concordance between the formulated examination objectives concerning spinal joint motion function and the actual use of PIVM assessment will be presented as frequencies.

For each pair of therapists, 2×2 tables will be constructed and reliability for the dichotomous positive or negative decisions about whether or not SMT is indicated will be calculated as chance-corrected reliability using Cohen's kappa [68]. As recommended by Cicchetti and Feinstein [69] and Byrt et al. [70], observed agreement (%), prevalence of positive decisions (mobilisations and/or manipulations indicated) relative to the total number of indications, prevalence index (PI), bias index (BI), and specific agreement (%) in positive (p_{pos}) and negative (p_{neg}) decisions will be calculated in order to evaluate whether kappa was influenced by high prevalence of positive or negative decisions, or by systematic bias between examiners. PI reflects the difference between the proportion of agreement on positive indications as compared to that of negative indications. PI ranges between 0 and 1, and is high when the prevalence of concordant positive (or negative) indications is high, chance agreement is consequently also high, and kappa is reduced accordingly (prevalence effect) [71]. BI provides a quantification of the extent to which examiners disagree on the proportions of positive (or negative) indications. BI also ranges between 0 and 1, and is high when the difference between the discordant indications is high, chance agreement is consequently low, and kappa is inflated accordingly (bias) [71]. P_{pos} and P_{neg} are the proportions of agreement on positive and negative indications, respectively, relative to the total number of positive and negative indications, respectively, from both therapists. Overall kappa (95% CI) will be calculated as a generalized chance-corrected reliability across all pairs of therapists. See Additional file 1 for formulas.

In addition, for each pair of therapists, separate 2×2 tables will be presented for judgements about the indication for PIVM assessment and for judgements about mobility, end-feel, and pain provocation obtained from PIVM assessment (four tables in total). Observed agreement, prevalence of positive decisions, PI, BI, p_{pos}, p_{neg}, and overall kappa (95% CI) will also be calculated. Analyses will be conducted using DAG_Stat [72].

Kappa (95% CI) is interpreted in accordance with value labels as assigned by Landis & Koch [73]: <0.00: poor, 0.00-0.20: slight, 0.21-0.40: fair, 0.41-0.60: moderate, 0.61-0.80: substantial, 0.81-1.00: almost perfect. We arbitrarily assume a lower bound of the 95% CI around overall kappa of 0.60 to indicate acceptable reliability.

Univariable logistic regression analysis will be performed to explore which demographic, professional, and clinical factors contributed to the reliability of therapists' decision-making. Firstly, patients' demographic and clinical factors at baseline will concern their gender, age, type of complaints, duration of complaints (less or more than three months), radiation, traumatic origin, comorbidity, pain intensity, and disability. Such factors are associated with variation in diagnostic accuracy [74], but evidence in the context of reliability is lacking. Secondly, therapists' professional factors will include their clinical experience and weekly amount of work related to spinal disorders. Weekly amount of work related to spinal disorders was positively associated with perceived importance and confidence related to the use and interpretation of PIVM assessment [20] and may, therefore, contribute to variation in diagnostic decision-making. In addition, other clinical factors will be explored involving PIVM assessment (indicated or not, and judgements on mobility, resistance, and pain provocation), the diagnostic conclusion (specific or non-specific neck or low-back pain), therapists' level of certainty of their decision about the treatment indication, and the concordance between examination objectives and the use of PIVM assessment. Factors will be entered in the model as single covariates with the concordant decisions, either positive or negative, as the dependent variable. Concordant decisions will be coded as 1 while the discordant decisions will be coded 0. Therapists' experience and work related to spinal disorders will be entered as mean scores from each pair. A p-value <0.05 indicates a statistically significant association between a factor and a concordant decision about whether or not SMT is indicated.

With a sample size of 165, a two-sided 95% CI around kappa would extend ±0.109 from the observed value of kappa, assuming a true value of kappa of 0.70, and a prevalence of positive decisions of 50%. Consequently, each pair of examiners will be asked to include 12 patients. Multiple imputation will be used to handle records with data points missing at random. If, for any reason, data on the primary outcome measure are not available or obtainable from one or both therapists, all data from this patient will be excluded from the analysis and the pair of therapists will be asked to include a new patient. Analyses will be conducted using IBM SPSS Statistics for Windows version 22.

Discussion

The results of this study will provide 1) an estimate of the inter-examiner reliability among manual therapists of indicating SMT in patients with neck or low-back pain based on a multivariable diagnostic reasoning and decision-making process, as opposed to reliability of individual clinical tests, and 2) a first exploration of which demographic, professional, or clinical factors can explain variation in the reliability of therapists' decision-making with specific attention to the contribution of PIVM assessment. We do not aim or hypothesise that reliability from a multivariable approach to clinical diagnostics will be higher than that from individual test diagnostics. Rather, we believe that such an estimate will be a more real resemblance of the reliability among therapists of making decisions in daily practice concerning the distinction between patients who are indicated for SMT and those who are not. In addition, this approach will add to the ongoing discussion of the identification of specific subgroups of patients that may be more likely to respond to SMT and we propose alternative research strategies for establishing treatment effects.

It has been recognised that treatment effects of SMT, or any other physiotherapy modality for that matter, especially in patients with low-back pain, are, on average, small which may be due to heterogeneity of patients obscuring a wide range of individual treatment responses and variation of treatment effects [75]. Ever since the mid-nineties of the last century, identifying subgroups of patients that may benefit more from specific or targeted interventions has had the highest research priority [76-81]. As a result, there has been a proliferation of subgrouping systems aiming to identify people with a particular pathoanatomical condition, a particular prognosis, or those that are more likely to respond favorably to treatment [82]. Primary care clinicians themselves do not believe that low-back pain is one condition and they treat patients differently based on patterns of clinical signs and symptoms [83]. Moreover, they classify patients predominantly based on pathoanatomy, but they show little consensus regarding these related patterns [84]. With the aim to identify patients that may be more likely to show a positive response to spinal manipulation, clinical prediction rules have been derived to identify predictors in patients with neck and low-back pain [44-47,50-55]. Unfortunately, systematic reviews have consistently concluded that there is, as yet, insufficient evidence to support the general application of these rules [85-89]. Another systematic review found significant treatment effects favoring subgroup-specific SMT over a number of comparison treatments for pain and disability at short and intermediate follow-up based on low-quality trials [90]. Foster et al. [75] concluded that no subgrouping approaches have yet passed the tests for clinical value and robustness of evidence, and there is still a long way to go before closer matching of treatments to patient characteristics becomes a clinical reality. Indeed, two decades after the derivation of the Ottawa Ankle Rules [91], their validation and implementation is still an ongoing research process worldwide and it can be assumed that following a similar pathway for far more complex problems such as the treatment of non-specific neck and low-back pain may be even more time-consuming.

When determining treatment effects of SMT, randomised clinical trials currently do not make use of patients' full clinical health profile according to the domains of the ICF for targeting treatment. For instance, Cochrane Reviews consider primary studies including participants only based on their age and the presence of pain with or without radiation [11,13,14]. The resulting heterogeneity among trial participants and the subsequent dilution of treatment effects may be deleterious to SMT as its effectiveness may be underestimated for certain groups of patients. The majority of primary studies in patients with neck pain do not apply well-defined clinical criteria to select patients for SMT and if they do, they use only one physical test, such as a mobility test or a pain provocation test, in order to diagnose neck pain from a mechanical origin [92]. It is stated that clinical tests are not valid or reliable to allow targeting treatment in clinical trials [84]. This is certainly true when the reliability of individual physical tests is considered [26-30]. However, several of the increasingly popular predication rules also contain clinical variables that are unreliable, including PIVM assessment [42,46,88]. Targeting SMT to a more homogeneous group of patients with neck or low-back pain, based on a multivariable diagnostic process resembling daily practice, may outweigh the disadvantages of the current selection procedures in randomised clinical trials.

Awaiting evidence from the further validation of prediction rules and other classification systems, our study could offer an initial step toward a faster and easier development of an alternative approach to the identification of those patients with spinal disorders that may show a better response to SMT based on a multivariable decision process. A satisfactory level of reliability is a prerequisite for incorporating such decision-making into the design of randomised clinical trials for establishing treatment effects of SMT and thereby validating the approach. When reliability (lower bound of 95% CI around kappa) exceeds 0.60 and with BI, arbitrarily, <0.10, patients with neck or low-back pain with a positive indication can be randomised to receive, for instance, either manual mobilisations or manipulations, or both, within a multimodal treatment on the one hand or multimodal treatment without mobilisations or manipulations on the other (Figure 1A). Should reliability be below this cut-off but with p_{pos} (or p_{neg}), arbitrarily, >60%, this strategy can still be used by randomising only those patients of which the indication was agreed upon by two manual therapists (Figure 1B). P_{pos} and p_{neg} here indicate the absolute specific agreement on positive or negative indications, respectively, between therapists [25].

With respect to our second research objective, it is important to note that empirical evidence for sources of bias and variation in reliability studies is lacking contrary to studies of diagnostic accuracy [74,93-95]. Variation arises from differences between studies, for example, in terms of demographic and disease features of study participants, characteristics of examiners, setting, or test protocol. As such, it does not lead to biased estimates of reliability, but it can limit the applicability of study results [94]. Knowledge of factors that explain variation in reliability may inform ways to improve reliability. For instance, examiner training and choosing a group of more heterogeneous study participants have been mentioned as improvement strategies, but both have their limitations and lack supporting evidence [24]. Systematic reviews may reveal subgroups of participants, examiners, or tests that consistently show higher or lower reliability. In systematic reviews, between-study comparisons are conducted to search for these subgroups as sources of variation. However, these comparisons are less valid as they are hampered by the often strong clinical and methodological heterogeneity between studies [96]. In addition, the identification of these sources of variation becomes even more troublesome when reliability is consistently low (or high) across studies. Within-study comparisons are the preferred method to explore variation in reliability. To date, very few studies have been undertaken in the field of manual therapy with this aim and method. Cook et al. [97] investigated factors related to the large variability of forces used during passive accessory intervertebral movements and they found that examiners' age, gender, experience, background and education, and frequency of use did not contribute to this variation. We present simple logistic regression analysis of concordant decisions as a flexible method that can easily be incorporated in any reliability study to explore and

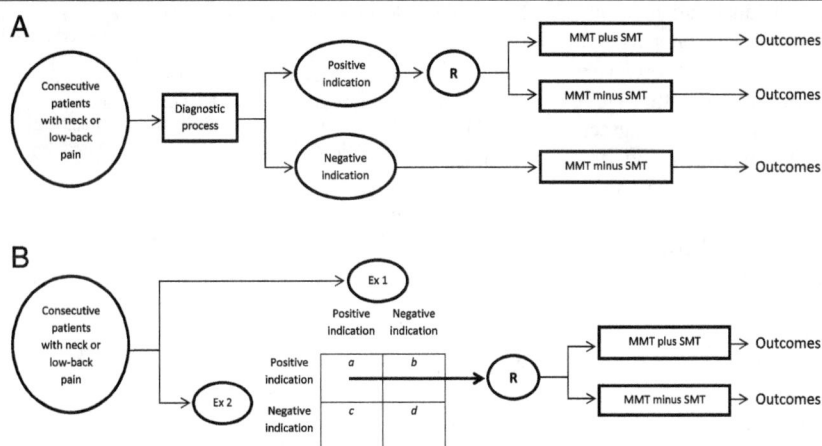

Figure 1 A. Design of an RCT including patients positively indicated for SMT when lower bound of 95% CI around kappa >0.60 and BI <0.10. B. Design of an RCT including only patients positively indicated for SMT by two examiners when kappa <0.60 but p_{pos} (or p_{neg}) >60%.

explain variation in reliability from a large number of demographic, professional, and clinical factors.

Potential limitations of this study

This study protocol presents several new approaches to investigating and analysing decision-making in manual therapy and to reliability research in general. Several of its methods need further discussion in order to appraise their effect on the validity and generalisability of the study's results. First, establishing examination objectives for physical examination by physiotherapists has been used in earlier studies [98,99]. However, the prospective formulation and registration of examination objectives is far from common practice for physiotherapists in the Netherlands [100]. The specific training of our examiners in the formulation and digital registration of these objectives may diminish the generalisability of the estimated reliability of indicating SMT. We encourage that establishing and prospectively registering of examination objectives become an integral part of daily practice in physiotherapy.

Stability of participants' characteristics is a prerequisite for the valid estimation of reliability [23]. However, very few empirical data are available as to the minimum length of the time period between test procedures that ensures that patients' responses to questions and physical tests, such as joint motion assessment, will remain unchanged. Shirley et al. [101] reported that stiffness responses to repeated mechanical posteroanterior loading of lumbar motion segments returned to the pre-testing state within five minutes. On the other hand, a 30-minute recovery period after 30 minutes of *in vitro* creep loading of the lumbar spine was not sufficient to return to the baseline situation [102]. By incorporating a 10 minute break for patients between examinations and limiting the number of movement repetitions during PIVM assessment, we are more confident that underestimation of reliability will be avoided. Research into the natural variation over time within and between individuals regarding joint mobility and other body functions, as well as into the variation induced by the physical examination itself, is needed.

Our sample size calculation strongly depends on the assumed prevalence of positive indications which was based on data from the numerous studies on practice patterns among physiotherapists in the treatment of patients with neck and low back pain [103-113]. Within the large variation in choices of treatment options by therapists, mobilisations and manipulations were only rarely among the most preferred options and their frequency of use ranged from 16% to 83% and from 2% to 37%, respectively. These figures were not substantially different for specific subgroups of manual therapists who reported remarkably low frequencies of use of manipulations in the cervical region [36,114-116]. As we will consider reliability of indicating either mobilisations or manipulations, or both, we assume a 50% prevalence of positive indications. Choosing a higher or lower prevalence would have resulted in a larger required sample [117].

In our sample of manual therapists and patients, we cannot rule out the possibility of a substantially higher (or lower) prevalence of positive indications for SMT. Because of such a skewed distribution of decisions, a distorted interpretation of kappa could then occur. Recently, kappa, as a relative measure of reliability, has been criticised because it can only provide information about the ability to distinguish between patients on a sample level [25]. The authors suggest using the specific agreement parameters (p_{pos} and p_{neg}) as absolute measures to quantify observer variation regarding a certain diagnosis or decision on an individual patient level [25]. No single omnibus index, however, can be satisfactory for all purpose and situations [69,70]. Therefore, we will calculate all recommended parameters from the 2×2 tables to allow full interpretation of reliability and agreement as related to the prevalence of concordant and discordant indications. We will not, however, correct kappa for prevalence effects and bias, for instance by calculating prevalence-adjusted bias-adjusted kappa, because this would generate values of reliability that no longer relate to the original situation [117,118].

We will select pairs of manual therapists as examiners that share a common educational background. With this background from the largest institute for manual therapy education in the Netherlands, they likely form a representative sample from the Dutch population of manual therapists registered with the Dutch Association for Manual Therapy or the Royal Dutch Society for Physical Therapy. Manual therapy education in the Netherlands is strongly embedded within international concepts. In these traditional concepts, especially passive joint motion assessment takes a prominent place [15]. Therefore, we suppose that the results of this study will to a certain extent be generalisable to populations of manual therapists outside the Netherlands. We do, however, suggest that this study be replicated over different countries and concepts to account for local idiosyncrasies in clinical reasoning and decision-making. In addition, for practical reasons, we will choose pairs of manual therapists that work in the same practice. This may inflate reliability and by pairing therapists with different levels of experience, we aim to minimise this potential threat to the validity of the study.

Finally, when analysing the reliability of indicating SMT, we will not distinguish specifically between mobilisations or manipulations. Despite the disparate mechanisms of these interventions [9,119], no evidence is available on whether one or the other, or both, should be preferred in any clinical situation. Results of randomised controlled trials have been conflicting so far [120-123]. New research should focus on the relationship between clinical findings, the choice for either mobilisation or manipulation, and subsequent clinical outcomes.

Additional file

Additional file 1: Formulas for kappa and associated measures.

Abbreviations

ICF: International Classification of Functioning, Disability and Health; PIVM: Passive intervertebral motion; SMT: Spinal manual therapy.

Competing interests

The authors declare that they have no competing interests.

Authors' contributions

EvT is the principal investigator of the study, developed the research questions and methods, obtained ethical approval, and drafted the article. RL, MS, CL, BK, RO assisted in the development of the methods and wrote the study protocol. RL, EvT, PB developed the statistical plan for this protocol. PB, RO supervised the project. All authors assisted with revisions to the study protocol and methods, and approved the final version of the article.

Author details

[1]Department of Clinical Epidemiology, Biostatistics & Bioinformatics, Academic Medical Centre, University of Amsterdam, Amsterdam, the Netherlands. [2]Institute for Master Education in Musculoskeletal Therapy, Amersfoort, the Netherlands. [3]Department of General Practice, Erasmus MC University Medical Centre, Rotterdam, the Netherlands. [4]Scientific Institute for Quality of Healthcare, Radboud University Nijmegen Medical Centre, Nijmegen, the Netherlands. [5]Department of Rehabilitation, Physiotherapy and Manual Therapy, Faculty of Medicine and Pharmacology, Free University of Brussels, Brussels, Belgium.

References

1. Borghouts JAJ, Koes BW, Bouter LM: Cost-of-illness in neck pain in the Netherlands in 1996. Pain 1999, 80:629-636.
2. Côte P, Cassidy D, Carroll L: The Saskatchewan health and back pain survey. The prevalence of neck pain and related disability in Saskatchewan adults. Spine 1998, 23:1689-1698.
3. Hogg-Johnson S, van der Velde G, Carroll LJ, Holm LW, Cassidy JD, Guzman J, Côte P, Haldeman S, Ammendolia C, Carragee E, Hurwitz E, Nordin M, Peloso P: The burden and determinants of neck pain in the general population: results of the Bone and Joint Decade 2000-2010 Task Force on Neck Pain and Its Associated Disorders. Spine 2008, 33(Suppl 4):39-51.
4. Linton SJ, Hellsing AL, Hallden K: A population-based study of spinal pain among 35-45 year old individuals. Prevalence, sick leave and health care use. Spine 1998, 23:1457-1463.
5. van Tulder MW, Koes BW, Bouter LM: A cost-of-illness study of back pain in The Netherlands. Pain 1995, 62:233-240.
6. Waddell G: Low back pain: a twentieth century health care enigma. Spine 1996, 21:2820-2825.
7. Assendelft WJ, Morton SC, Yu EI, Suttorp MJ, Shekelle PG: Spinal manipulative therapy for low back pain. A meta-analysis of effectiveness relative to other therapies. Ann Intern Med 2003, 138:871-881.
8. Gross A, Miller J, D'Sylva J, Burnie SJ, Goldsmith CH, Graham N, Haines T, Brønfort G, Hoving JL: Manipulation or mobilization for neck pain: a Cochrane Review. Man Ther 2010, 15:315-333.
9. Bialosky JE, Bishop MD, Price DD, Robinson ME, George SZ: The mechanisms of manual therapy in the treatment of musculoskeletal pain: A comprehensive model. Man Ther 2009, 14:531-538.
10. Bronfort G, Haas M, Evans R, Leininger B, Triano J: Effectiveness of manual therapies: The UK evidence report. Chiropr Osteopat 2010, 18:3.
11. Gross A, Miller J, D'Sylva J, Burnie SJ, Goldsmith CH, Graham N, Haines T, Brønfort G, Hoving JL: Manipulation or mobilisation for neck pain. Cochrane Database Syst Rev 2010, (Issue 1): Art. No.: CD004249. doi:10.1002/14651858.CD004249.pub3.
12. Michaleff ZA, Lin C-WC, Maher CG, van Tulder MW: Spinal manipulation epidemiology: Systematic review of cost-effectiveness studies. J Electromyogr Kinesiol 2012, 22:655-662.
13. Rubinstein SM, van Middelkoop M, Assendelft WJJ, de Boer MR, van Tulder MW: Spinal manipulative therapy for chronic low-back pain. Cochrane Database Syst Rev 2011, (Issue 2): Art. No.: CD008112. doi:10.1002/14651858.CD008112.pub2.
14. Rubinstein SM, Terwee CB, Assendelft WJJ, de Boer MR, van Tulder MW: Spinal manipulative therapy for acute low-back pain. Cochrane Database Syst Rev 2012, (Issue 9): Art. No.: CD008880. doi:10.1002/14651858.CD008880.pub2.
15. Farrell JP, Jensen GM: Manual therapy: A critical assessment of role in the profession of physical therapy. Phys Ther 1992, 72:843-852.
16. Maher C, Latimer J: Pain or resistance – the manual therapists' dilemma. Austr J Physiotherapy 1992, 38:257-260.

17. van Ravensberg CDD, Oostendorp RAB, van Berkel LM, Scholten-Peeters GGM, Pool JJM, Swinkels RAHM, Huijbregts PA: Physical therapy and manual physical therapy: Differences in patient characteristics. *J Man Manip Ther* 2005, 13:113–124.

18. Jull G, Treleaven J, Versace G: Manual examination: Is pain provocation a major cue for spinal dysfunction? *Austr J Physiotherapy* 1994, 40:159–165.

19. Abbott JH, Flynn TW, Fritz JM, Hing WA, Reid D, Whitman JM: Manual physical assessment of spinal segmental motion: Intent and validity. *Man Ther* 2009, 14:36–44.

20. van Trijffel E, Oostendorp RAB, Lindeboom R, Bossuyt PMM, Lucas C: Perceptions and use of passive intervertebral motion assessment of the spine. A survey of Dutch physiotherapists specializing in manual therapy. *Man Ther* 2009, 14:243–251.

21. MacDermid JC, Walton DM, Côté P, Lina Santaguida P, Gross A, Carlesso L: Use of outcome measures in managing neck pain: An international multidisciplinary survey. *Open Orthop J* 2013, 7:440–460.

22. Bartko JJ, Carpenter WT: On the methods and theory of reliability. *J Nerv Ment Dis* 1976, 163:307–317.

23. de Vet HC, Terwee CB, Knol DL, Bouter LM: When to use agreement versus reliability measures. *J Clin Epidemiol* 2006, 59:1033–1039.

24. Streiner DL, Norman GR: *Health measurement scales. A practical guide to their development and use.* 4th edition. Oxford, UK: Oxford University Press; 2008:167–210.

25. de Vet HCW, Mokkink LB, Terwee CB, Hoekstra OS, Knol DL: Clinicians are right not to like Cohen's κ. *BMJ* 2013, 346:f2125.

26. Haneline MT, Cooperstein R, Young M, Birkeland K: Spinal motion palpation: A comparison of studies that assessed intersegmental end feel vs excursion. *J Manipulative Physiol Ther* 2008, 31:616–626.

27. May S, Littlewood C, Bishop A: Reliability of procedures used in the physical examination of non-specific low back pain: a systematic review. *Austr J Physiother* 2006, 52:91–102.

28. Seffinger MA, Najm WI, Mishra SI, Adams A, Dickerson VM, Murphy LS, Reinsch S: Reliability of spinal palpation for diagnosis of back and neck pain: a systematic review of the literature. *Spine* 2004, 29:E413–E425.

29. Stochkendahl MJ, Christensen HW, Hartvigsen J, Vach W, Haas M, Hestbæk L, Adams A, Bronfort G: Manual examination of the spine: a systematic critical literature review of reproducibility. *J Manipulative Physiol Ther* 2006, 29:475–485.

30. van Trijffel E, Anderegg Q, Bossuyt PM, Lucas C: Inter-examiner reliability of passive assessment of intervertebral motion in the cervical and lumbar spine: a systematic review. *Man Ther* 2005, 10:256–269.

31. Moons KG, Biesheuvel CJ, Grobbee DE: Test research versus diagnostic research. *Clin Chem* 2004, 50:473–476.

32. Jones MA, Jensen G, Edwards I: Clinical reasoning in physiotherapy. In *Clinical Reasoning in the Health Professions.* 3rd edition. Edited by Higgs J, Jones MA, Loftus S, Christensen N. Edinburgh, UK: Elsevier/Butterworth Heinemann; 2008:245–256.

33. Rothstein JM, Echternach JL, Riddle DL: The hypothesis-oriented algorithm for clinicians II (HOAC II): a guide for patient management. *Phys Ther* 2003, 83:455–470.

34. Rivett DA, Higgs J: Hypothesis generation in the clinical reasoning behaviour of manual therapists. *J Phys Ther Educ* 1997, 11:40–45.

35. van Trijffel E, Plochg T, van Hartingsveld F, Lucas C, Oostendorp RAB: The role and position of passive intervertebral motion assessment within clinical reasoning and decision-making in manual physical therapy: a qualitative interview study. *J Man Manip Ther* 2010, 18:111–118.

36. Carlesso LC, Macdermid JC, Santaguida PL, Thabane L, Giulekas K, Larocque L, Millard J, Williams C, Miller J, Chesworth BM: Beliefs and practice patterns in spinal manipulation and spinal motion palpation reported by Canadian manipulative therapists. *Physiother Canada* 2013, 65:167–175.

37. Riddle DL: Classification and low back pain: A review of the literature and critical analysis of selected systems. *Phys Ther* 1996, 78:708–737.

38. Fairbank J, Gwilym SE, France JC, Daffner SD, Dettori J, Hermsmeyer J, Andersson G: The role of classification of chronic low back pain. *Spine* 2011, 36(Suppl 2):19–42.

39. Arab AM, Abdollahi I, Joghataei MT, Golafshani Z, Kazemnejad A: Inter- and intra-examiner reliability of single and composites of selected motion palpation and pain provocation tests for sacroiliac joint. *Man Ther* 2009, 14:213–221.

40. Kokmeyer DJ, van der Wurff P, Aufdemkampe G, Fickenscher TC: The reliability of multitest regimens with sacroiliac pain provocation tests. *J Manipulative Physiol Ther* 2002, 25:42–48.

41. Robinson HS, Brox JI, Robinson R, Bjelland E, Solem S, Telje T: The reliability of selected motion- and pain provocation tests for the sacroiliac joint. *Man Ther* 2007, 12:72–79.

42. Fritz JM, Brennan GP, Clifford SN, Hunter SJ, Thackeray A: An examination of the reliability of a classification algorithm for subgrouping patients with low back pain. *Spine* 2006, 31:77–82.

43. Stanton TR, Fritz JM, Hancock MJ, Latimer J, Maher CG, Wand BM, Parent EC: Evaluation of a treatment-based classification algorithm for low back pain: A cross-sectional study. *Phys Ther* 2011, 91:496–509.

44. Childs JD, Fritz JM, Flynn TW, Irrgang JJ, Johnson KK, Majkowski GR, Delitto A: A clinical prediction rule to identify patients with low back pain most likely to benefit from spinal manipulation: A validation study. *Ann Intern Med* 2004, 141:920–928.

45. Flynn T, Fritz J, Whitman J, Wainner R, Magel J, Rendeiro D, Butler D, Garber M, Allison S: A clinical prediction rule for classifying patients with low back pain who demonstrate short-term improvement with spinal manipulation. *Spine* 2002, 27:2835–2843.

46. Fritz JM, Whitman JM, Flynn TW, Wainner RS, Childs JD: Factors related to the inability of individuals with low back pain to improve with a spinal manipulation. *Phys Ther* 2004, 84:173–190.

47. Hicks GE, Fritz JM, Delitto A, McGill SM: Preliminary development of a clinical prediction rule for determining which patients with low back pain will respond to a stabilization exercise program. *Arch Phys Med Rehabil* 2005, 89:1753–1762.

48. Cook C: Key issues for manual therapy clinical practice and research in North America. *Man Ther* 2013, 18:269–270.

49. Fritz JM, Brennan GP: Preliminary examination of a proposed treatment-based classification system for patients receiving physical therapy interventions for neck pain. *Phys Ther* 2007, 87:513–524.

50. Cleland JA, Childs JD, Fritz JM, Whitman JM, Eberhart SL: Development of a clinical prediction rule for guiding treatment of a subgroup of patients with neck pain: Use of thoracic spine manipulation, exercise, and patient education. *Phys Ther* 2007, 87:9–23.

51. Cleland JA, Fritz JM, Whitman JM, Heath R: Predictors of short-term outcome in people with a clinical diagnosis of cervical radiculopathy. *Phys Ther* 2007, 87:1619–1632.

52. Puentedura EJ, Cleland JA, Landers MR, Mintken PE, Louw A, Fernándes-de-las-Peñas C: Development of a clinical prediction rule to identify patients with neck pain likely to benefit from thrust joint manipulation to the cervical spine. *J Orthop Sports Phys Ther* 2012, 42:577–592.

53. Schellingerhout JM, Verhagen AP, Heymans MW, Pool JJ, Vonk F, Koes B, de Vet HCW: Which subgroups of patients with non-specific neck pain are more likely to benefit from spinal manipulation, physiotherapy, or usual care? *Pain* 2008, 139:670–680.

54. Thiel HW, Bolton JE: Predictors for immediate and global responses to chiropractic manipulation of the cervical spine. *J Manipulative Physiol Ther* 2008, 31:172–183.

55. Tseng Y-L, Wang WTJ, Chen W-Y, Hou T-J, Chen T-C, Lieu F-K: Predictors for the immediate responders to cervical manipulation in patients with neck pain. *Man Ther* 2006, 11:306–315.

56. Gemmell H, Miller P: Interexaminer reliability of multidimensional examination regimens for detecting spinal manipulable lesions: a systematic review. *Clin Chiropr* 2005, 8:199–204.

57. de Hertogh WJ, Vaes PH, Vijverman V, de Cordt A, Duquet W: The clinical examination of neck pain patients: the validity of a group of tests. *Man Ther* 2007, 12:50–55.

58. Guzman J, Hurwitz EL, Carroll LJ, Haldeman S, Côté P, Carragee EJ, Peloso PM, van der Velde G, Holm LW, Hogg-Johnson S, Nordin M, Cassidy JD: A new conceptual model of neck pain: linking onset, course, and care. The Bone and Joint Decade 2000–2010 Task Force on Neck Pain and Its Associated Disorders. *Spine* 2008, 33(Suppl 4):14–23.

59. Airaksinen O, Brox JI, Cedraschi C, Hildebrandt J, Klaber-Moffet J, Kovacs F, Mannion AF, Reis S, Staal JB, Ursin H, Zanoli G: Chapter 4 European guidelines for the management of chronic nonspecific low back pain. *Eur Spine J* 2006, 15(Suppl 2):192–300.

60. Hawker GA, Mian S, Kendzerska T, French M: Measures of adult pain. Visual Analog Scale for Pain (VAS Pain), Numeric Rating Scale for Pain (NRS Pain), McGill Pain Questionnaire (MPQ), Short-Form McGill Pain Questionnaire (SF-MPQ), Chronic Pain Grade Scale (CPGS), Short Form-36 Bodily Pain Scale (SF-36 BPS), and Measure of Intermittent and Constant Osteoarthritis Pain (ICOAP). *Arthritis Care Res* 2011, 63(Suppl 11):240–252.

61. Schoppink LE, van Tulder MW, Koes BW, Beurskens SA, de Bie RA: **Reliability and validity of the Dutch adaptation of the Quebec Back Pain Disability Scale.** *Phys Ther* 1996, **76:**268–275.
62. Schellingerhout JM, Heymans MW, Verhagen AP, de Vet HC, Koes BW, Terwee CB: **Measurement properties of translated versions of neck-specific questionnaires: A systematic review.** *BMC Med Res Methodol* 2011, **11:**87.
63. Greenhalgh S, Selfe J: *Red flags. A guide to identifying serious pathology of the spine.* Amsterdam/New York: Elsevier/Churchill Livingstone; 2006:5–48.
64. **KNGF Guideline Low-back Pain.** 2013, [http://www.fysionet-evidencebased.nl/index.php/component/kngf/richtlijnen/lage-rugpijn-2013] [In Dutch] Last accessed 30 December 2013.
65. van der El A: *Orthopaedic manual therapy diagnosis. Spine and temperomandibular joints.* London, UK: Jones and Bartlett Publishers; 2010:351–498.
66. Macfadyen N, Maher CG, Adams R: **Number of sampling movements and manual stiffness judgements.** *J Manipulative Physiol Ther* 1998, **21:**604–610.
67. International classification of functioning, disability and health (ICF). [http://www.who.int/classifications/icf/en/] Last accessed 30 December 2013.
68. Cohen J: **A coefficient of agreement for nominal scales.** *Educ Psychol Meas* 1960, **20:**37–46.
69. Cicchetti DV, Feinstein AR: **High agreement but low Kappa: II. Resolving the paradoxes.** *J Clin Epidemiol* 1990, **43:**551–558.
70. Byrt T, Bishop J, Carlin JB: **Bias, prevalence and Kappa.** *J Clin Epidemiol* 1993, **46:**423–429.
71. Feinstein AR, Cicchetti DV: **High agreement but low kappa: I. The problems of two paradoxes.** *J Clin Epidemiol* 1990, **43:**543–549.
72. MacKinnon A: **A spreadsheet for the calculation of comprehensive statistics for the assessment of diagnostic tests and inter-rater agreement.** *Comput Biol Med* 2000, **30:**127–134.
73. Landis JR, Koch DG: **The measurement of observer agreement for categorical data.** *Biometrica* 1977, **33:**159–164.
74. Whiting PF, Rutjes AWS, Westwood ME, Mallett S, and the QUADAS-2 Steering Group: **A systematic review classifies sources of bias and variation in diagnostic test accuracy studies.** *J Clin Epidemiol* 2013, **66:**1093–1104.
75. Foster NE, Hill JC, Hay EM: **Subgrouping patients with low back pain in primary care: Are we getting any better at it?** *Man Ther* 2011, **16:**3–8.
76. Borkan JM, Cherkin DC: **An agenda for primary care research on low back pain.** *Spine* 1996, **21:**2880–2884.
77. Borkan JM, Koes B, Reis S, Cherkin DC: **A report from the Second International Forum for Primary Care Research on Low Back Pain. Examining priorities.** *Spine* 1998, **23:**1992–1996.
78. Bouter LM, van Tulder MW, Koes BW: **Methodologic issues in low back pain research in primary care.** *Spine* 1998, **23:**2014–2020.
79. Clinical research agenda for physical therapy. *Phys Ther* 2000, **80:**499–513. http://www.ncbi.nlm.nih.gov/pubmed/10792860.
80. Foster NE, Dziedzic KS, van der Windt DAWM, Fritz JM, Hay EM: **Research priorities for non-pharmacological therapies for common musculoskeletal problem: Nationally and internationally agreed recommendations.** *BMC Musculoskelet Disord* 2009, **10:**3.
81. Goldstein MS, Scalzitti DA, Craik RL, Dunn SL, Irion JM, Irrgang J, Kolobe THA, McDonough CM, Shields RK: **The revised research agenda for physical therapy.** *Phys Ther* 2011, **91:**165–174.
82. Kent P, Keating JL, Leboeuf-Yde C: **Research methods for subgrouping low back pain.** *BMC Med Res Methodol* 2010, **10:**62.
83. Kent P, Keating J: **Do primary care clinicians think that nonspecific low back pain is one condition?** *Spine* 2004, **29:**1022–1031.
84. Kent P, Keating J: **Classification in nonspecific low back pain: What methods do primary care clinicians currently use?** *Spine* 2005, **30:**1433–1440.
85. Beneciuk JM, Bishop MD, George SZ: **Clinical prediction rules for physical therapy interventions: A systematic review.** *Phys Ther* 2009, **89:**114–124.
86. May S, Rosedale R: **Prescriptive clinical prediction rules in back pain research: A systematic review.** *J Man Manip Ther* 2009, **17:**36–45.
87. Kent P, Mjøsund HL, Petersen DHD: **Does targeting manual therapy and/or exercise improve patient outcomes in nonspecific low back pain. A systematic review.** *BMC Med* 2010, **8:**22.
88. Stanton TR, Hancock MJ, Maher CG, Koes BW: **Critical appraisal of clinical prediction rules that aim to optimize treatment selection for musculoskeletal conditions.** *Phys Ther* 2010, **90:**843–854.
89. Patel S, Friede T, Froud R, Evans DW, Underwood M: **Systematic review of randomized controlled trials of clinical prediction rules for physical therapy in low back pain.** *Spine* 2013, **38:**762–769.
90. Slater SL, Ford JJ, Richards MC, Taylor NF, Surkitt LD, Hahne AJ: **The effectiveness of sub-group specific manual therapy for low back pain: A systematic review.** *Man Ther* 2012, **17:**201–212.
91. Stiell IG, Greenberg GH, McKnight RD, Nair RC, McDowell I, Worthington JR: **A study to develop clinical decision rules for the use of radiography in acute ankle injuries.** *Ann Emerg Med* 1992, **21:**384–390.
92. Smith J, Bolton PS: **What are the clinical criteria justifying spinal manipulative therapy for neck pain? A systematic review of randomized controlled trials.** *Pain Med* 2013, **14:**460–468.
93. Lijmer JG, Mol BW, Heisterkamp S, Bonsel GJ, Prins MH, van der Meulen JHP, Bossuyt PMM: **Empirical evidence of design-related bias in studies of diagnostic tests.** *JAMA* 1999, **282:**1061–1066.
94. Whiting P, Rutjes AWS, Reitsma JB, Glas AS, Bossuyt PMM, Kleijnen J: **Sources of variation and bias in studies of diagnostic accuracy. A systematic review.** *Ann Intern Med* 2004, **140:**189–202.
95. Rutjes AW, Reitsma JB, di Nisio M, Smidt N, van Rijn JC, Bossuyt PM: **Evidence of bias and variation in diagnostic accuracy studies.** *CMAJ* 2006, **174:**469–476.
96. Scales CD Jr, Canfield SE: **Advanced topics in evidence-based urological oncology: Using results of a subgroup analysis.** *Urol Oncol* 2011, **29:**462–466.
97. Cook C, Turney L, Ramirez L, Miles A, Haas S, Karakostas T: **Predictive factors in poor inter-rater reliability among physical therapists.** *J Man Manip Ther* 2002, **10:**200–205.
98. Riddle DL, Rothstein JM, Echternach JL: **Application of the HOAC II: An episode of care for a patient with low back pain.** *Phys Ther* 2003, **83:**471–485.
99. Thoomes EJ, Schmitt MS: **Practical use of the HOAC II for clinical decision making and subsequent therapeutic interventions in an elite athlete with low back pain.** *J Orthop Sports Phys Ther* 2011, **41:**108–117.
100. Oostendorp RAB, Rutten GM, Dommerholt J, Nijhuis-van der Sanden MW, Harting J: **Guideline-based development and practice test of quality indicators for physiotherapy care in patients with neck pain.** *J Eval Clin Prac* 2013, **13:**194.
101. Shirley D, Ellis E, Lee M: **The response of posteroanterior lumbar stiffness to repeated loading.** *Man Ther* 2002, **7:**19–25.
102. Busscher I, van Dieën JH, van der Veen AJ, Kingma I, Meijer GJM, Verkerke GJ, Veldhuizen AG: **The effects of creep and recovery on the *in vitro* biomechanical characteristics of human multi-level thoracolumbar spinal segments.** *Clin Biomech* 2011, **26:**438–444.
103. Battlé MC, Cherkin DC, Dunn R, Ciol MA, Wheeler KJ: **Managing low back pain: Attitudes and treatment preferences of physical therapists.** *Phys Ther* 1994, **74:**219–226.
104. Carey TS, Freburger JK, Holmes GM, Castel L, Darter J, Agans R, Kalsbeek W, Jackman A: **A long way to go. Practice patterns and evidence in chronic low back pain care.** *Spine* 2009, **34:**718–724.
105. Freburger JK, Carey TS, Holmes GM: **Physical therapy for chronic low back pain in North Carolina: Overuse, underuse, or misuse?** *Phys Ther* 2011, **91:**484–495.
106. Goode AP, Freburger J, Carey T: **Prevalence, practice patterns, and evidence for chronic neck pain.** *Arthritis Care Res* 2010, **62:**1594–1601.
107. Gracey JH, McDonough SM, Baxter GD: **Physiotherapy management of low back pain. A survey of current practice in Northern Ireland.** *Spine* 2002, **27:**406–411.
108. Jette AM, Delitto A: **Physical therapy treatment choices for musculoskeletal impairments.** *Phys Ther* 1997, **77:**145–154.
109. Li LC, Bombardier C: **Physical therapy management of low back pain: An exploratory survey of therapist approaches.** *Phys Ther* 2001, **81:**1018–1028.
110. Liddle SD, Baxter GD, Gracey JH: **Physiotherapists' use of advice and exercise for the management of chronic low back pain: A national survey.** *Man Ther* 2009, **14:**189–196.
111. Mikhail C, Korner-Bitensky N, Rossignol M, Dumas J-P: **Physical therapists' use of interventions with high evidence of effectiveness in the management of a hypothetical typical patient with acute low back pain.** *Phys Ther* 2005, **85:**1151–1167.
112. Mielenz TJ, Carey TS, Dyrek DA, Harris BA, Garrett JM, Darter JD: **Physical therapy utilization by patients with acute low back pain.** *Phys Ther* 1997, **77:**1040–1051.

Indicating spinal joint mobilisations or manipulations in patients with neck or low-back pain: protocol...

67

113. van Baar ME, Dekker J, Bosveld W: A survey of physical therapy goals and interventions for patients with back and knee pain. *Phys Ther* 1998, **78**:33–42.

114. Adams G, Sim J: A survey of UK manual therapists' practice of and attitudes towards manipulation and its complications. *Physiother Res Int* 1998, **3**:206–227.

115. Jull G: Use of high and low velocity cervical manipulative therapy procedures by Australian manipulative physiotherapists. *Aust J Physiother* 2002, **48**:189–193.

116. Hurley L, Yardley K, Gross AR, Hendry L, McLaughlin L: A survey to examine attitudes and patterns of practice of physiotherapists who perform cervical spinal manipulation. *Man Ther* 2002, **7**:10–18.

117. Sim J, Wright CC: The Kappa statistic in reliability studies: use, interpretation, and sample size requirements. *Phys Ther* 2005, **85**:257–268.

118. Hoehler FK: Bias and prevalence effects on kappa viewed in terms of sensitivity and specificity. *J Clin Epidemiol* 2000, **53**:499–503.

119. Zusman M: There's something about passive movement. *Med Hypotheses* 2010, **75**:106–110.

120. Hurwitz EL, Morgenstern H, Harber P, Kominski GF, Yu F, Adams AH: A randomized trial of chiropractic manipulation and mobilization for patients with neck pain: Clinical outcomes from the UCLA neck-pain study. *Am J Public Health* 2002, **92**:1634–1641.

121. Leaver AM, Maher CG, Herbert RD, Latimer J, McAuley JH, Jull G, Refshauge KM: A randomized controlled trial comparing manipulation with mobilization for recent onset neck pain. *Arch Phys Med Rehabil* 2010, **91**:1313–1318.

122. Dunning JR, Cleland JA, Waldrop MA, Arnot C, Young I, Turner M, Sigurdsson G: Upper cervical and upper thoracic thrust manipulation versus mobilization in patients with mechanical neck pain: A multicenter randomized clinical trial. *J Orthop Sports Phys Ther* 2012, **42**:5–18.

123. Cook C, Learman K, Showalter C, Kabbaz V, O'Halloran B: Early use of thrust manipulation versus non-thrust manipulation: a randomized clinical trial. *Man Ther* 2013, **18**:191–198.

Current preventative and health promotional care offered to patients by chiropractors in the United Kingdom: a survey

Patricia E Fikar[1]*, Kent A Edlund[2] and Dave Newell[2]

Abstract

Background: With increasing morbidity and mortality attributable to non-communicable disease, primary healthcare providers are urged to increasingly support people in making healthy lifestyle choices. Many chronic physical diseases associated with lifestyle behaviours have been linked to neuromusculoskeletal disorders and pain. Chiropractors, as primary healthcare professionals, are in a position to provide preventative and promotional healthcare to patients, however, it is unknown to what extent such care is provided, particularly in the United Kingdom (UK).

Method: This study was a cross sectional online questionnaire distributed to four UK chiropractic associations. The responses were collected over a period of two months from March 26th 2012 to May 25th 2012. Descriptive analyses were performed to identify the trends in current practice of chiropractors in the UK. Additionally, subgroup analyses of all items were performed using Pearson Chi-Square tests to determine statistically significant differences between respondents based on gender, years in practice, educational institution and association membership.

Results: Of the 2,448 members in the four participating associations, 509 chiropractors (approximately 21%) completed the survey. The great majority of UK chiropractors surveyed report evaluating and monitoring patients in regards to posture (97.1%), inactivity/overactivity (90.8%) and movement patterns (88.6%). Slightly fewer provide this type of care for psychosocial stress (82.3%), nutrition (74.1%) and disturbed sleep (72.9%). Still fewer do so for smoking (60.7%) and over-consumption of alcohol (56.4%). Verbal advice given by the chiropractor was reported as the most successful resource to encourage positive lifestyle changes as reported by 68.8% of respondents. Goal-setting is utilised by 70.7% to 80.4% of respondents concerning physical fitness issues. For all other lifestyle issues, goal-setting is used by approximately two-fifths (41.7%) or less. For smoking and over-consumption of alcohol, a mere one-fifth (20.0% and 20.6% respectively) of the responding chiropractors set goals.

Conclusions: UK chiropractors are participating in promoting positive lifestyle changes in areas common to preventative healthcare and health promotion areas; however, more can be done, particularly in the areas of smoking and over-consumption of alcohol. In addition, goal-setting to support patient-provider relationships should be more widespread, potentially increasing the utility of such valuable advice and resources.

Keywords: Chiropractic, Health promotion, Health prevention, Wellness, Non-communicable disease, Goal-setting

* Correspondence: patricia.fikar@gmail.com
[1]Private Practice, Vienna, Austria
Full list of author information is available at the end of the article

Background

One of the greatest challenges facing global public health is the burden of non-communicable diseases (NCDs). NCDs are non-infectious and non-transmittable which include chronic, slow progressing diseases. Statistics show that in 2008, of the 57 million deaths globally, 36 million where due to NCDs of which 80% were preventable [1]. Top on the list are cardiovascular disease (most especially coronary heart disease and stroke), cancer, chronic respiratory disease and diabetes. Additionally, many countries report mental health issues as contributors to the burden by increasing the instance of the other NCDs [2]. Consequently, the World Health Organization (WHO), in its Global Strategy on Diet, Physical Activity and Health [3], is encouraging individuals to make appropriate lifestyle changes and is looking to healthcare professionals of all disciplines to be facilitators in this task on both an individual patient basis and for society as a whole. It emphasised that primary care providers have an important duty to make routine inquiries regarding these issues, helping individuals where possible to develop sustained behavioural change.

In 2006, the Council on Chiropractic Education (CCE) in the United States of America (USA) suggested a set of standards indicating specific health promotional efforts that every chiropractor should perform and health promotion and prevention methods that ideally should be part of the curriculum at accredited USA chiropractic colleges [4]. According to this standard, accepted principles of health promotion include assessing the patients' health status, screening for risky lifestyle behaviours, and using multiple health outcome instruments. Preventative care includes educating patients regarding the impact of lifestyle on health, providing appropriate recommendations and counselling, and providing the necessary resources to promote health and wellness. For the purpose of this paper, health promotion and preventative care will take these two definitions.

Acknowledging the debate within the chiropractic profession as to whether chiropractors serve as primary care providers or spine specialists, Evans and Rupert [5] argue that health promotion and prevention are important to all chiropractors regardless of their view on their role in healthcare. They state that since many chiropractic patients seek care as part of a health maintenance programme, chiropractors are well-positioned to make routine inquiry and initiate preventative care and health promotion. In a study by Von Korff et al. [6], the authors concluded that chronic spinal pain may be co morbid with another conditions including stroke, hypertension, asthma, COPD, irritable bowel syndrome, ulcers, HIV/AIDS, epilepsy and vision problems, which are by association relevant to chiropractors. In a systematic review by Goldberg et al. [7], it was found that smoking is likely to be associated with the

incidence and prevalence of non-specific back pain. Additionally, in a multiphase cross-sectional survey of muscu loskeletal pain in the United Kingdom (UK) general population, Webb et al. [8] reported obesity as an important independent predictor of back pain and its severity. Furthermore, Fishbain et al. [9] found depression to be more common in chronic pain patients than in healthy controls as a consequence of the presence of chronic pain, further highlighting the importance of addressing these issues in all types of chiropractic practices.

Although some patients seek chiropractic care for pain relief and end treatment when they become asymptomatic, Evans and Rupert [5] suggest that if a patient indicates willingness to attempt to change any unhealthy behaviour, chiropractors should not simply stress personal empowerment, but be able to provide specific information and resources. UK chiropractic education not only consists of chiropractic technique and diagnosis, but provides chiropractors with a broad base in health knowledge including nutrition, physical fitness and psychosocial considerations in patient care [10]. Additionally, UK chiropractors can further their knowledge in these areas by completing continuing professional development hours through self-directed study, continuing post-graduate education or by attending national and international seminars [11].

Preventative health care and health promotion are of emerging importance to the chiropractic profession. Previous work in this area has been done by Evans et al. [12] who focused on the patients' perspective of health promotional advice in a chiropractic teaching clinic in the USA, however, the chiropractors' perspective on providing this type of care to their patients is unknown. Therefore, the purpose of this UK-based study is two-fold. Firstly, to determine if care is being provided by UK chiropractors in regards to preventative healthcare and health promotion, particularly in the areas of nutrition, physical fitness and exercise, psychosocial well-being, smoking and alcohol consumption. Secondly, to identify to what extent such care is provided.

Methods

The survey questionnaire was generated from November, 2011 to March, 2012. The items were organised into categories, namely, nutrition, physical activity, psychosocial well-being, smoking and alcohol consumption. Additionally, every item on the questionnaire had a comment box where the participants could leave additional issues that did not appear on the item lists. The information submitted in these comment boxes were not included in the data analysis, but rather used for interpretation and to direct future research.

To reach a large number of chiropractors throughout the UK, the survey was distributed electronically through four UK chiropractic associations. The four participating

UK associations were the British Chiropractic Association (BCA) [13], the McTimoney Chiropractic Association (MCA) [14], the Scottish Chiropractic Association (SCA) [15], and the United Chiropractic Association (UCA) [16]. The survey items were entered into the open source on-line survey application Limesurvey® [17]. An email bulletin with a link to the survey requesting members to participate was sent to the chiropractors by the associations' secretaries. The survey ran once for a two-month period from the 26th of March, 2012 to the 25th of May, 2012. A reminder bulletin was sent at the end of April 2012 to all members regardless if they had already completed the survey or not, however, the bulletin indicated that they should only complete the survey once. Descriptive analyses were performed to identify the trends in current practice of chiropractors in the UK. Additionally, with the use of Statistical Package for the Social Sciences (SPSS 21.0), subgroup analyses of all items were performed using Pearson Chi-Square tests to determine statistically significant differences between respondents based on gender, years in practice, educational institution and association membership.

Ethics

This research was ethically approved by the Anglo-European College of Chiropractic undergraduate ethics panel in March 2012.

Results

Cohort characteristics

Five hundred and nine participants returned fully completed surveys. The total number of members of the four participating associations, which was provided through email request by the associations' secretaries, sums up to 2,448 member chiropractors. The 509 respondents represent approximately 21% of chiropractic membership in these four associations; however, as individual chiropractors can be members of multiple associations, the response rate is potentially higher than 21%. Furthermore, the associations' secretaries where unable to determine the number

of members on their mailing lists, so the exact number of bulletin recipients as well as the actual response rate is unknown. Of the total respondents, 63% were BCA members, with another 25% representing the UCA, 11% representing the MCA, 3% representing the SCA and 4% representing other associations. Table 1 shows the total number of members of each association at the time the study was conducted and the proportion of chiropractors in those associations who completed the survey.

Just under half of all respondents (44.6%) were female. Most (52.1%) had practiced for 10 years or less and the majority (54.2%) were trained at the AECC. Table 2 illustrates the demographic and professional characteristics of the entire cohort.

Of all respondents, 89.0% consider themselves to be evidence informed practitioners. Depending on the issue, 61.7 to 97.1% of the respondents agreed that the items associated with lifestyle issues were their responsibility to discuss. These issues included decreasing alcohol consumption, decreasing psychosocial stress, regular exercise, improving eating habits, improving posture, improving movement patterns, normalising sleep patterns and smoking cessation. The specific values for each issue are shown in Table 3. Similar proportions of chiropractors indicated they would evaluate/monitor (56.4-97.1%) or give advice/resources (53.8-96.3%), again depending on the specific issues listed. However, respondents' perceived responsibility to discuss lifestyle issues with patients and the actual proportion that evaluate/monitor, give advice/resources or set goals in practice differed across all categories. These differences are visually highlighted in Figure 1. In this survey, the highest number (70.7-80.4%) of chiropractors who incorporate goal-setting and re-evaluation of goals did so in regards to physical activity. However, in all of the other areas, up to approximately two-fifths (20.0-41.7%) of the chiropractors set goals and re-evaluate. For over-consumption of alcohol and smoking, merely one-fifth (20.0% and 20.6% respectively) provide this service. Additionally, fewer chiropractors indicated they "set goals" or "re-

Table 1 Association membership and survey response rate

Association	Members[1]	Respondents	Survey respondents[2] (%)	Membership (%)
BCA	1352	319	63	24
MCA	544	55	11	10
SCA	145	15	3	10
UCA	407	127	25	31
Other*	unknown	19	4	N/A
Total	2448	516	106	21

[1]The number of members in each association was obtained through email request and the figures shown were given directly by each association.
[2]Multiplicity of membership included.
*Other associations indicated: American Chiropractic Association, Associazione Italiana Chiropratici, China Hong Kong Macao Chiropractic' Association, Chiropractic Association of South Africa, Chiropractors' Association of Australia, College of Chiropractors, Danish Chiropractors Association, European Chiropractors' Union, International Chiropractic Pediatric Association, International Chiropractors Association, SOTO Europe, Swedish Chiropractic Association.

Table 2 Demographic and professional characteristics of whole cohort (N= 509)

Variable	Proportion (%)	N
Gender (F)	44.6	227
Years in practice		
0-5	27.1	138
6-10	25.0	127
11-15	14.5	74
16-20	11.6	59
>20	21.8	111
Chiropractic education		
AECC	54.2	276
McTimoney	12.2	62
WIOC	19.4	99
Other*	14.2	72

*Other countries indicated for chiropractic education: Australia, Canada, New Zealand, South Africa, Sweden, UK, USA.

evaluated goals", with less than half (41.6%) setting/re-evaluating goals at the majority of visits. When asked which resource the respondents think is the most successful to prevent illness and promote their patients' health, the majority (68.8%) indicated verbal advice, followed in descending order by written advice (10.6%), referral to another health professional (internal or external) (6.3%), brochures and pamphlets (3.3%), internet website address (1.4%) and a place address or contact number (0.2%). Table 3 summarises the respondents' practice characteristics and behaviours.

Subgroup analysis

In order to determine any differences between subgroups, analyses were carried out using Pearson Chi-Square tests. This revealed that there was a statistically significant greater proportion of males with >20 years in practice, χ^2 (4, N =489) =13.85, p = .008) reflecting an increasing female representation in the profession over the most recent decades. Additionally, in regards to years in practice and association membership, the UCA had a statistically significant over-representation of respondents with fewer years in practice, χ^2 (4, N =489) =17.18, p = .002), while the BCA was over-represented by respondents with greater years in practice, χ^2 (4, N =489) =16.66, p = .002). This was not seen in the MCA or SCA.

In relation to patient behaviours, a significantly greater number of female respondents reported disturbed sleep, χ^2 (1, N =489) =9.74, p = .002), and psychosocial stress, χ^2 (1, N =489) =6.99, p = .008), as being behaviours they evaluate and/or monitor. Conversely, males reported poor posture, χ^2 (1, N =489) =5.98, p = .014), with higher frequency than females. In regards to the lifestyle changes for which the respondents set and/or re-

evaluate goals with their patients, respondents in practice for ≤20 years reported doing so more frequently in regards to poor posture, χ^2 (4, N =489) =12.97, p = .011). On the other hand, respondents in practice for >20 years reported with higher frequency goal setting/re-evaluation for smoking, χ^2 (4, N =489) =11.35, p = .023).

Discussion

This study indicates that the surveyed UK chiropractors are participating in preventative healthcare and health promotion activities, encouraging patients to make positive lifestyle changes especially in regards to physical activity and fitness. Although less in comparison to physical activity, our findings indicate that a fair degree of nutritional and psychosocial care is provided. These are potentially important components not only to individual patients, but to public health initiatives as highlighted by O'Connor et al. [18]. The authors suggest that chiropractors, given the practicalities of their work, have the opportunity to be opportunistic screeners and referrers for a variety of conditions that can potentially decrease mortality and morbidity at minimal cost, an important consideration emerging across the global health care sector.

The results also show that just over half of the chiropractors reported smoking and over-consumption of alcohol as their responsibility to discuss. However, less of these same clinicians evaluate and monitor their patients for these behaviours. This is surprising as over-consumption of alcohol and smoking are not only known to lead directly to the development of NCDs, but additionally have quite severe consequences on skeletal and nervous system health [19-21]. Nevertheless, the proportion of UK chiropractors reporting that they provide advice for smoking cessation is similar to the amount of advice being offered by other healthcare professionals to patients in the USA [22,23]. In the UK, Coleman et al. [24] states that many opportunities to discuss smoking with patients are not being utilised by general practitioners in order to avoid negative responses from patients and many practitioners do not raise the topic unless the patients present with smoking-related problems. It appears to be an area of care that needs more attention from healthcare professionals as a whole and chiropractors could have a positive role to play.

As preventative care and health promotion focus on the daily choices an individual makes regarding their long-term health objectives, goal-setting should be a core component. In a study by Holliday et al. [25], neurological rehabilitation patients in the UK who were encouraged to participate in goal-setting found such goals to be more relevant than those set primarily by the providers as they felt a greater sense of autonomy and satisfaction when they were part of the process. Goal-setting where patients and providers co-create health by focusing on a specific problem, setting realistic objectives, and developing action

Table 3 Practice characteristics and behaviours of whole cohort (N= 509)

Question	Proportion (%)	N
Evidence informed?		
Yes	89.0	453
No	2.4	12
No answer	8.6	44
Lifestyle issues considered responsible to discuss		
Decrease alcohol consumption	61.7	314
Decrease psychosocial stress	80.4	409
Regular exercise	95.9	488
Improve eating	81.1	413
Improve posture	97.1	494
Improve movement patterns	90.2	459
Normalise sleep patterns	71.9	366
Smoking cessation	65.8	335
Other	11.8	60
Behaviours Evaluated/monitored		
Over-consumption alcohol	56.4	787
Psychosocial stress	82.3	419
Inactivity/Over activity	90.8	462
Poor diet	74.1	377
Poor posture	97.1	494
Faulty movement patterns	88.6	451
Disturbed sleep	72.9	371
Smoking	60.7	309
Other	7.7	39
Advice/resources given		
Over-consumption alcohol	53.8	274
Psychosocial stress	82.3	419
Inactivity/Over activity	91.6	466
Poor diet	78.6	400
Poor posture	96.3	490
Faulty movement patterns	88.0	448
Disturbed sleep	75.4	384
Smoking	56.6	288
Other	8.8	45
Set goals/re-evaluate progress		
Over-consumption alcohol	20.6	105
Psychosocial stress	40.5	206
Inactivity/Over activity	72.7	370
Poor diet	41.7	212
Poor posture	80.4	409
Faulty movement patterns	70.7	360

Table 3 Practice characteristics and behaviours of whole cohort (N= 509) *(Continued)*

Disturbed sleep	34.8	177
Smoking	20.0	102
Other	6.7	34
Frequency of setting/review goals		
Up to 50% of visits	48.5	247
51-100% of visits	41.6	212
Never	4.7	24
Only per patient request	5.1	26
Successful resources to prevent disease/promote health		
Verbal advice from chiropractor	68.8	350
Written advice from chiropractor	10.6	54
Brochures/Pamphlets	3.3	17
Internal/External referral	6.3	32
Internet website address	1.4	7
Place address/contact number	0.2	1
No answer	9.4	48

plans should be viewed as a core service according to Von Korff et al. [26]. In our study, other than for physical fitness issues, goal-setting appears to be under-utilised with only up to two-fifths (41.7%) of the chiropractors setting and re-evaluating goals depending on the specific lifestyle issue and only one-fifth doing so for issues of over-consumption of alcohol (20.0%) and smoking (20.6%). A case therefore could be made to encourage more chiropractors to adopt goal-setting in key areas of preventative healthcare and health promotion.

Study limitations

A significant limitation of this study is the estimated 79% non-response rate from the UK chiropractors in this survey. Although the approximate 21% response rate allows us to draw conclusions regarding the practices of those who responded, the UK chiropractic profession is not represented in its entirety. This leads to less than robust confidence in the generalisability of these attitudes and practices to the wider profession.

Additionally, the chiropractors were asked to report general tendencies, not specific patient encounters, and interpretation between chiropractors may differ. This is particularly important where clinicians were asked to report the number of patient visits where goal-setting and re-evaluation of goals took place. Additionally, false reports, conscious or subconscious, might have occurred; however, this is an unavoidable limitation of the study design.

Lastly, some issues were not included in the survey, but may have an impact on decreasing NCDs as suggested by the respondents in the comment boxes. These included

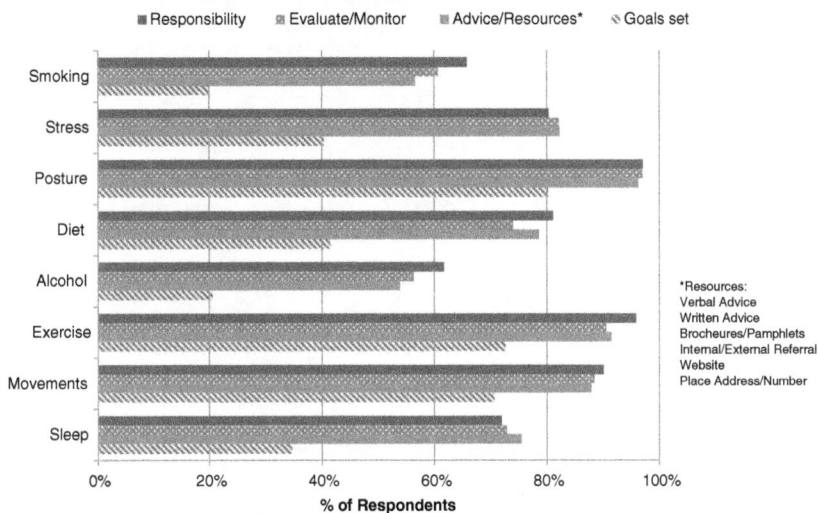

Figure 1 Proportion of respondents who perceived responsibility to discuss lifestyle issues and proportion who evaluate/monitor, give advice/resources or set goals for lifestyle issues in practice.

pregnancy and birth plans, regular weight checks, work-life balance, supplements, prescription drugs, vaccinations, ergonomics, exposing oneself to adequate sunlight and spiritual pursuits.

Future research
This survey explored the degree with which UK chiropractors engage with patients concerning efforts to support the potential reduction in the burden of NCDs. While being only a snapshot of the current situation for the chiropractors who responded, this study could serve as a starting point for further work in this area in the UK. Future studies in this field will not only be of interest to patients and chiropractors, but potentially to other health care professionals as well as policy makers. Further exploration of the patients' perspective and the reasons why chiropractors do or do not consider it their responsibility to incorporate such care into their practices as well as seeking insight into successful methods being utilised in chiropractic practices should be explored.

Conclusion
Links have been shown between chronic disease, smoking, obesity and depression with pain, particularly spinal pain. With the WHO calling on primary healthcare professionals to assist patients in developing sustained lifestyle changes, the goal of this study was to explore the chiropractic professions' engagement with preventative healthcare and health promotion. This survey of a subset of UK chiropractors shows that a good degree of preventative healthcare and health promotion is already provided, especially in regards to physical activity, nutrition and psychosocial stress. However, goal-setting and re-evaluation of

goals could be incorporated more routinely by UK chiropractors into their practices. The chiropractic profession has a valuable role in preventative healthcare and health promotion and many of those surveyed are already participating in decreasing the burden of NCDs in various aspects of patient care. However, as in most things, there is considerable room for improvement if desired.

Abbreviations
BCA: British Chiropractic Association; CAM: Complementary and alternative medicine; MCA: McTimoney Chiropractic Association; NCD: Non-communicable disease; SCA: Scottish Chiropractic Association; SPSS: Statistical Package for the Social Sciences; UCA: United Chiropractic Association; UK: United Kingdom; USA: United States of America; WHO: World Health Organization.

Competing interests
The authors declare that this paper is original and has not been published nor is being considered elsewhere for publication. The authors, individually and collectively, declare no conflicts of interests.

Authors' contributions
The corresponding author, PEF, planned the design, was responsible for the concept development, communication with the chiropractic associations, data collection/processing, analysis/interpretation, literature search, and writing of this manuscript. KAE was integral for concept development, survey supervision, and critical review of this manuscript. DN also helped with concept development, data analysis/interpretation and critical review of this manuscript. All authors read and approved the final manuscript.

Authors' information
Patricia E Fikar, MChiro, BA, CNA, Chiropractor, Private Practice, Vienna, Austria. Kent A Edlund, DC, BSc, ICSSD, Senior Clinical Tutor, Anglo-European College of Chiropractic, 13–15 Parkwood Road, Bournemouth, Dorset, BH5 2DF, UK. Dave Newell, BSc MSc PhD FRCC (Hon) FEAC, Director of Research, Anglo-European College of Chiropractic, 13–15 Parkwood Road, Bournemouth, Dorset, BH5 2DF, UK.

Acknowledgements
The authors would like to acknowledge the members of the AECC faculty and staff who participated in the pilot survey and gave feedback. Additionally, the authors would like to acknowledge the secretaries of the four participating chiropractic associations (BCA, MCA, SCA and UCA) who were most helpful in distributing the survey to their members and sending reminder bulletins.

Author details
[1]Private Practice, Vienna, Austria. [2]AECC-Anglo-European College of Chiropractic, 13-15 Parkwood Road, Bournemouth, Dorset BH5 2DF, UK.

References
1. WHO. Global Status Report on Noncommunicable Diseases 2010. Geneva, Switzerland: World Health Organization; 2011.
2. Beaglehole R, Yach D. Globalisation and the prevention and control of non-communicable disease: the neglected chronic diseases of adults. Lancet. 2003;362(9387):903–8.
3. WHO. Global strategy on diet, physical activity and health. Geneva, Switzerland: World Health Organization; 2004.
4. The Council on Chiropractic Education. Standards for Doctor of Chiropractic Programs and Requirements for Institutional Status Scottsdale, AZ. 2007; 45–47.
5. Evans MW, Rupert R. The council on chiropractic education's new wellness standard: a call to action for the chiropractic profession. Chiropr Osteopat. 2006;14:23.
6. Von Korff M, Crance P, Lane M, Miglioretti, Simon G, Saunders K, et al. Chronic spinal pain and physical-mental comorbidity in the United States: results from the national comorbidity survey replication. Pain. 2005;113:331–9.
7. Goldberg MS, Scott SC, Mayo NE. A review of the association between cigarette smoking and the development of nonspecific back pain and related outcomes. Spine. 2000;25(8):995–1014.
8. Webb R, Brammah T, Lunt M, Urwin M, Allison T, Symmons D. Prevalence and predictors of intense, chronic, and disabling neck and back pain in the UK general population. Spine. 2003;28(11):1195–202.
9. Fishbain DA, Cutler R, Rosomoff HL, Rosomoff RS. Chronic pain-associated depression: antecedent or consequence of chronic pain? A review. Clin J Pain. 1997;13(2):116–37.
10. CCE. Standards for doctor of chiropractic programs and requirements for institutional status. Scottsdale: Council on Chiropractic Education; 2007.
11. Stuber KJ, Grod JP, Smith DL, Powers P. An online survey of chiropractors' opinions of continuing education. Chiropr Osteopat. 2005;13:22.
12. Evans MW, Page G, Ndetan H, Martinez D, Brandon P, Daniel D, et al. Are patients receiving health promotional advice in the chiropractic teaching clinic setting? An impact assessment of a brief intervention to increase advising rates and goal setting. J Chiropract Educ. 2011;25(2):132–41.
13. British Chiropractic Association [http://www.chiropractic-uk.co.uk/]
14. McTimoney Chiropractic Association [http://www.mctimoneychiropractic.org/]
15. Scottish Chiropractic Association [http://www.sca-chiropractic.org/]
16. United Chiropractic Association [http://www.united-chiropractic.org/]
17. Limesurvey® [www.limesurvey.org]
18. O'Connor L, Walker BF, Watts C. The early detection and prevention of skin cancer by complementary health professionals. COMSIG Rev. 1994;3(2):54–60.
19. Hollenbach KA, Barrett-Connor E, Edelstein SL, Holbrook T. Cigarette smoking and bone mineral density in older men and women. Am J Public Health. 1993;83(9):1265–70.
20. Laitinen K, Välimäki M. Factors affecting bone metabolism and osteoporosis: alcohol and bone. Calcif Tissue Int. 1991;49(1):70–3.
21. Thomas VS, Rockwood KJ. Alcohol abuse, cognitive impairment, and mortality among older people. J Am Geriatr Soc. 2001;49(4):415–20.
22. Kruger J, Shaw L, Kahende J, Frank E. Health care providers' advice to quit smoking, National health interview survey, 2000, 2005, and 2010 CME. Prev Chronic Dis. 2012;9:110340.
23. Fiore MC, Bailey WC, Cohen SJ. Treating Tobacco Use and Dependence: Quick Reference Guide for Clinicians. Rockville, MD: US Department of Health and Human Services. The Public Health Service; 2000.
24. Coleman T, Murphy E, Cheater F. Factors influencing discussion of smoking between general practitioners and patients who smoke: a qualitative study. Br J Gen Pract. 2000;50(452):207–10.
25. Holliday RC, Cano S, Freeman JA, Playford ED. Should patients participate in clinical decision making? An optimised balance block design controlled study of goal setting in a rehabilitation unit. J Neurol Neurosurg Psychiatry. 2007;78(6):576–80.
26. Von Korff M, Gruman J, Schaefer J, Curry SJ, Wagner EH. Collaborative management of chronic illness. Ann Intern Med. 1997;127(12):1097–102.

Chiropractic treatment approaches for spinal musculoskeletal conditions: a cross-sectional survey

Mattijs Clijsters[1], Francesco Fronzoni[1] and Hazel Jenkins[2*]

Abstract

Background: There are several chiropractic spinal manipulative technique systems. However, there is limited research differentiating the efficacy of these techniques. Additionally, chiropractors may also use ancillary procedures in the treatment of musculoskeletal pain, a variable that also needs to be considered when measuring the efficacy of chiropractic therapy. No data is currently available regarding the frequency of usage of chiropractic technique systems or ancillary procedures for the treatment of specific musculoskeletal conditions. Knowing which technique systems and ancillary procedures are used most frequently may help to direct future research. The aim of this research was to provide insight into which treatment approaches are used most frequently by Australian chiropractors to treat spinal musculoskeletal conditions.

Methods: Cross-sectional survey design. The survey was sent online to the members of the two main Australian chiropractic associations between 30th June 2013 and 7th August 2013. The participants were asked to provide information on treatment choices for specific spinal musculoskeletal conditions.

Results: 280 respondents. Diversified manipulative technique was the first choice of treatment for most of the included conditions. Diversified was used significantly less in 4 conditions; cervical disc syndrome with radiculopathy and cervical central stenosis were more likely to be treated with Activator; flexion distraction technique was used almost as much as Diversified in the treatment of lumbar disc syndrome with radiculopathy and lumbar central stenosis. More experienced Australian chiropractors use more Activator and soft tissue therapy and less Diversified technique compared to their less experienced peers. The majority of responding chiropractors used ancillary procedures such as soft tissue techniques and exercise prescription in the treatment of spinal musculoskeletal conditions.

Conclusion: This survey provides information on commonly used treatment choices to the chiropractic profession. Treatment choices changed based on the region of disorder and whether neurological symptoms were present rather than with specific diagnoses. Diversified technique was the most commonly used spinal manipulative therapy, however, ancillary procedures such as soft tissue techniques and exercise prescription were also commonly utilised. This information may help direct future studies into the efficacy of chiropractic treatment for spinal musculoskeletal disorders.

Keywords: Chiropractic, Technique systems, Manipulation, Manual therapy, Musculoskeletal, Treatment, Prevalence

* Correspondence: hazel.jenkins@mq.edu.au
[2]Department of Chiropractic, Macquarie University Sydney, Sydney NSW 2109, Australia
Full list of author information is available at the end of the article

Background

One of the main tools chiropractors use to treat patients is the chiropractic manipulation, which can be manually applied or instrument-assisted. In the chiropractic profession there are several technique systems with regard to spinal manipulative therapy [1]. Curiously, in studies that examine the effect of spinal manipulation the technique system used is often not described, or a variety of techniques are applied in the intervention [2,3]. As different chiropractic techniques might cause distinct effects, the results of such intervention studies do not reveal information of the effectiveness of a single technique system. Furthermore, a particular system might be more or less effective depending on the musculoskeletal condition it is used for. In chiropractic research studies the targeted musculoskeletal condition is often not specified. General symptomatic areas such as neck pain are researched instead of more defined conditions such as cervical facet syndrome or cervical disc syndrome. In medicine, the condition to be treated and the exact drug are specifically described and tested. For example "the efficacy of ...acyclovir...in the treatment of post-herpetic pain" [4]. By doing this they know the exact effectiveness of the drug for that specific condition. If future chiropractic studies could administer manipulations from only one chiropractic technique system targeted to a specific musculoskeletal condition, it would enhance the study's clinical relevancy.

There are several commonly used chiropractic technique systems [1] and many different spinal musculoskeletal conditions, therefore a myriad of specific intervention studies would have to be executed to cover all clinical situations. To aid in this process our survey aims to explore which techniques graduate chiropractors most frequently use to treat common musculoskeletal conditions. Frequency of use of a certain technique system in the treatment of a particular condition is not evidence of its effectiveness. However, it indicates that further research needs to be prioritised to these techniques to produce resultant data that will be relevant to a large group of chiropractors. As chiropractors do not only use manipulation in their treatment approaches [5-12], this study will also explore the usage of ancillary treatment techniques such as soft tissue therapy and exercise prescription.

Previous published studies have already explored the frequency of usage of chiropractic technique systems in general in clinical practice [5,13,14]. Our study will explore the frequency of usage of these technique systems in particular musculoskeletal conditions. With regards to the specific conditions we surveyed there is only limited positive evidence available in the literature for manipulative treatment (in isolation or as part of the therapy) of cervicogenic headache [15], myofascial pain syndrome

[10], cervical radiculopathy [16], lumbar disc syndrome [2], lumbar stenosis [17], lumbar disc herniation [18,19] and sacroiliac dysfunction [20]. However, the evidence is weak due to lack of randomised controlled trials. Most studies included in the referenced reviews did not include any specification of the used technique system for manipulation.

The purpose of this survey is to provide descriptive information to help inform researchers and chiropractors about the patterns of use of chiropractic techniques by Australian chiropractors in specific musculoskeletal conditions. In particular, this study aims to provide a starting point for future intervention studies.

Methods

The study, an online cross-sectional survey of Australian chiropractors, was approved by the Macquarie University Human Research Ethics Committee (Medical Sciences) (reference no.: 5201300295) prior to the commencement of the study.

Survey development

The research being undertaken has not been previously performed in the literature and as such a relevant validated survey could not be found. Therefore, the survey questions were developed for initial use in this study. A list of commonly treated musculoskeletal conditions and commonly used chiropractic modalities was created based on literature review and consultation with practicing chiropractors. This process resulted in a list of 18 common spinal musculoskeletal conditions and eight chiropractic technique systems or ancillary procedures.

The final survey included background demographic questions and questions regarding most commonly used treatment modalities. For each of the spinal musculoskeletal conditions the participants were asked to select their first, second and third most commonly used treatment modalities. Where less than three modalities were used for a particular condition, participants were instructed to leave the additional modalities blank. Participants were given the opportunity to select 'other' as a treatment modality and any additional techniques used could be specified at the end of the survey. The survey questions used in this research can be found in Additional file 1.

The survey was pilot-tested in the Department of Chiropractic at Macquarie University. Eight staff members (graduate chiropractors involved in education) completed the online survey and provided feedback about the content and accessibility of the survey, with subsequent minor amendments made. The final version of the online survey was structured to allow participants to complete it within a five to ten minute time period.

Survey administration and data management

The online survey was emailed via the professional associations COCA and CAA to their members. They have approximately 1000 and 2700 members respectively [21,22]. An initial email to the participants was followed by a reminder email after three weeks. The survey was open from the 30th of June 2013 until the 7th of August 2013. All potential participants were notified that participation was voluntary and that confidentiality would be maintained. No identifying information was requested.

The survey was designed and administered online using the Qualtrics software of the Qualtrics Research Suite (Qualtrics, Provo, UT) [23].

Survey response rates were calculated compared to the number of chiropractors in the professional associations and the number of chiropractors within Australia. Demographic data from survey respondents was compared to national demographic data from the Chiropractic Board of Australia. Descriptive statistics were used to describe the style of practice reported and the main techniques generally used by respondents. Descriptive statistics were also used to summarise the overall frequency of individual techniques used for each musculoskeletal condition and the most commonly used techniques as first choice of treatment. Finally responses were subdivided into those from practitioners with more than ten years' experience and those from practitioners with less than ten years' experience. Descriptive statistics were used to describe any differences in treatment techniques between these two groups.

Results

Response rates

Two hundred and eighty practitioners completed the on-line survey, giving a response rate of 7%. However, this is likely to be an underestimation of the true response rate. It is unknown how many chiropractors are members of both professional associations, therefore, the total number of chiropractors who received the email is likely to be less than 3700. In addition, it is unknown how many members successfully received and opened the email invitation to participate in the survey. The number of total practicing registered chiropractors in Australia is 4399 [24], the available data, therefore, represented 6% of the total number of chiropractors working in Australia.

Demographics and background data

As reported in Table 1, 58% of the respondents were under 40 years old and half of the respondents have been in practice for ten years or less. Fifty-seven percent of the participants received their education in New South Wales (NSW). Almost half of the respondents

Table 1 Demographic and background data

	Responses (n)	%
Age of the participants (n = 263)		
<26	24	9%
26-30	57	22%
31-35	44	17%
36-40	27	10%
41-45	26	10%
46-50	21	8%
51-55	27	10%
56-60	20	8%
61-65	8	3%
>65	9	3%
Place of Chiropractic Education (n = 263)		
NSW	151	57%
VIC	64	24%
WA	15	6%
New Zealand	3	1%
Other (please specify)	30	11%
Place of Practice (n = 267)		
NSW	122	47%
VIC	43	16%
SA	20	8%
ACT	5	2%
QLD	35	13%
TAS	4	2%
WA	23	9%
NT	0	0%
New Zealand	2	1%
Other (Please specify)	13	5%
Years in Practice (n = 264)		
<6	96	36%
6-10	37	14%
11-15	38	14%
16-20	24	9%
21-30	39	15%
31-40	25	9%
>40	5	2%

Key: NSW = New South Wales; VIC = Victoria; WA = Western Australia; SA = South Australia; ACT = Australian Capital Territory; QLD = Queensland; TAS = Tasmania; NT = Northern Territory.

(47%) are practising in NSW, whereas only 16% are practising in Victoria. Only 3 respondents were from New Zealand.

When compared to chiropractic registrant data from the Chiropractic Board of Australia [24], demographic distribution of the survey respondents is skewed towards younger practitioners and those practising in NSW; and away from those practising in Victoria. Chiropractic registrant data reports 34% of Australian chiropractors practicing in NSW, 27% in Victoria and 50% less than 40 years old. The percentages of respondents from other states are similar to reports from the Chiropractic Board of Australia [24].

Scope of practice and main technique used in practice

The survey also included a question on scope of practice. As seen in Table 2, 97% of respondents described their scope of practice to be based on treatment of musculoskeletal pain and/or dysfunction. Ninety-six percent of the respondents reported use of rehabilitation or exercise prescription in their treatments. Ninety-seven percent of the respondents declared they used an evidence informed approach in their daily practice.

Chiropractors were also asked about the main technique system they used in practice. The majority of them (67%) used Diversified, followed by instrument adjusting (5%), Gonstead technique (5%) and Thompson or table assisted drop piece technique (4%). Seventeen percent of respondents reported that they used 'other' techniques. On analysis of their responses no clear technique systems were being repetitively used and a number of respondents had used the 'other' response to account for using more than one of the technique systems listed in the survey.

Techniques used for specific musculoskeletal disorders

Table 3 summarises the overall frequency of use of each technique for the musculoskeletal conditions surveyed. Diversified technique, soft tissue therapy, instrument adjusting and exercise prescription are the most commonly used techniques throughout the cervical and thoracic spinal regions, regardless of condition. In the lumbar spine instrument adjusting is less commonly used and table assisted drop piece/Thompson technique and 'other' techniques become more common. Flexion distraction also demonstrates increased usage in the lumbar spine, particularly with disorders associated with neurological change including lumbar disc syndrome

(with radiculopathy), lumbar lateral canal stenosis and lumbar central canal stenosis.

Table 4 gives an overview of the techniques that were most commonly selected as the first treatment choice for each musculoskeletal disorder investigated. Diversified technique is the first choice of treatment modality for the majority of listed conditions. There were four conditions where there was a significant decrease in the use of Diversified as the first choice of treatment. Instrument adjusting was the first choice of treatment modality for cervical disc syndrome with radiculopathy and cervical central stenosis. Diversified technique was the preferred first treatment modality for lumbar disc syndrome with radiculopathy and lumbar central stenosis, however, flexion distraction was used with similar frequency. Soft tissue therapy and instrument adjusting were the most commonly chosen treatment modalities in combination with Diversified technique.

To explore the possible role of experience in choice of technique system a comparison was made between practitioners of 10 years or less in practice (n = 133) and practitioners of more than ten years in practice (n = 131) (Figure 1). Practitioners who have been in practice ten years or less use more Diversified technique in all the conditions except for sacroiliac joint dysfunction for which Diversified was used in equal amount between the two groups. The chiropractors that have been practicing for more than a decade, use more instrument adjusting and more soft tissue therapy across all of the 18 conditions, compared to their less experienced colleagues.

Discussion

There are many different chiropractic technique systems that have been developed. To our knowledge there is no current information available regarding which technique systems are the most effective in the management of specific musculoskeletal conditions. Developing studies to evaluate the effect of every technique system on every specific condition is not feasible at this stage. This survey describes the techniques commonly used by chiropractors in the treatment of specific spinal musculoskeletal

Table 2 Scope of practice

	Always	Most of the time	Sometimes	Rarely	Never	Total responses
Wellness care	51 (20%)	74 (29%)	63 (25%)	35 (14%)	28 (11%)	251
Subluxation-based care	42 (17%)	49 (20%)	37 (15%)	33 (13%)	89 (36%)	250
Treatment of musculoskeletal dysfunction	169 (65%)	72 (29%)	11 (4%)	4 (2%)	3 (1%)	259
Treatment of musculoskeletal pain	142 (55%)	84 (33%)	25 (10%)	2 (1%)	5 (2%)	258
Evidence informed practice	112 (44%)	112 (44%)	25 (10%)	4 (2%)	3 (1%)	256
Rehabilitation or exercise prescription	92 (36%)	104 (41%)	49 (19%)	9 (4%)	2 (1%)	256
Other (Please specify)	13 (31%)	14 (33%)	8 (19%)	1 (2%)	6 (14%)	42

Table 3 Overall frequency of use of each technique for specific musculoskeletal conditions*

Musculoskeletal condition	Overall order of use of techniques								
	1st	2nd	3rd	4th	5th	6th	7th	8th	9th
Cervical myofascial pain syndrome	STT (84%)	Div (78%)	Ex (52%)	Instr (36%)	Other (21%)	Gon (8%)	TPT (6%)	EPT (4%)	FlexDist (<1%)
Torticollis	STT (82%)	Div (76%)	Instr (43%)	Ex (38%)	Other (25%)	Gon (7%)	EPT (5%)	TPT (5%)	FlexDist (2%)
Cervical facet syndrome	Div (85%)	STT (66%)	Ex (44%)	Instr (42%)	Other (18%)	Gon (9%)	TPT (7%)	EPT (4%)	FlexDist (2%)
Cervical disc syndrome (without radiculopathy)	Div (66%)	STT (65%)	Instr (45%)	Ex (45%)	Other (25%)	TPT (8%)	FlexDist (7%)	Gon (7%)	EPT (7%)
Cervical disc syndrome (with radiculopathy)	STT (65%)	Instr (50%)	Div (46%)	Ex (45%)	Other (36%)	FlexDist (11%)	EPT (9%)	TPT (7%)	Gon (6%)
Cervical lateral stenosis	STT (67%)	Div (59%)	Ex (50%)	Instr (44%)	Other (28%)	FlexDist (6%)	TPT (6%)	Gon (5%)	EPT (5%)
Cervical central stenosis	STT (62%)	Ex (46%)	Instr (46%)	Div (38%)	Other (38%)	FlexDist (9%)	Gon (6%)	TPT (6%)	EPT (5%)
Cervical related headache	Div (85%)	STT (81%)	Ex (41%)	Instr (34%)	Other (19%)	TPT (8%)	Gon (8%)	EPT (4%)	FlexDist (1%)
Thoracic myofascial pain syndrome	Div (85%)	STT (81%)	Ex (44%)	Instr (26%)	Other (18%)	TPT (11%)	Gon (9%)	EPT (4%)	FlexDist (1%)
Thoracic facet syndrome	Div (86%)	STT (66%)	Ex (38%)	Instr (30%)	Other (17%)	TPT (16%)	Gon (13%)	EPT (4%)	FlexDist (2%)
Rib dysfunction	Div (90%)	STT (63%)	Instr (41%)	Ex (30%)	TPT (17%)	Other (15%)	Gon (7%)	EPT (4%)	FlexDist (<1%)
Lumbar myofascial pain syndrome	STT (80%)	Div (73%)	Ex (45%)	Other (23%)	Instr (23%)	TPT (20%)	Gon (12%)	EPT (5%)	FlexDist (4%)
Lumbar facet syndrome	Div (81%)	STT (61%)	Ex (42%)	TPT (27%)	Instr (25%)	Other (18%)	Gon (14%)	FlexDist (8%)	EPT (34%)
Lumbar disc syndrome (without radiculopathy)	Div (62%)	STT (53%)	Ex (47%)	TPT (29%)	Other (28%)	Instr (25%)	FlexDist (20%)	Gon (11%)	EPT (5%)
Lumbar disc syndrome (with radiculopathy)	STT (47%)	Ex (47%)	Div (43%)	Other (38%)	Instr (29%)	FlexDist (29%)	TPT (26%)	Gon (10%)	EPT (9%)
Lumbar lateral stenosis	Div (55%)	STT (55%)	Ex (45%)	Instr (28%)	TPT (28%)	Other (26%)	FlexDist (21%)	Gon (10%)	EPT (4%)
Lumbar central stenosis	STT (52%)	Ex (49%)	Div (39%)	Other (35%)	Inst (29%)	FlexDist (26%)	TPT (22%)	Gon (8%)	EPT (5%)
Sacroiliac dysfunction	Div (77%)	STT (53%)	TPT (42%)	Ex (40%)	Other (30%)	Instr (20%)	Gon (13%)	EPT (2%)	FlexDist (1%)

*Percentages add up to more than 100% as up to 3 treatment options could be selected per condition.
Key: STT = soft tissue therapy. TPT = Table assisted drop piece/Thompson technique. Instr = Instrument adjusting (Activator or similar). Ex = Exercise program/ rehabilitation. Div = Diversified. Gon = Gonstead. FlexDist = Flexion distraction. EPT = Electrophysical therapy. Other = techniques not listed in survey.

conditions with the aim to help researchers make clinically relevant choices for future research.

Scope of practice

The majority of respondents primarily focus their treatments on musculoskeletal conditions and apply an evidence informed approach to their clinical practice (Table 2). Therefore, the scope of practice reported by the respondents is consistent with the focus of the survey. The positive attitude of many Australian chiropractors towards evidence based practice was also found in a study from Walker et al., where 78% of the respondents agreed that the application of evidence based practice is necessary [25].

Diversified technique was reported to be the most commonly used technique system amongst Australian chiropractors. The high frequency of use of Diversified technique is in line with previous studies from Australia and overseas [4-6,13,26]. A Canadian study from 2009 found that Diversified was the main technique used in

private practice, followed by Activator and Thompson technique [14]. In North America, Diversified technique is by far the most common (over 92%), followed by flexion distraction, Gonstead and Activator [5]. In 1994 a large chiropractic job analysis was done in Australia and New Zealand [13]. At that time Diversified was the most commonly used technique, followed by Activator, Gonstead, SOT, AK, Thompson and flexion distraction. In 2005, Walker et al. [26] conducted a telephone survey in Australia and New Zealand. In this study the most common technique system used by Australasian practitioners was Activator (49%), followed by Diversified (44%) and Gonstead (29%). However, additional categories of 'manual adjustment' and 'manipulation' were used in Walker's survey that may have skewed the results.

The survey results indicate that Australian chiropractors often include exercise prescription and soft tissue therapy in their treatments but rarely use electrophysical therapies. This is in contrast to chiropractic care in North America [5,27] but similar to European studies

Table 4 Techniques reported as first choice to treat specific musculoskeletal disorders

Musculoskeletal condition	Most commonly reported first choice	2nd most commonly reported first choice	3rd most commonly reported first choice
Cervical myofascial pain syndrome	Div (46%)	STT (32%)	Instr (9%)
Torticollis	Div (40%)	STT (32%)	Instr (13%)
Cervical facet syndrome	Div (70%)	Instr (12%)	STT (7%)
Cervical disc syndrome (without radiculopathy)	Div (36%)	Instr (21%)	STT (18%)
Cervical disc syndrome (with radiculopathy)	Instr (26%)	STT (20%)	Div (18%)
Cervical lateral stenosis	Div (35%)	Instr (21%)	STT (18%)
Cervical central stenosis	Instr (23%)	Div (22%)	STT (20%)
Cervical related headache	Div (68%)	STT (12%)	Instr (8%)
Thoracic myofascial pain syndrome	Div (46%)	STT (31%)	Instr (7%)
Thoracic facet syndrome	Div (73%)	Gon (8%)	Instr (8%)
Rib dysfunction	Div (70%)	Instr (10%)	STT (8%)
Lumbar myofascial pain syndrome	Div (34%)	STT (32%)	Instr (8%)
Lumbar facet syndrome	Div (59%)	TPT (10%)	Instr (8%)
Lumbar disc syndrome (without radiculopathy)	Div (30%)	FlexDist (14%)	TPT (13%)
Lumbar disc syndrome (with radiculopathy)	Div (18%)	FlexDist (18%)	STT (16%)
Lumbar lateral stenosis	Div (30%)	FlexDist (13%)	STT (12%)
Lumbar central stenosis	Div (20%)	FlexDist (18%)	Instr (12%)
Sacroiliac dysfunction	Div (49%)	TPT (18%)	Gon (8%)

Key: STT = soft tissue therapy. TPT = Table assisted drop piece/Thompson technique. Instr = Instrument adjusting (Activator or similar). Gon = Gonstead. Div = Diversified. FlexDist = Flexion distraction.

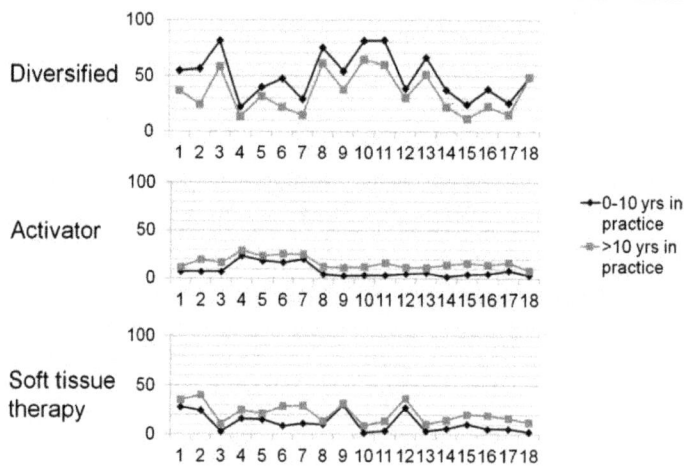

Figure 1 Differences in first choice of treatment (in %) between chiropractors in practice less than 10 years versus chiropractors in practice more than 10 years. Key: 1 Cervical myofascial pain syndrome, 2 Torticollis, 3 Cervical facet syndrome, 4 Cervical disc syndrome (without radiculopathy), 5 Cervical disc syndrome (with radiculopathy), 6 Cervical lateral stenosis, 7 Cervical central stenosis, 8 Cervical related headache, 9 Thoracic myofascial pain syndrome, 10 Thoracic facet syndrome, 11 Rib dysfunction, 12 Lumbar myofascial pain syndrome, 13 Lumbar facet syndrome, 14 Lumbar disc syndrome (without radiculopathy), 15 Lumbar disc syndrome (with radiculopathy), 16 Lumbar lateral stenosis, 17 Lumbar central stenosis, 18 Sacroiliac dysfunction.

[6,28]. French et al. [29] performed an observation and analysis study of Australian chiropractors. They found a high use of manipulative technique, soft tissue techniques and exercise prescription consistent with the results of this survey.

Technique selection for specific musculoskeletal conditions

Manipulative therapy (Diversified technique), soft tissue techniques and exercise prescription were reported as the most commonly used treatment techniques in the management of spinal musculoskeletal disorders. Instrument adjusting (Activator or similar) was commonly used in the cervical spine, however, use decreased in the thoracic and lumbar spinal regions. Table assisted drop piece and flexion distraction techniques were more commonly used in the lumbar spine. Small changes were noted in the frequency of use of different techniques between specific musculoskeletal conditions, however, the predominant differences were region rather than condition specific.

Diversified manipulative technique is the most frequent initial treatment of choice for the majority of musculoskeletal conditions surveyed. In 16 of the listed 18 conditions, it was reported to be used as the most frequent first choice of treatment. Conditions with a neural component such as: cervical disc syndrome (with radiculopathy); cervical central stenosis; lumbar disc syndrome (with radiculopathy); and lumbar central stenosis were associated with less use of Diversified technique as the first treatment choice. In these conditions more practitioners reported the use of instrument adjusting in the cervical spine and flexion distraction in the lumbar spine. It is unknown whether the increased use of instrument adjustment and flexion distraction in these conditions may be related to safety concerns or belief of increased efficacy. Instrument adjusting and flexion distraction are viewed as lower force techniques, however, no clinical evidence exists indicating that the use of these techniques is safer than Diversified technique [30]. Further research to determine risk versus treatment benefit is important in these cases.

A higher use of instrument adjusting (Activator or similar) was reported for musculoskeletal conditions in the cervical spine compared to conditions in other spinal regions. Similar findings were reported in a British study where chiropractors reported cervical pain as the predominant reason for using Activator [31]. Our data suggests an increased use of flexion distraction in conditions such as lumbar disc syndrome with radiculopathy and lumbar central stenosis. A review by Gay et al. [32] also reported that lumbar dysfunction was the main indication for the use of flexion distraction. In light of these data, controlled studies are needed to determine if instrument adjusting is more effective or safer than other treatments for cervical conditions and if flexion distraction is more effective or safer than other treatments for lumbar conditions.

Table assisted drop piece technique was rarely used for cervical and thoracic conditions, but there was an increase in use for lumbar and sacroiliac conditions. To our knowledge, no randomised trials evaluating the effectiveness of table assisted drop piece technique are available and evaluation of this technique in the treatment of sacroiliac dysfunction may be indicated.

Factors influencing treatment choice

Chiropractors may choose to use a specific technique system in certain conditions for several different reasons. As a result of clinical experience and therapeutic trial and error in similar situations, practitioners may have developed an understanding of what techniques work better with specific presentations. Practitioners may find one technique system easier to apply than others because of their own physical characteristics or the complexity of the technique system. In addition, they may have been guided by their education and apply technique systems to a degree which they were taught in their chiropractic course.

Practitioners might choose a certain technique system, based on their clinical experience in managing patients with a similar musculoskeletal condition. A trend was noted when chiropractic practitioners of more than ten years' of clinical experience were compared to those of less than ten years' experience. In general, the more experienced practitioners tended to use more instrument adjusting and soft tissue therapy, whereas, the less experienced practitioners tended to use more Diversified technique. Possible reasons may be that the more experienced chiropractors have found better results with these techniques or it may relate to the fact that these techniques are less physical demanding. Also, instrument adjusting is not taught in pre-professional courses in Australia, but can be learnt after graduation. Therefore, new graduate chiropractors may use instrument adjusting less frequently due to reduced exposure to this treatment modality.

Implications for further research

It is hard to determine which chiropractic techniques are most effective. To do this, randomised controlled trials (RCTs) have to be executed. Unfortunately, it is very difficult to provide a placebo treatment for a manipulation. RCTs comparing the clinical effectiveness of two different technique systems on specific musculoskeletal disorders may help to inform practitioners' treatment choices. However, reaching a conclusive musculoskeletal diagnosis in a clinical setting may limit the ability to perform this research. Subgrouping musculoskeletal disorders into those with and without neurological involvement would be more achievable in a clinical setting, and would capture the differences in preferred treatment technique found in this survey. As evidenced by our data and data from other studies [5-12], a chiropractor often uses a combination of manipulative techniques and ancillary treatment methods in the clinical setting. Although this does not provide evidence of efficacy of a single technique, RCTs investigating a combined approach would more closely mimic clinical practice.

The data from this study can be used to inform future studies and direct formulation of research questions. After analysing our data we suggest seven future research questions (see 'Proposed future research questions for major RCTs' list below) that might directly influence decision making in clinical practice for Australian chiropractors. These seven research questions have been formulated based on the trends we described in the above sections.

Proposed future research questions for major RCTs

- Clinical effectiveness of Diversified technique in the management of any of our listed musculoskeletal conditions.
- Clinical effectiveness of instrument adjusting (Activator or similar) in the management of cervical disc syndrome with radiculopathy.
- Clinical effectiveness of instrument adjusting (Activator or similar) in the management of cervical central stenosis.
- Clinical effectiveness of the flexion distraction technique in the management of lumbar disc syndrome with radiculopathy.
- Clinical effectiveness of the flexion distraction technique in the management of lumbar central stenosis.
- Clinical effectiveness of table assisted drop piece technique in the management of sacroiliac joint dysfunction.
- Clinical effectiveness of soft tissue therapy and/or exercise prescription in combination with Diversified technique in the management of any of our listed conditions

Limitations

The main limitation of this research is that of low response rate. Surveys were distributed through emails from the two main Australian chiropractic associations and it is impossible to know how many chiropractors actually received and read the emails. Therefore, true response rate, and assessment of potential non-response bias, cannot be determined. Non-response bias is of concern if only subjects interested in the subject complete

the survey. The results of this survey were compared to demographic data from the chiropractic registration board and previous research to try and establish how reflective the respondents of this survey were to the chiropractic population as a whole. Demographic data was similar to survey respondents except for an increase in the number of respondents working in New South Wales with a decrease in those working in Victoria and an increase in the number of respondents from a younger age group. Scope of practice among survey respondents was heavily skewed to those treating muscular pain and dysfunction, possibly indicating respondant bias. However, previous research conducted by French et al. [29] also indicated that Australian chiropractic practice primarily focuses on the treatment of musculoskeletal pain. Therefore, this result may be reflective of the chiropractic population as a whole. There was also a high proportion of respondents who used Diversified as their primary therapeutic technique as opposed to other chiropractic techniques. However, similar trends are noted in previous studies done in Australia [13,29] and the United States [5], indicating that our sample population responded fairly consistently with other, larger scaled, studies. Although we do have some similarities between the survey responses and previously published data we cannot eliminate the possiblity of non-response bias skewing the results of this survey. Therefore, the results of this survey should be interpreted with caution as they may not be reflective of the Australian chiropractic population as a whole.

Epidemiological data was to be used to help formulate the list of musculoskeletal conditions included in the survey. However, data regarding the prevalence of specific musculoskeletal conditions presenting to chiropractic practices is lacking. There is some data available regarding presenting symptomatic regions [7,26,33], but not related to specific musculoskeletal diagnoses. Therefore, selection of musculoskeletal conditions based on specific epidemiological data was not possible.

The survey instrument was not validated, however, it was based on questionnaires used in similar studies that focused on technique systems in general [5,13,14]. These questionnaires were reformed to suit our condition-specific questions. In addition, the survey was not exhaustive, with only five chiropractic technique systems included. Although the option was provided to select and specify any other technique system, the setup of the question may have influenced respondents to select one of the five listed technique systems. These five technique systems were chosen as previous research had shown them to be the main techniques used in Australia [13]. Reviewing comments from practitioners who specified "other techniques" in the survey failed to demonstrate any consistent trends in additional technique systems used.

Recall bias may also be a concern in this survey. Practitioners may over- or under-estimate the degree that they use certain techniques for specific conditions. Although we cannot rule out recall bias we feel that the general nature of the questions asked limit this as a particular concern. The survey questions asked for preferred first, second and third treatment techniques rather than the frequency of usage of those techniques to reduce the effect of recall bias.

Lastly, it may be possible that the musculoskeletal conditions listed in the survey were interpreted differently by different respondents. The aim of the survey was not to test diagnostic abilities in the practitioners, but rather to gain information about which chiropractic technique they would use to treat a specific textbook condition. Gradations in severity of the conditions were not provided, nor were many other variables that may change decision making.

Conclusion

This survey provides information on commonly used treatment choices to the chiropractic profession. Treatment choices changed based on the region of disorder and whether neurological symptoms were present rather than with specific diagnoses. Diversified technique was the most commonly used manipulative therapy, however, ancillary procedures such as soft tissue therapy and exercise prescription were also commonly utilised. This information may help direct future studies into the efficacy of chiropractic treatment for spinal musculoskeletal disorders.

Additional file

Additional file 1: Survey Questions: copy of the survey questions used in the research.

Competing interests
The authors declared that they have no competing interests.

Authors' contributions
All authors contributed to the research design, survey design and administration. MC and FF performed the data analysis and initial drafting of the manuscript. HJ supervised the research and edited the final manuscript. All authors read and approved the final manuscript.

Author details
[1]Macquarie University Sydney, Sydney NSW 2109, Australia. [2]Department of Chiropractic, Macquarie University Sydney, Sydney NSW 2109, Australia.

References

1. Cooperstein R, Gleberzon BJ: *Technique systems in chiropractic.* 1st edition. London: Elsevier Health Sciences; 2004.
2. Lisi AJ, Holmes EJ, Ammendolia C: High-velocity low-amplitude spinal manipulation for symptomatic lumbar disk disease: a systematic review of the literature. *J Manipulative Physiol Ther* 2005, 28(6):429–442.
3. Gross A, Miller J, D'Sylva J, Burnie SJ, Goldsmith CH, Graham N, Haines T, Bronfort G, Hoving JL: Manipulation or mobilisation for neck pain. *Cochrane Database Syst Rev* 2010, 1:CD004249.
4. Rasi A, Heshmatzade Behzadi A, Rabet M, Nejat AA, Haghshenas A, Hassanloo J, Honarbakhsh Y, Dehghan N, Kamrava SK: The efficacy of time-based short-course acyclovir therapy in treatment of postherpetic pain. *J Infect Dev Ctries* 2010, 4(11):754–760.
5. Coulter ID, Shekelle PG: Chiropractic in North America: a descriptive analysis. *J Manipulative Physiol Ther* 2005, 28(2):83–89.
6. Ailliet L, Rubinstein SM, de Vet HC: Characteristics of chiropractors and their patients in Belgium. *J Manipulative Physiol Ther* 2010, 33(8):618–625.
7. Hurwitz EL: Epidemiology: spinal manipulation utilization. *J Electromyogr Kinesiol* 2012, 22(5):648–654.
8. Sihawong R, Janwantanakul P, Sitthipornvorakul E, Pensri P: Exercise therapy for office workers with nonspecific neck pain: a systematic review. *J Manipulative Physiol Ther* 2011, 34(1):62–71.
9. Schneider M, Vernon H, Ko G, Lawson G, Perera J: Chiropractic management of fibromyalgia syndrome: a systematic review of the literature. *J Manipulative Physiol Ther* 2009, 32(1):25–40.
10. Vernon H, Schneider M: Chiropractic management of myofascial trigger points and myofascial pain syndrome: a systematic review of the literature. *J Manipulative Physiol Ther* 2009, 32(1):14–24.
11. Slade SC, Keating JL: Trunk-strengthening exercises for chronic low back pain: a systematic review. *J Manipulative Physiol Ther* 2006, 29(2):163–173.
12. Mayer J, Mooney V, Dagenais S: Evidence-informed management of chronic low back pain with lumbar extensor strengthening exercises. *Spine J* 2008, 8(1):96–113.
13. National Board of Chiropractic Examiners: *Job analysis of chiropractic in Australia and New Zealand.* Colorado: NBCE; 1994.
14. Mykietiuk C, Wambolt M, Pillipow T, Mallay C, Gleberzon BJ: Technique Systems used by post-1980 graduates of the Canadian Memorial Chiropractic College practicing in five Canadian provinces: a preliminary survey. *J Can Chiropr Assoc* 2009, 53(1):32–39.
15. Racicki S, Gerwin S, DiClaudio S, Reinmann S, Donaldson M: Conservative physical therapy management for the treatment of cervicogenic headache: a systematic review. *J Man Manip Ther* 2013, 21(2):113–124.
16. Rodine RJ, Vernon H: Cervical radiculopathy: a systematic review on treatment by spinal manipulation and measurement with the Neck Disability Index. *J Can Chiropr Assoc* 2012, 56(1):18–28.
17. Stuber K, Sajko S, Kristmanson K: Chiropractic treatment of lumbar spinal stenosis: a review of the literature. *J Chiropr Med* 2009, 8(2):77–85.
18. Hahne AJ, Ford JJ, McMeeken JM: Conservative management of lumbar disc herniation with associated radiculopathy: a systematic review. *Spine* 2010, 35(11):E488–E504.
19. Snelling NJ: Spinal manipulation in patients with disc herniation: a critical review of risk and benefit. *Int J Osteopath Med* 2006, 9:77–84.
20. Zelle BA, Gruen GS, Brown S, George S: Sacroiliac joint dysfunction: evaluation and management. *Clin J Pain* 2005, 21(5):446–455.
21. COCA: [http://www.coca.com.au/about/coca-history/2013] accessed 07/10/2013.
22. CAA: [http://www.chiropractors.asn.au/index.php?option=com_k2&view=item&id=140:joining-caa&Itemid=2552013] accessed 07/10/2013.
23. Qualtrics: [http://www.qualtrics.com].
24. AHPRA: [http://www.chiropracticboard.gov.au/About-the-Board/Statistics.aspx] accessed 07/10/2013.
25. Walker BF, Stomski NJ, Herbert JJ, French SD: A survey of Australian chiropractors' attitudes and beliefs about evidence-based practice and their use of research literature and clinical practice guidelines. *Chiropr Man Ther* 2013, 21:44.
26. Walker S, Bablis P, Pollard H, McHardy A: Practitioner perceptions of emotions associated with pain: a survey. *J Chiropr Med* 2005, 4(1):11–18.
27. Mootz RD, Cherkin DC, Odegard CE, Eisenberg DM, Barassi JP, Deyo RA: Characteristics of chiropractic practitioners, patients, and encounters in Massachusetts and Arizona. *J Manipulative Physiol Ther* 2005, 28(9):645–653.
28. Malmqvist S, Leboeuf-Yde C: Chiropractors in Finland–a demographic survey. *Chiropr Osteopat* 2008, 16:9.
29. French SD, Charity MJ, Fordslke K, Gunn JM, Polus BI, Walker BF, Chondros P, Britt HC: Chiropractic observation and analysis study (COAST): providing an understanding of current chiropractic practice. *Med J Aust* 2012, 199(10):687–691.

30. Huggins T, Boras AL, Gleberzon BJ, Popescu M, Bahry LA: **Clinical effectiveness of the activator adjusting instrument in the management of musculoskeletal disorders: a systematic review of the literature.** *J Can Chiropr Assoc* 2012, **56**(1):49–57.

31. Read D, Wilson JH, Gemmell A: **Activator as a therapeutic instrument: Survey of usage and opinions amongst members of the British Chiropractic Association.** *Clin Chiropractic* 2006, **9**(2):70–75.

32. Gay RE, Bronfort G, Evans RL: **Distraction manipulation of the lumbar spine: a review of the literature.** *J Manipulative Physiol Ther* 2005, **28**(4):266–273.

33. Cherkin DC, Deyo RA, Sherman KJ, Hart LG, Street JH, Hrbek A, Davis RB, Cramer E, Miliman B, Booker J, Mootz R, Barassi J, Kahn JR, Kaptchuk TJ, Eisenberg DM: **Characteristics of visits to licensed acupuncturists, chiropractors, massage therapists, and naturopathic physicians.** *J Am Board Fam Pract* 2002, **15**(6):463–472.

US chiropractors' attitudes, skills and use of evidence-based practice: A cross-sectional national survey

Michael J Schneider[1*], Roni Evans[2], Mitchell Haas[3], Matthew Leach[4], Cheryl Hawk[5], Cynthia Long[6], Gregory D Cramer[7], Oakland Walters[8], Corrie Vihstadt[2] and Lauren Terhorst[9]

Abstract

Background: Evidence based practice (EBP) is being increasingly utilized by health care professionals as a means of improving the quality of health care. The introduction of EBP principles into the chiropractic profession is a relatively recent phenomenon. There is currently a lack of information about the EBP literacy level of US chiropractors and the barriers/facilitators to the use of EBP in the chiropractic profession.

Methods: A nationwide EBP survey of US chiropractors was administered online (Nov 2012-Mar 2013) utilizing a validated self-report instrument (EBASE) in which three sub-scores are reported: attitudes, skills and use. Means, medians, and frequency distributions for each of the sub-scores were generated. Descriptive statistics were used to analyze the demographic characteristics of the sample. Means and proportions were calculated for all of the responses to each of the questions in the survey.

Results: A total of 1,314 US chiropractors completed the EBASE survey; the sample appeared to be representative of the US chiropractic profession. Respondents were predominantly white (94.3%), male (75%), 47 (+/− 11.6) years of age, and in practice for more than 10 years (60%). EBASE sub-score means (possible ranges) were: attitudes, 31.4 (8–40); skills, 44.3 (13–65); and use, 10.3 (0–24). Survey participants generally held favorable attitudes toward EBP, but reported less use of EBP. A minority of participants indicated that EBP coursework (17%) and critical thinking (29%) were a major part of their chiropractic education. The most commonly reported barrier to the use of EBP was "lack of time". Almost 90% of the sample indicated that they were interested in improving their EBP skills.

Conclusion: American chiropractors appear similar to chiropractors in other countries, and other health professionals regarding their favorable attitudes towards EBP, while expressing barriers related to EBP skills such as research relevance and lack of time. This suggests that the design of future EBP educational interventions should capitalize on the growing body of EBP implementation research developing in other health disciplines. This will likely include broadening the approach beyond a sole focus on EBP education, and taking a multilevel approach that also targets professional, organizational and health policy domains.

Keywords: Evidence-based medicine, Chiropractic, Complementary and alternative medicine, Survey research, Dissemination and implementation, Knowledge translation

* Correspondence: mjs5@pitt.edu
[1]Department of Physical Therapy, School of Health and Rehabilitation Sciences, Clinical and Translational Science Institute, University of Pittsburgh, Pittsburgh, PA, USA
Full list of author information is available at the end of the article

Background

Evidence-based practice (EBP) has been steadily advocated since the mid 1990's [1,2] and has increasingly been adopted as a foundational framework for improving the quality of healthcare delivery systems [3,4]. Despite the growing awareness of EBP, there still remains a large gap between this appreciation of EBP and the actual uptake and application of EBP in clinical settings. This gap between knowledge and awareness of EBP - and actual clinical use of EBP - is found in almost all healthcare fields, including medicine, nursing, and physical therapy [5,6].

Over the past decade the chiropractic profession has also embraced EBP, as evidenced by new EBP educational programs at chiropractic institutions [7-11] and the creation of professional evidence-based chiropractic guidelines [12-16]. However, while the enthusiasm for EBP in chiropractic is encouraging, a key aspect of its success will be whether or not it translates to changes in clinical practice. These changes would include the reduced use of unsupported clinical tests and procedures, as well as increased emphasis on those with an evidence base [17].

Dissemination and implementation research provides the means to bridge the gap between EBP principles and their application in clinical practice. This is accomplished by examining the mechanisms by which research evidence is spread and affects change in healthcare providers' attitudes and beliefs, and by evaluating strategies for changing healthcare professionals' behaviors to include the uptake of evidence-based clinical practices [18].

Chiropractic is one of the largest complementary and alternative medicine (CAM) professions in the United States. An important step for addressing the EBP gap in the chiropractic profession is to first understand chiropractors' attitudes and knowledge related to EBP, as well as the perceived barriers and facilitators to its application. Much of what is currently known is based on studies performed outside the United States. Walker et al. reported the results of an EBP survey showing that most of the 584 Australian chiropractors surveyed held positive attitudes towards EBP, thought EBP was useful, and were interested in improving their EBP skills [19]. However, despite their favorable inclination toward EBP, many Australian chiropractors stated they did not routinely use clinical practice guidelines. The three main barriers to the uptake of EBP identified in this study were: insufficient time, lack of generalizability of evidence to patient population, and inability to apply research findings to individual patients [19]. Similarly, researchers from Canada [20] and Great Britain [21] have found that accessibility to research, knowledge of how to access research, and critical appraisal skills are poor amongst chiropractors.

A study in a sub-specialty of 144 chiropractic orthopedists in the US also found favorable attitudes towards EBP, and a desire for EBP post-graduate continuing education [22]. The most frequently reported barriers to EBP in this study were lack of relevant clinical evidence and lack of time. Facilitators to EBP included internet and database access, online EBP educational materials, critical reviews of chiropractic research, and ability to download full-text articles. The findings of this study are limited however by its small and specialized sample; consequently, the factors associated with the uptake of EBP by the US chiropractic profession still remain poorly understood.

The purpose of this article is to describe the results of a cross-sectional survey of US chiropractors' attitudes, skills and use of research evidence in clinical practice, as well as the barriers and facilitators to use of EBP.

Methods

Study design and setting

This was a cross-sectional survey conducted online between November 17, 2012 and March 5, 2013. The survey was administered electronically through the University of Pittsburgh (UPitt), Pittsburgh, Pennsylvania, using the UPitt web platform.

Ethics

Ethical approval (PRO12060417) was obtained through the University of Pittsburgh's (UPitt) institutional review board (IRB), which granted "exempt status" in June 2012. Informed consent was secured from all subjects on the homepage of the research website, prior to participation in the survey.

Context

The *Distance Education Online Intervention for Evidence-Based Practice Literacy (DELIVER)* project is a two-phase NIH/NCCAM-funded study (R21 AT007547) designed to evaluate the effectiveness of an online EBP educational program on chiropractors' attitudes, skill, and use of EBP. This cross-sectional survey comprised the first phase of the DELIVER study and served as a baseline measure of EBP literacy against which to analyze the effectiveness of an online EBP educational program (second phase).

Participants & recruitment

The survey was open to all Doctors of Chiropractic (DCs) in the US who had internet access and a valid email address. A convenience sample of DCs were recruited primarily by emails forwarded to the membership rosters of several cooperating organizations including the following: American Chiropractic Association, Council on Chiropractic Guidelines and Practice Parameters, Congress of Chiropractic State Associations, Sacro Occipital Research Society International, Activator Methods, US ChiroDirectory, International College of Applied Kinesiology, the Pediatric

Councils of the American Chiropractic Association and International Chiropractors Association.

These organizations provided email-forwarding services through their respective membership lists, which created a potential pool of over 30,000 DCs. The forwarded email message described a unique opportunity to participate in an online survey; participation was incentivized by offering participants the opportunity to enter a drawing to win an Apple iPad™. Recipients of the email were encouraged to forward the message on to their colleagues. Articles announcing the study and inviting readers to participate were published in two national chiropractic publications; Dynamic Chiropractic [23] and the Journal of American Chiropractic Association [24]. Another national chiropractic publication - The American Chiropractor - announced the study by sending an email blast to its national circulation of DCs.

Questionnaire and outcomes

The Evidence-Based Practice Attitude and Utilization SurvEy (EBASE) is a self-administered instrument designed to measure CAM providers' attitudes, skills and use of EBP [25]. The instrument has demonstrated good internal consistency, content validity, and acceptable test-retest reliability [26]. Minor modifications of a few EBASE items were required to ensure the language was appropriate for use with chiropractors [22]. These changes were made in consultation with the survey developer (ML) to ensure the structure and intent of the modified questions were not altered in any manner that would jeopardize the validity of the original survey. Only the demographics section (Part G) required major modifications to be relevant to the chiropractic profession.

Our modified version of the EBASE contains 75 items and is divided into 7 parts (Parts A-G); Parts A-F each address a different EBP construct, and Part G contains demographic items only. Each question within these parts allowed the participant 5 possible responses, which were rated numerically from 1 to 5 for Parts A and B, and from 0 to 4 for Part D. Although there are 7 parts to this survey, only 3 parts generate sub-scores: Parts A (Attitudes), B (Skill), and D (Use). The 4 remaining parts of the EBASE are not scored, including Part C (Training & Education), Part E (Barriers), Part F (Facilitators) and Part G (Demographics). The completion time of the online EBASE is approximately 10–12 minutes (see Additional file 1 for a copy of the modified EBASE survey and the scoring rubric used for calculating the three sub-scores).

Survey administration and data collection

Interested DCs were invited to follow a link to a dedicated UPitt website where they could obtain detailed information about the study procedures and register for the study by submitting an email address. Participants were subsequently emailed a password to enter the survey site, an effort aimed at preventing multiple responses from the same individual. To encourage honest and transparent responses, anonymity was insured by assigning a unique identification number to each registered DC, which was used to identify the respondent's survey data. As participants completed the survey, responses were captured through a secure data capturing feature/system, Web Data Xpress, an interface that allows for direct entry and storage of data within a designated SQL Server database. This method of data capture is resource-efficient and minimizes human error by avoiding the need for manual data entry.

Data analysis

Data were analyzed using SPSS version 22 (SPSS Inc., Chicago, IL, USA). Since this was a cross-sectional survey we calculated descriptive statistics including response frequencies and means for each item in Parts A, B, D, E and F and response frequencies for Parts C and G. The attitudes, skills, and use sub-scores were calculated using the scoring rubric (see Additional file 1) developed with the original EBASE. This involves summing the first eight items of Parts A (response range 1–5; total score range of 8–40), all 13 of the items of Part B (response range 1–5; total score range of 13–65), and the first 6 items of Part D (response range 0–4; total score range of 0–24). Frequency distributions for the group sub-score means for Part A, B and D were also calculated. Higher sub-scores indicate higher self-reported levels of attitudes (Part A), skills (Part B) and use (Part D) of EBP.

Results

Sample Size

A total of 1,314 US chiropractors responded to the survey.

Participant characteristics (Demographics and Education/Training)

Table 1 provides a summary of the frequencies of the demographic characteristics of the participants. The majority of the sample were male (75%), Caucasian (94%), practiced as sole proprietors (72%) and held a Bachelor's or higher level graduate degree in addition to their chiropractic degree (>80%). The average age of our sample was 47 years (range: 24 to 85 years), and the mean number of years in practice was 17 years (range: 0 to 30 years or more).

Only a small minority of the sample indicated that the following topics were major parts of their chiropractic education: coursework about EBP (17%), applying research evidence to clinical practice (13%), and critical thinking/analysis (29%) (Table 2). Eleven percent of the

Table 1 Demographic characteristics of the 1,314 American chiropractors who completed the online evidence-based practice survey

Variable	Characteristic	n (%)
Gender	Male	989 (75.3)
	Female	325 (24.7)
Age	Mean = 46.7 yrs (SD = 11.6); Range = 24-85 yrs	
Race	White	1239 (94.3)
	Black	13 (1.0)
	Asian	33 (2.5)
	Mixed Race/Other	29 (2.2)
Years since chiropractic graduation	0-5	273 (20.8)
	6-10	146 (11.1)
	11-15	187 (14.2)
	16-20	159 (12.1)
	21-25	170 (12.9)
	26-29	144 (11.0)
	30 or more Mean = 17 yrs; Range = 0-30 or more yrs	235 (17.9)
Highest education level	High School	17 (1.3)
	Associate's Degree	214 (16.3)
	Bachelor's Degree	821 (62.5)
	Master's Degree	226 (17.2)
	Doctorate	36 (2.7)
Region of practice	Midwest	380 (28.9)
	Northeast	287 (21.8)
	West	264 (20.1)
	Southeast	245 (18.6)
	Southwest	131 (10.0)
	Non-continental US	7 (0.5)
Geographic setting	Suburban	629 (47.9)
	City	449 (34.2)
	Rural	236 (18.0)
Patients seen daily	0-10	367 (27.9)
	11-20	455 (34.6)
	21-30	259 (19.7)
	31-40	126 (9.6)
	41-50	60 (4.6)
	51 or more Median = 20/day; (IQR = 10-30) Range = 0-100/day	47 (3.6)
Focus of clinical practice	**Musculoskeletal focus**	**869 (66.1)**
	Spine and extremities	742 (56.5)
	Spine	72 (5.5)
	Sports	55 (4.2)
	Non-musculoskeletal focus	**445 (33.9)**
	Family care	192 (14.6)
	Subluxation-based	114 (8.7)

Table 1 Demographic characteristics of the 1,314 American chiropractors who completed the online evidence-based practice survey *(Continued)*

	Wellness/Prevention	105 (8.0)
	Non-musculoskeletal	20 (1.5)
	Pediatrics	14 (1.1)
Clinical role	Sole Proprietor	946 (72.0)
	Partner or group practice	171 (13.0)
	Associate or employee	144 (11.0)
	Hospital-based practice	53 (4.0)
Organizational membership	Unaffiliated	722 (55.0)
	American Chiropractic Assoc. (ACA)	526 (40.0)
	International Chiropractors Assoc. (ICA)	66 (5.0)

SD = Standard Deviation. IQR = Interquartile Range. Yrs = Years.

sample indicated they never had any critical thinking/analysis included in their chiropractic education. Almost half the sample reported that they had never received any education/training on conducting systematic reviews (48%) or clinical research (42%).

Descriptive results for parts A, B and D (Attitudes, Skills and Use)

Participants held a generally favorable attitude (Part A) toward EBP, with a mean attitude sub-score of 31.4 (range 8–40); while the frequency distribution was skewed to the left, the median sub-score (32.0) was close to the mean (Figure 1). The majority (>75%) of participants gave responses of "agree" or "strongly agree" to most questions (Table 3). There were two individual attitude related items with which a smaller proportion of the respondents agreed: 1) "EBP takes into account a patient's preference for treatment" (42% agree/strongly agree); and 2) "EBP takes into account my clinical experience when making clinical decisions" (65% agree/strongly agree). It was also very interesting to note that the vast majority of our sample (89.5%) agreed or strongly agreed with the statement "I am interested in learning or improving the skills necessary to incorporate EBP into my practice".

For self-reported skills in EBP (Part B) the mean sub-score was 44.3 (range of 13–65) with a left skewed frequency distribution, and a median sub-score (44.0) similar to the mean (Figure 2). For the majority of skill items, more than half of respondents indicated a generally high level ('4' or '5') of self-reported skill in EBP (Table 4); however nearly a third of respondents rated their skills in the mid-range ('3' on 1–5 scale) for 11 of the 13 skill items. The two skills rated poorest were: 1) "conducting clinical research" (66% of respondents) and 2) "conducting systematic reviews" (47% of respondents).

Table 2 Response frequency of Training/Education items (Part C of E-BASE)

PART C Item	None	Seminar (<1 day)	Short course (<1 week)	Minor part of chiropractic education	Major part of chiropractic education	Minor part of diplomate education	Major part of diplomate education	Academic diploma	Informal personal study
Applying research evidence to clinical practice	8.1%	23.4%	5.7%	23.4%	13.1%	3.7%	3.9%	1.8%	17.0%
Critical thinking/critical analysis	10.8%	8.4%	5.3%	21.7%	29.0%	2.7%	3.8%	3.4%	14.9%
Evidence-based clinical practice/evidence-based chiropractic	4.8%	25.5%	5.5%	22.8%	17.0%	5.6%	4.9%	1.8%	12.1%
Conducting systematic reviews or meta-analysis	47.6%	6.3%	6.5%	21.8%	3.7%	1.9%	0.6%	1.2%	10.4%
Conducting clinical research	42.2%	6.3%	6.1%	26.5%	4.0%	2.4%	0.9%	1.8%	9.8%

These are responses to the question "Please indicate the highest level of training/education you have received in the following areas".

The mean sub-score for use of EBP (Part D) was 10.3 (range of 0–24). The frequency distribution was skewed to the right, with a median sub-score of 8.0 (Figure 3). While 36% reported not consulting magazines, laypersons or self-help books for clinical decision making in the previous month, 23% also reported not using research findings to change their clinical practice and 29% did not use an online database to search for practice-based literature or research findings. About 45% of the sample indicated that only a small, very small, or no proportion of their practice was based on clinical research evidence (Table 5).

Descriptive results for parts E and F (Barriers and Facilitators to EBP Uptake)

When presented with a list of potential barriers to EBP uptake (Part E), most (>75%) participants indicated that the majority of the factors were either "not a barrier" or a "minor barrier" (Table 6), with a few notable exceptions. Items rated as being moderate or major barriers to EBP uptake included: 1) 'lack of time' (48%); 2) 'lack of clinical evidence about CAM' (44%); 3), 'lack of industry support' (37%); and 4) 'lack of incentive' (36%). Approximately a quarter of respondents cited insufficient skills for interpreting (27%); locating (23%) and critically appraising research (24%); lack of colleague support for EBP (23%); and lack of relevance to chiropractic practice (24%).

In terms of the perceived usefulness of various factors in facilitating the uptake of EBP (Part F) in clinical practice, over 70% of respondents indicated all 10 items as either "moderately useful" or "very useful" (Table 7). The two items that received the greatest percentage of "very useful" responses were "access to the internet" (78%) and "access to free online databases" (70%). Items

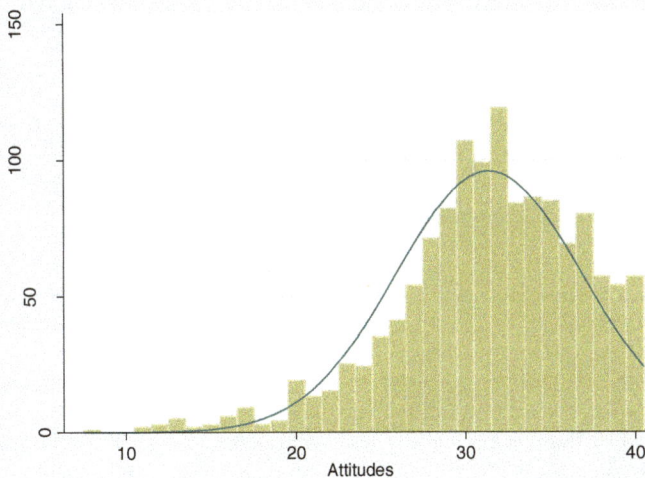

Figure 1 Frequency distribution of Attitudes sub-scores. The Y-axis indicates the number of survey participants and the X-axis indicates the Attitudes subscores. The mean sub-score was 31.4 (sd = 5.5) with a possible range of 8 to 40 (8 items scored 1–5). Median = 32.0 (IQR = 28-35).

Table 3 Response frequency and means of Attitudes toward EBP items (Part A of E-BASE)

Part A Items	Strongly Disagree(1)	Disagree(2)	Neutral(3)	Agree(4)	Strongly Agree(5)	Mean (Range=1-5)
*I am interested in learning or improving the skills necessary to incorporate EBP into my practice	0.9%	2.1%	7.5%	42.8%	46.7%	4.3
*Evidence based practice (EBP) is necessary in the practice of chiropractic	2.1%	3.5%	9.1%	39.6%	45.7%	4.2
*Professional literature (i.e. journals & textbooks) and research findings are useful in my day-to-day practice	0.9%	3.4%	9.6%	53.4%	32.7%	4.1
*EBP improves the quality of my patient's care	2.1%	4.4%	14.4%	43.2%	35.9%	4.1
*EBP assists me in making decisions about patient care	1.2%	3.7%	10.6%	48.6%	35.9%	4.1
Prioritizing EBP within chiropractic practice is fundamental to the advancement of the profession	2.4%	7.8%	13.3%	39.8%	36.7%	4.0
*EBP takes into account my clinical experience when making clinical decisions	2.3%	14.8%	17.7%	41.5%	23.7%	3.7
*The adoption of EBP places an unreasonable demand on my practice **[Note: Item is reverse coded]**	14.4%[5]	43.2[4]	29.1%[3]	10.6% [2]	2.7%[1]	3.6
*EBP takes into account a patient's preference for treatment	5.3%	24.1%	28.5%	27.1%	15.0%	3.2
There is a lack of evidence from clinical trials to support most of the treatments I use in my practice	13.5%	42.2%	17.7%	22.6%	4.0%	2.6

*The sum of the 8 items with asterisks comprises the "Attitudes" sub-score, which ranges from 8-40. See Figure 1 for frequency distribution graph of attitudes sub-scores. These are responses to the question "On a scale ranging from strongly disagree to strongly agree, how would you rate your opinion on the following statements?"

most frequently reported as "not useful" or "slightly useful" included: 1) "access to online tools to assist you to conduct your own critical appraisals of multiple research papers" (30%), and 2) "access to research rating tools that facilitate critical appraisal of single research papers" (26%).

Discussion

This is one of the largest studies to examine chiropractors' perspectives relative to EBP, and to our knowledge, the first national survey to be conducted in the United States. One other EBP study was performed in the US, however the sample was limited to mid-western chiropractors with advanced training in orthopedics [22]. Despite the large absolute sample size of our survey (n = 1,314), it represents only a small relative cross-sectional sample of the American chiropractic profession (n = 60,000) [27-29]. However, the demographic characteristics of our sample (Table 1) are strikingly similar to those reported by three National Board of Chiropractic Examiners' Job Analysis Reports [27-29]. This provides support for the generalizability of our survey results and makes us more confident that we have obtained a representative sample of US chiropractors.

The results suggest that our respondents generally have positive attitudes about evidence-based practice and a high level of self-reported skills in EBP, but only a modest level of EBP uptake in their clinical practices. These results are relatively similar to those reported from a recent EBP survey of Australian chiropractors [19] and are consistent with the observation that passive diffusion of knowledge does not automatically translate

into clinical implementation [6]. Further, it emphasizes the need for high quality EBP continuing education programs to meet the needs of the chiropractic profession.

Our participants reported generally positive attitudes toward EBP, with most agreeing that EBP is important for improving practice, patient care, and advancing the profession. Noteworthy was that nearly a third strongly agreed that there is a 'lack of evidence from clinical trials to support most of the treatments I use in my practice'. Similarly, only 42% agreed or strongly agreed that 'EBP takes into account a patient's preference for treatment'. These findings suggest that the basic principles of EBP may be misunderstood by DCs given the original definition of EBP clearly states that clinical expertise, patient values and best available research evidence are all integral components of evidence-based practice [1]. However, these opinions might also reflect what has become a growing recognition across healthcare fields; that clinical research needs to become more patient-oriented, pragmatic and generalizable to "real life" clinical practice [30].

Our sample of DCs reported that their poorest EBP skills were in conducting clinical research and/or systematic reviews; given that this survey was of practicing DCs without academic or research affiliation, this is not surprising. Distinctions have been drawn between the expectation for practitioners to be 'consumers' who 'use' research rather than 'manufacturers' who 'produce' research [31]; future studies should take this into consideration by ensuring that data collection instruments reflect this thinking.

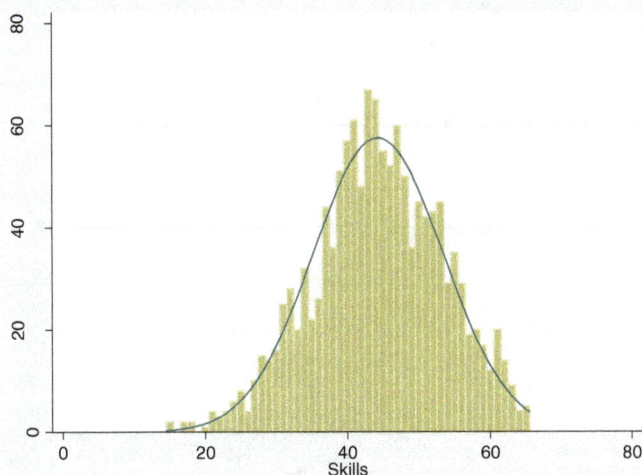

Figure 2 Frequency distribution of Skills sub-scores. The Y-axis indicates the number of survey participants and the X-axis indicates the Skills subscores. The mean sub-score was 44.3 (sd = 9.1) with a possible range of 13 to 65 (13 items scored 1–5). Median = 44.0 (IQR = 39-51).

Most of our sample reported above average skills in EBP, particularly in relation to identifying answerable clinical questions, identifying knowledge gaps in practice, locating professional literature and online database searching. However, nearly a third of respondents rated themselves only in the mid-range on nearly all of the EBP skill items. Some of these skills included the ability to synthesize research evidence, sharing evidence with colleagues, and using the findings from systematic reviews. Interestingly, while almost two-thirds reported above-average to advanced skills in using findings from clinical research, less than half reported the same level of skill in using findings from systematic reviews. This suggests that DCs have a limited understanding of the value and availability of systematic reviews, which is problem shared by many health professionals [32].

The introduction of EBP into the curricula of US chiropractic colleges is a relatively new phenomenon that has largely occurred over the past decade. The National Center for Complementary and Integrative Health (formerly NCCAM) has provided funding through its R25 mechanism to nine CAM colleges - four of them with chiropractic education programs - to develop institutional programs focused on teaching EBP. An

Table 4 Response frequency and means of Skills in EBP items (Part B of E-BASE)

PART B Items	Poor (1)	(2)	(3)	(4)	Advanced(5)	Mean (Range=1-5)
Identifying answerable clinical questions	0.3%	3.0%	18.6%	52.5%	25.6%	4.0
Identifying knowledge gaps in practice	0.4%	3.5%	29.5%	50.0%	16.7%	3.8
Locating professional literature	1.7%	8.6%	25.5%	38.7%	25.5%	3.8
Online database searching	3.7%	12.1%	25.3%	35.2%	23.7%	3.6
Retrieving evidence	3.0%	11.4%	28.5%	38.5%	18.6%	3.6
Critical appraisal of evidence	1.9%	10.6%	31.2%	42.4%	13.9%	3.6
Synthesis of research evidence	3.7%	15.8%	34.6%	36.6%	9.3%	3.3
Applying research evidence to patient cases	1.7%	8.0%	27.2%	48.9%	14.2%	3.7
Using findings from clinical research	1.5%	7.1%	29.1%	47.4%	14.9%	3.7
Sharing evidence with colleagues	4.8%	18.0%	30.6%	33.3%	13.3%	3.3
Using findings from systematic reviews	6.3%	19.2%	30.7%	34.0%	9.8%	3.2
Conducting systematic reviews	17.0%	29.9%	29.9%	18.4%	4.8%	2.6
Conducting clinical research	36.8%	29.5%	20.9%	10.3%	2.5%	2.1

The sum of all 13 items comprises the "skills" sub-score, which ranges from 13-65. See Figure 2 for frequency distribution graph of skills sub-scores. These are responses to the question "On a scale from 1 to 5, with 1 being poor and 5 being advanced, how would you rate your skills in the following areas"?

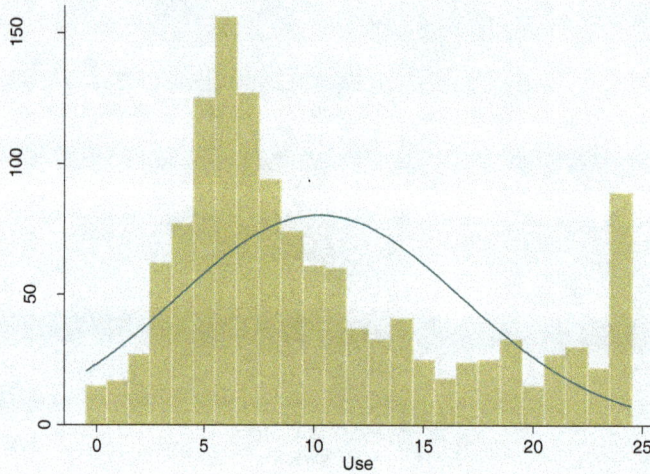

Figure 3 Frequency distribution of Use sub-scores. The Y-axis indicates the number of survey participants and the X-axis indicates the Use subscores. The mean sub-score was 10.3 (sd = 6.5) with a possible range of 0 to 24 (6 items scored 0–4). Median value = 8.0 (IQR = 6-14).

overarching goal of these R25 research education grants was to provide CAM faculty and students with the skills they need to apply a rigorous evidence-based perspective to their training and practice. Adding research literacy and EBP competencies to the curricula at these CAM colleges has led to changes in their institutional cultures, such as increased faculty use of EBP case studies in the classroom and student-led research/journal clubs [33-35]. However, with approximately two thirds of our sample receiving their chiropractic training 11 to 30 years ago, it is

Table 5 Response frequency and means of Use of EBP items (Part D of E-BASE)

PART D Item	None (0)	Very small (1-25%) (1)	Small (26-50%) (2)	Moderate (51-75%) (3)	Large (76-99%) (4)	All (100%) (5)	Mean (Range=1-5)
What percentage of your practice do you estimate is based on clinical research evidence (i.e. evidence from clinical trials)?	2.7%	21.2%	21.0%	32.3%	21.0%	1.8%	2.5

PART D Items	0 times (0)	1-5 times (1)	6-10 times (2)	11-15 times (3)	16+ times (4)		Mean (Range=0-4)
*I have read/reviewed professional literature (i.e. professional journals & textbooks) related to my practice	3.4%	41.9%	22.6%	8.7%	23.4%		2.1
*I have used an online search engine to search for practice related literature or research	7.9%	39.0%	23.5%	9.9%	19.7%		1.9
*I have read/reviewed clinical research findings related to my practice	7.8%	48.3%	17.4%	7.5%	19.0%		1.8
*I have used professional literature or research findings to assist my clinical decision making	11.0%	52.1%	14.8%	6.3%	15.8%		1.6
*I have used an online database to search for practice related literature or research	28.6%	36.5%	12.4%	6.4%	16.1%		1.4
*I have used professional literature or research findings to change my clinical Practice	23.2%	48.9%	11.3%	4.3%	12.3%		1.3
I have consulted a colleague or industry expert to assist my clinical decision making	22.5%	51.8%	13.5%	4.7%	7.5%		1.2
I have referred to magazines, layperson/ self-help books, or non-government/ non-education institution websites to assist my clinical decision making	35.6%	43.8%	11.1%	4.2%	5.3%		1.0

*The sum of the 6 items with asterisks comprises the "Use" sub-score, which ranges from 0-24. See Figure 3 for frequency distribution graph of the "use" sub-scores. These are responses to the question "Indicate how often you have performed the following activities over the last month".

Table 6 Response frequency and means of Barriers to EBP uptake items (Part E of E-BASE)

PART E Items	Not a barrier (1)	Minor barrier (2)	Moderate barrier (3)	Major barrier (4)	Mean (Range = 1-4)
Lack of time	19.2%	33.0%	34.1%	13.7%	2.4
Lack of clinical evidence in complementary and alternative medicine	18.9%	37.2%	32.2%	11.7%	2.4
Lack of industry support for EBP	31.4%	31.6%	26.3%	10.7%	2.2
Lack of incentive to participate in EBP	34.6%	29.2%	26.2%	10.0%	2.1
Insufficient skills for interpreting research	34.3%	38.7%	19.9%	7.1%	2.0
Insufficient skills for locating research	39.7%	37.3%	16.8%	6.2%	1.9
Insufficient skills to critically appraise/evaluate the literature	35.8%	39.8%	18.8%	5.6%	1.9
Lack of colleague support for EBP	44.1%	32.7%	17.0%	6.2%	1.9
Insufficient skills to apply research findings to clinical practice	39.9%	41.5%	15.8%	2.8%	1.8
Lack of relevance to chiropractic practice	47.1%	29.1%	17.8%	6.0%	1.8
Patient preference for treatment	41.5%	38.0%	16.8%	3.7%	1.8
Lack of interest in EBP	52.5%	30.5%	12.6%	4.4%	1.7
Lack of resources (i.e. access to a computer, the internet or online databases)	60.0%	26.8%	10.4%	2.8%	1.6

These are responses to the question "On a scale ranging from 'not a barrier' to 'major barrier', to what extent do the following factors prevent you from participating in EBP"?

likely that many of our participants never received what would now be considered foundational training in EBP.

Additionally, our results suggest that educational emphasis should be focused on improving the skills of appraising and applying research evidence in clinical practice. This needs to be done in a way that provides clinicians with 'real life' clinical examples, in order to overcome the barriers of lack of interest or clinical relevance to chiropractic practice. This issue was addressed in the second phase of our project, which explores the effectiveness of online EBP educational modules and "booster exercises" that incorporate clinical examples

Table 7 Response frequency and means of Facilitators of EBP uptake items (Part F of E-BASE)

PART F Items	Not useful (1)	Slightly useful (2)	Moderately useful (3)	Very useful (4)	Mean (Range = 1-4)
Access to the Internet in your workplace	3.4%	5.2%	13.5%	77.9%	3.7
Access to free online databases in the workplace, such as Cochrane and PubMed	2.0%	8.9%	18.9%	70.2%	3.6
Ability to download full-text / full-length journal articles	2.1%	11.5%	20.9%	65.5%	3.5
Access to online education materials related to evidence based practice	1.4%	9.3%	23.7%	65.6%	3.5
Access to critical reviews of research evidence relevant to your field (these are critical reviews of multiple research papers addressing a single topic)	1.8%	11.3%	31.4%	55.5%	3.4
Free access to online databases that usually require license fees, such as DynaMed and CINAHL	6.9%	15.1%	19.7%	58.3%	3.3
Access to critically appraised topics relevant to your field (these are critical appraisals of single research papers)	2.2%	15.6%	35.2%	47.0%	3.3
Access to tools used to assist the critical appraisal/evaluation of research evidence	3.4%	17.6%	36.7%	42.3%	3.2
Access to research rating tools that facilitate critical appraisal of single research papers	4.3%	21.9%	35.5%	38.3%	3.1
Access to online tools that assist you to conduct your own critical appraisals of multiple research papers related to a single topic	6.8%	22.9%	30.4%	39.9%	3.0

These are responses to the question "On a scale ranging from 'not useful' to 'very useful', to what extent would the following strategies assist you in participating in EBP"?

relevant to chiropractors. Results of the second phase of this project will be reported in a future publication.

The results of this survey also indicate that there are serious gaps in the uptake of research evidence into chiropractic practice, with nearly half reporting only a very small proportion of what they do in their clinical practice is based on research evidence. DCs appear to have challenges with performing online searches of the literature and interpreting the results of systematic reviews. Although most DCs in our sample reported they had above average skills in locating literature online, they also indicated that they did not engage in the uptake of EBP on a frequent basis (> six times a month). This apparent contradiction may be associated with the issues of time and lack of evidence, as discussed in the next paragraph. However, almost 90% of our sample indicated that they were interested in learning or improving the skills necessary to incorporate EBP into their practices (Table 3). Educational interventions and strategies are more likely to be successful if they are informed by known barriers and facilitators [36-39].

On the whole, most DCs indicated there were few barriers to their uptake of EBP, which is consistent with their generally positive attitudes toward EBP. It is worth noting however, that almost half of DCs indicated that the two biggest barriers to EBP uptake were 'lack of time' and 'lack of clinical evidence in CAM'. A sizeable proportion (a quarter to one third) also cited: 'lack of industry support'; 'lack of incentive'; 'insufficient skills for interpreting research'; 'locating and critically appraising research'; 'lack of colleague support for EBP'; and 'lack of relevance to chiropractic practice'. Many of the barriers identified in this study are similar to those found for chiropractors in Australia [19], Canada [20] and Great Britain [21] as well as a sub-specialty of chiropractic orthopedists in the US [22]. Interestingly, many of the same barriers are encountered in the medical and nursing professions [5,6], leading us to conclude that the challenges facing the chiropractic profession in implementing EBP are not unique.

Interestingly, very few DCs indicated that computer, internet, or database access were barriers to their uptake of EBP. Coupled with our sample's perceived usefulness of all of the listed facilitator items, these findings underscore the importance of providing clinicians with training in EBP skills, particularly through online resources. Our findings also suggest a need for greater support from professional organizations to facilitate collegial support of EBP, as well as better collaboration between scientists and practitioners in the design of clinically applicable research. Indeed, while educational strategies are an important part of narrowing the gap between science and practice for chiropractic and other health disciplines, they will likely be insufficient on their own to accomplish true

change. Comprehensive and multi-faceted approaches that take into account all the relevant levels affecting EBP, including professional, managerial, organizational and health systems, will likely be needed to integrate research into practice [41].

There were several limitations to this study. The first is inherent to any type of survey design, which is reliance on self-reporting. For example, the 'skills' sub-score was based upon the participants' self-perceived level of skill; we did not directly test a participant's knowledge or skills in EBP. It would be useful in future studies to correlate an actual "grade" from tests or quizzes of EBP knowledge with the self-reported survey data. Another inherent limitation is selection bias; it is possible that the 'attitudes' sub-scores were skewed toward higher values because participants were already in favor of an evidence-based practice paradigm prior to commencing the survey.

Although we had a relatively large number of survey responders (n = 1,314), this number represents only a small proportion of the approximately 60,000 licensed chiropractors in the US. We made some minor modifications in the original EBASE questionnaire, chiefly to use the word "chiropractic" in certain questions. We do not believe these minor changes altered the intrinsic properties of the EBASE, however we did not formally conduct a psychometric evaluation of this modified version.

Conclusion

The results of this survey have provided new insights into the attitudes, skills and use of EBP among US chiropractors. The information gained from this survey will be most helpful in informing the design of future educational interventions for chiropractors to improve their level of EBP literacy and use of evidence in clinical practice. Overall, American chiropractors appear very similar to chiropractors in other countries, as well as other health professionals in terms of their favorable attitudes towards EBP, while expressing limitations and barriers related to EBP skills, research relevance, and lack of time. This suggests that the design of future EBP interventions for chiropractic should capitalize on the growing body of EBP implementation research evidence developing in other health disciplines. This will likely include broadening the approach beyond a sole focus on EBP education, and taking a multilevel approach that also targets professional, organizational and health policy domains.

Additional file

Additional file 1: EBASE Questionnaire and Scoring Rubric.

Abbreviations
ACA: American Chiropractic Association; CAM: Complementary and
Alternative Medicine; DELIVER: Distance Education Online Intervention for

Evidence-Based Practice Literacy; DC: Doctor of Chiropractic; EBP: Evidence-Based Practice; EBASE: Evidence-Based Practice Attitude and Utilization Survey; UPitt: University of Pittsburgh; NCCAM: National Center for Complementary and Alternative Medicine.

Competing interests
The authors declare that they have no competing interests.

Authors' contributions
MS was the principal investigator of the DELIVER study and was responsible for securing the funding and administration of the research grant. He was responsible for data collection, analysis, and a majority of the manuscript preparation. RE contributed to the conceptualization, design and funding acquisition of this work; she participated in data collection implementation and monitoring as well as decisions regarding data analysis and interpretation of results. She worked with the primary author to prepare the manuscript for publication and contributed content to the background and discussion sections. MH was responsible for assisting in designing the study, and interpretation of findings, as well as drafting and editing the manuscript. GC contributed to the initial concept and design of the study, was involved in meetings assessing progress, and critically reviewed the drafts of the manuscript, including data analyses. CH contributed to the initial concept and design of the study, interpretation of findings, as well as editing the manuscript. ML was involved in the design and funding of the study, development of the outcome measure, drafting of the methods, and editing of the draft and final manuscript. CL contributed to the initial concept and design of the study, was involved in meetings assessing progress, and critically reviewed the drafts of the manuscript, including data analyses. CV worked with the primary author and co-authors to prepare the manuscript. She also participated in the implementation of Phase II of the DELIVER study. OW made significant contributions to the conception and design, acquisition and analysis of data; he was involved in drafting/revising the manuscript and gave final approval of the version to be published. LT performed the statistical analyses of the data and assisted with the interpretations of the results. She prepared the tables and worked with the primary author to write the methods, statistical analyses, and results sections of the manuscript. All authors read and approved the final manuscript.

Acknowledgements
This research was made possible by Grant Number R21AT007547 from the National Center for Complementary and Integrative Health (NCCIH; formerly NCCAM) at the National Institutes of Health (NIH). The views expressed in this article are solely those of the authors and do not necessarily represent the official views of the NCCIH, NCCAM or NIH.
The authors would like to acknowledge the hard work and assistance of our senior research associate Kris Gongaware and our research coordinator Christine McFarland. We would also like to acknowledge the important contributions of our database and information technology consultant Jack Doman.

Author details
[1]Department of Physical Therapy, School of Health and Rehabilitation Sciences, Clinical and Translational Science Institute, University of Pittsburgh, Pittsburgh, PA, USA. [2]Center for Spirituality and Healing, Integrative Health and Wellbeing Research Program, University of Minnesota, Minneapolis, MN, USA. [3]University of Western States, Portland, OR, USA. [4]School of Nursing and Midwifery, University of South Australia, Adelaide, SA, Australia. [5]Logan College of Chiropractic, Chesterfield, MO, USA. [6]Palmer Center for Chiropractic Research, Palmer College of Chiropractic, Davenport, IA, USA. [7]National University of Health Sciences, Lombard, IL, USA. [8]The Commonwealth Medical College, Scranton, PA, USA. [9]Department of Occupational Therapy, School of Health and Rehabilitation Sciences, University of Pittsburgh, Pittsburgh, PA, USA.

References
1. Sackett DL, Rosenberg WM, Gray JA, Haynes RB, Richardson WS. Evidence based medicine: what it is and what it isn't. BMJ. 1996;312:71–2.

2. Claridge JA, Fabian TC. History and development of evidence-based medicine. World J Surg. 2005;29:547–53.

3. Balakas K, Potter P, Pratt E, Rea G, Williams J. Evidence equals excellence: the application of an evidence-based practice model in an academic medical center. Nurs Clin North Am. 2009;44:1–10.

4. Glasziou P, Ogrinc G, Goodman S. Can evidence-based medicine and clinical quality improvement learn from each other? BMJ Qual Saf. 2011;20:13–7.

5. Ubbink DT, Guyatt GH, Vermeulen H. Framework of policy recommendations for implementation of evidence-based practice: a systematic scoping review. BMJ Open. 2013; doi:10.1136/bmjopen-2012-001881.

6. Cabana MD, Rand C, Powe N, Wu A, Wilson M, Abboud P, et al. Why don't physicians follow clinical practice guidelines? A framework for improvement. JAMA. 1999;282(15):1458–65.

7. Academic Consortium for Complementary & Alternative Health Care, Competencies for Optimal Practice in Integrated Environments. 2011. http://accahc.org/images/stories/accahc_competencies_optimal_february2012.pdf. Accessed 3 February 2015.

8. Evans R, Maiers M, Delagran L, Kreitzer MJ, Sierpina V. Evidence informed practice as the catalyst for culture change in CAM. Explore. 2012;8(1):68–72.

9. Haas M, Leo M, Peterson D, Lefebvre R, Vavrek D. Evaluation of the effects of an evidence-based practice curriculum on knowledge, attitudes, and self-assessed skills and behaviors in chiropractic students. J Manipulative Physiol Ther. 2012;35(9):701–9.

10. Sullivan BM, Furner SE, Cramer GD. Development of a Student Mentored Research Program between a Complementary and Alternative Medicine University and a Traditional, Research Intensive University. Acad Med. 2014;89(9):1220–6.

11. Cramer GD, Guiltinan J, Maiers M, Laird S, Goertz C, Furner SE, et al. Benefits, Challenges And Culture Change Related To Collaborations Between Complementary And Alternative Medicine And Traditional Research-Intensive Institutions. Med Sci Educator. 2014. doi:10.1007/s40670-014-0077-3.

12. Shaw L, Descarreaux M, Bryans R, Duranleau M, Marcoux H, Potter B, et al. A systematic review of chiropractic management of adults with Whiplash-Associated Disorders: recommendations for advancing evidence-based practice and research. Work. 2010;35(3):369–94.

13. Bussieres A, Stuber K. The Clinical Practice Guideline Initiative: A joint collaboration designed to improve the quality of care delivered by doctors of chiropractic. J Can Chiropr Assoc. 2013;57(4):279–84.

14. Hawk C, Schneider M, Evans Jr MW, Redwood D. Consensus Process to Develop a Best-Practice Document on the Role of Chiropractic Care in Health Promotion, Disease Prevention, and Wellness. J Manipulative Physiol Ther. 2012;35(7):556–67.

15. Hawk C, Schneider M, Dougherty P, Gleberzon B, Killinger L. Best practices recommendations for chiropractic care for older adults: results of a consensus process. J Manipulative Physiol Ther. 2010;33(6):464–73.

16. Hawk C, Schneider M, Ferrance R, Hewitt E, Van Loon M, Tanis L. Best practices recommendations for chiropractic care for infants, children, and adolescents: results of a consensus process. J Manipulative Physiol Ther. 2009;32(8):639–47.

17. Institute of Medicine Committee on Quality of Health Care in America. Crossing the quality chasm: a new health system for the 21st century. Washington, DC: National Academies Press; 2001.

18. Schillinger D. An Introduction to Effectiveness, Dissemination and Implementation Research. P. Fleisher and E. Goldstein, eds. From the Series: UCSF Clinical and Translational Science Institute (CTSI) Resource Manuals and Guides to Community-Engaged Research, P. Fleisher, editor. Published by Clinical Translational Science Institute Community Engagement Program, University of California San Francisco; 2010.

19. Walker BF, Stomski N, Hebert J, French S. A survey of Australian chiropractors' attitudes and beliefs about evidence-based practice and their use of research literature and clinical practice guidelines. Chiropr Man Therap. 2013;21(1):44.

20. Suter E, Vanderheyden L, Trojan L, Verhoef M, Armitage G. How important is research-based practice to chiropractors and massage therapists? J Manipulative Physiol Ther. 2007;30(2):109–15.

21. Hall G. Attitudes of chiropractors to evidence-based practice and how this compares to other healthcare professionals: a qualitative study. Clin Chiropractic. 2011;14:106–11.

22. Roecker CB, Long C, Vining R, Lawrence D. Attitudes toward evidence-based clinical practice among doctors of chiropractic with diplomate-level training in orthopedics. Chiropr Man Therap. 2013;21(1):43.

23. Putting evidence into practice: Dr. Michael Schneider talks about the DELIVER study. Dynamic Chiropractic. Feb 1, 2013. http://www.dynamicchiropractic.com/mpacms/dc/article.php?id=56343. Accessed 13 Feb 2015.

24. Your Opinion Counts. J Amer Chiropr Assoc. 2012;49(6):33. http://www.acatoday.org/content_css.cfm?CID=5060.

25. Leach MJ, Gillham D. Evaluation of the Evidence-Based practice Attitude and utilization SurvEy for complementary and alternative medicine practitioners. J Eval Clin Pract. 2008;14(5):792–8.

26. Leach MJ, Gillham D. Are complementary medicine practitioners implementing evidence based practice? Complement Ther Med. 2011;19(3):128–36.

27. Christensen MG, Kerkhoff D, Kollash M. Job Analysis of Chiropractic. Greeley, CO: National Board of Chiropractic Examiners; 2000.

28. Christensen MG, Kollash M, Ward R, Webb K, Day M. zum Brunnen J. Job Analysis of Chiropractic. Greeley, CO: National Board of Chiropractic Examiners; 2005.

29. Christensen MG, Kollash M, Hyland J. Job Analysis of Chiropractic. Greeley, CO: National Board of Chiropractic Examiners; 2010.

30. Gaglio B, Phillips SM, Heurtin-Roberts S, Sanchez MA, Glasgow RE. How pragmatic is it? Lessons learned using PRECIS and RE-AIM for determining pragmatic characteristics of research. Implement Sci. 2014;9:96.

31. Slawson DC, Shaughnessy A. Teaching evidence-based medicine: Should we be teaching information management instead? Acad Med. 2005;80:685–9.

32. Murthy L, Shepperd S, Clarke MJ, Garner SE, Lavis JN, Perrier L, Roberts NW, Straus SE. Interventions to improve the use of systematic reviews in decision-making by health system managers, policy makers and clinicians. Cochrane Database Syst Rev. 2012;Issue 9. Art. No.: CD009401. doi:10.1002/14651858.CD009401.pub2.

33. Zwickey H, Schiffke H, Fleishman S, Haas M, Cruser D, LeFebvre R, et al. Teaching Evidence-Based Medicine at Complementary and Alternative Medicine Institutions: Strategies, Competencies, and Evaluation. J Altern Complement Med. 2014;20(12):925–31.

34. Long CR, Ackerman D, Hammerschlag R, Delagran L, Peterson D, Berlin M, et al. Faculty development initiatives to advance research literacy and evidence-based practice at CAM academic institutions. J Altern Complement Med. 2014;20(7):563–70.

35. Clar C, Tsertsvadze A, Court R, Hundt GL, Clarke A, Sutcliffe P. Clinical effectiveness of manual therapy for the management of musculoskeletal and non-musculoskeletal conditions; systematic review and update of UK evidence report. Chiropr Man Therap. 2014;28(22):1.

36. Bartholomew LK, Parcel GS, Kok G, Gottlieb NH. Planning Health Promotion Program: An Intervention Mapping Approach. San Francisco, California: Jossey-Bass; 2006.

37. French SD, Green SE, O'Connor DA, McKenzie JE, Francis JJ, Michie S, et al. Developing theory-informed behaviour change interventions to implement evidence into practice: a systematic approach using the Theoretical Domains Framework. Implement Sci. 2012;7:38.

38. QUERI Implementation Guide Quality Enhancement Research Initiative. US Department of Veterans Affairs; 2014. http://www.queri.research.va.gov/implementation/default.cfm Accessed 4 December 2014.

39. Kawchuk G, Newton G, Srbely J, Passmore S, Bussières A, Busse J, et al. Knowledge transfer within the Canadian Chiropractic Community. Part 2: Narrowing the evidence-practice gap. J Can Chiropr Assoc. 2014;58(3):206–14.

Sick leave and healthcare utilisation in women reporting pregnancy related low back pain and/or pelvic girdle pain at 14 months postpartum

Cecilia Bergström[1*] ⓘ, Margareta Persson[2] and Ingrid Mogren[1]

Abstract

Background: Pregnancy related low back pain (PLBP) and pelvic girdle pain (PGP) are considered common complications of pregnancy. The long-term consequences for women with persistent PLBP/PGP postpartum are under-investigated. The main objective was to investigate the prevalence, pattern and degree of sick leave as well as healthcare utilisation and its perceived effect in women with persistent PLBP/PGP at 12 months postpartum.

Method: This is a follow-up study of a cohort involving of a sample of women, who delivered from January 1st 2002 to April 30th in 2002 at Umeå University Hospital and Sunderby Hospital, and who reported PLBP/PGP during pregnancy. A total of 639 women were followed-up by a second questionnaire (Q2) at approximately 6 months postpartum. Women with persistent PLBP/PGP at the second questionnaire ($N = 200$) were sent a third questionnaire (Q3) at approximately 12 months postpartum.

Results: The final study sample consisted of 176 women reporting PLBP/PGP postpartum where $N = 34$ (19.3 %) reported 'no' pain, $N = 115$ (65.3 %) 'recurrent' pain, and $N = 27$ (15.3 %) 'continuous' pain. The vast majority (92.4 %) of women reported that they had neither been on sick leave nor sought any healthcare services (64.1 %) during the past 6 months at Q3. Women with 'continuous' pain at Q3 reported a higher extent of sick leave and healthcare seeking behaviour compared to women with 'recurrent' pain at Q3. Most women with persistent PLBP/PGP had been on sick leave on a full-time basis. The most commonly sought healthcare was physiotherapy, followed by consultation with a medical doctor, acupuncture and chiropractic.

Conclusion: Most women did not report any sick leave or sought any healthcare due to PLBP/PGP the past 6 months at Q3. However, women with 'continuous' PLBP/PGP 14 months postpartum did report a higher prevalence and degree of sick leave and sought healthcare to a higher extent compared to women with 'recurrent' PLBP/PGP at Q3. Women with more pronounced symptoms might constitute a specific subgroup of patients with a less favourable long-term outcome, thus PLBP/PGP needs to be addressed early in pregnancy to reduce both individual suffering and the risk of transition into chronicity.

Keywords: Pelvic girdle pain, Pregnancy related low back pain, Sick leave, Healthcare utilisation, Postpartum period, Female, Pregnancy, Pregnancy complications, Cohort studies

* Correspondence: cecilia.bergstrom@umu.se
[1]Department of Clinical Sciences, Obstetrics and Gynecology, Umeå University, Umeå, Sweden
Full list of author information is available at the end of the article

Background

Pregnancy related low back pain (PLBP) and pelvic girdle pain (PGP) are common complications of pregnancy and represent a significant health problem among women both during and after pregnancy [1–3]. PLBP resembles low back pain (LBP) that occurs in a non-pregnant state while PGP is described as pain between the two posterior iliac crests in the proximity of the sacroiliac joints (SI-joints), the gluteal folds and with or without pain in the symphysis pubis and/or down the posterior thigh [4]. The prevalence of PLBP/PGP among pregnant women ranges from 4 to 76.4 % depending on definition used [5].

PLBP/PGP is not a self-limiting condition in some women [1]. Research has shown that among women developing PLBP/PGP during pregnancy about 80 % of women report mild complaints of PLBP/PGP postpartum, whereas 13 % of women report moderate and 7 % have very serious complaints [6]. In addition, women suffering from PGP postpartum seem to have a higher prevalence of depressive symptoms compared to women without postpartum PGP [7]. Predictors of poor outcome postpartum have shown to be: previous LBP, high levels of pain postpartum, high body mass index (BMI), high maternal age, hypermobility, physical strenuous work situation and low job satisfaction [1, 8–13]. Furthermore, there is an increased likelihood of reporting poorer health status in women reporting continuous pain postpartum [1]. Consequently, women with recurrent or continuous pain postpartum may have a poor prognosis in regard to future sick leave and disability.

The World Health Organization (WHO) considers musculoskeletal conditions to be the second greatest cause of years lived with disability (YLD), where low back pain ranks number one of the top 10 leading causes of global YLD [14]. Spine-related problems constitute large individual and societal costs as a result of chronic musculoskeletal pain. In Sweden, the cost has been estimated to SEK 87.5 billion (EUR 8.6 million), where over 90 % of the total costs are associated with indirect costs due to sickness absence and disability pension [15]. In addition, international studies have reported a higher utilisation of health services with regard to chronic pain [16–18].

Even though not all women with PLBP/PGP during pregnancy transition into a more chronic state postpartum, women with persistent problems are an understudied group of patients and relatively few studies have a longer follow-up time of more than 3 months [2, 3, 19–22]. Moreover, these women may constitute a specific subgroup of patients within the heterogeneous back pain population consuming a significant part of the allocated resources provided by the social security and healthcare systems. Therefore we wanted to investigate sick leave and healthcare utilisation in women with 'recurrent' or 'continuous' PLBP/PGP at approximately 12 months postpartum. More specifically, we wanted to determine the prevalence, pattern and degree of sick leave in women with 'recurrent' and 'continuous' PLBP/PGP during pregnancy, at 6 and 12 months postpartum. In addition, we wanted to investigate what type of healthcare had been sought the past 6 months at the 12 months postpartum follow-up and its perceived effect on symptoms.

Method
Design
This is a follow-up study that is part of a longitudinal cohort of pregnant women reporting persistent PLBP/PGP at 12 months postpartum and the project has been described in detail elsewhere [1]. Briefly, this is a longitudinal study consisting of a sample of women who delivered from January 1st 2002 to April 30th in 2002 at Umeå University Hospital (UUH) and Sunderby Hospital (SH), the largest hospitals situated in the two most northern counties of Sweden.

Data collection
Baseline data were collected through a questionnaire (Q1) in close proximity after delivery and women reporting PLBP/PGP at baseline (Q1) were thereafter invited to complete a second questionnaire (Q2) at 6 months postpartum. A third questionnaire (Q3) was distributed approximately 12 months postpartum to all women reporting persistent 'recurrent' or 'continuous' pain at Q2.

All questionnaires (Q1, Q2 and Q3) included issues such as persistence or remission of symptoms, use of medical services, family situation, SRH, sick leave, sexual life, physical activity, oral contraception and breastfeeding among other variables. Relevant background variables from Q1-Q3 for the research question in this study are presented in this paper.

Study participants
Detailed description of inclusion criteria and procedure are presented in another publication from this cohort [1]. The final study sample responding to Q3 comprised of 176 women (88.0 %) out of the 200 women who reported 'recurrent' or 'continuous' pain at 6 months postpartum (Q2). An overview of the entire cohort is illustrated in Fig. 1.

Validity of data
The validity of the data collected at Q1 has previously been discussed at length [23]. In brief, respondents and non-respondents did not differ concerning maternal age, gestational age, birth weight, mode of delivery, total experience of delivery, epidural or spinal anaesthesia

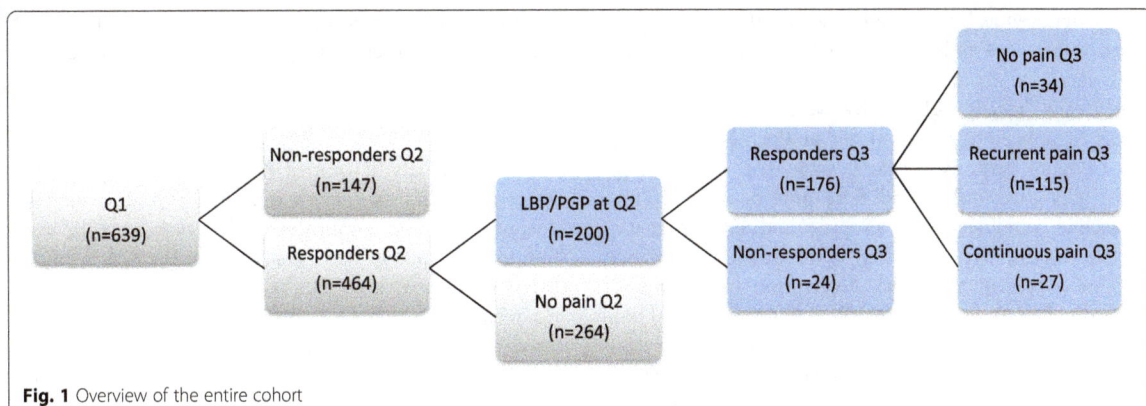

Fig. 1 Overview of the entire cohort

during delivery, and pre-pregnancy or end-pregnancy BMI. Moreover, no difference was found between respondents and non-respondents in regard to baseline variables except for smoking and maternal age at first delivery. Consequently, the conclusion was that the data collected through Q1 seem to be representative for Swedish women with persistent LBP and/or PGP postpartum [23]. Questions included in Q2 and Q3 were similar to those in Q1.

Definitions of variables

PLBP/PGP at Q3 was defined when the woman reported 'recurrent' pain or 'continuous' pain due to PLBP/PGP when responding to Q3. The response alternatives to the question: 'Do you experience low back pain or pelvic pain right now?' were 'yes, recurrent pain', 'yes, continuous pain' and 'no' pain. In addition, a pain drawing was included where marking of the affected area could be indicated. Women who reported a specific time point in Q3, at which PLBP/PGP had ceased (even though reporting 'recurrent' pain), were allocated to the 'no' pain group.

Sick leave. Information about sick leave was self-reported. The participants were asked if they had been on sick leave at all three time points (Q1-Q3) due to PLBP/PGP (response alternatives 'yes' or 'no'). In addition, at each time point (Q1 – Q3) they were asked to report how many weeks and to what degree (response options: full-time, part-time or both full- and part-time) they had been on sick leave. The participants were also asked to what degree they had been on sick leave during the pregnancy (Q1) and during the past 6 months at Q2 and Q3 due to PLBP/PGP. The response alternatives were 'full-time' or 'part-time'. Long-term sickness absence is often defined as more than 30 days [24, 25] as sick leave of less than 30 days is found to be a predictor of short-term recovery [26]. Consequently, sick leave was dichotomized into less or more than 4 weeks of self-

reported sick leave, irrespective of full-time or part-time sick leave.

Healthcare services were defined as healthcare provided by a practitioner in allopathic medicine or complementary and alternative medicine for the PLBP/PGP. Participants were asked to recall the total numbers of visits to a healthcare provider during the past 6 months at Q2 and Q3 and also, the perceived effect that a particular treatment had on their PLBP/PGP symptoms (response alternatives 'no effect', 'some effect', 'good effect').

Pre-pregnancy weight was defined as self-reported weight before the actual pregnancy and *end-pregnancy* weight was defined as reported weight before delivery. Self-reported weight was also asked for in kg at Q2 and Q3. *Height* was given in centimetres (cm). *Body Mass Index (BMI)* was defined as maternal weight in kilograms (kg)/height^2 (meters). WHO classification was used for the principal cut-off points for adult underweight, normal range, overweight and obesity: i.e. underweight <18.50 kg/m^2, normal range 18.50–24.99 kg/m^2, overweight ≥25.00 kg/m^2, and obesity ≥30.00 kg/m^2.

Work description. Participants were asked at Q1 about their primary employment status prior to the recent pregnancy with the response alternatives: 'gainfully employed', 'student', 'maternity leave', 'unemployed' and 'on sick leave'. They were also asked what kind of description that defined their job the best (with the possibility to give more than one option). The options were 'mainly sitting', 'physically active', 'alternatively sitting/ physically active', 'physically challenging', 'physically easy', 'alternatively physically challenging/easy', 'mentally challenging', 'mentally not challenging', 'alternatively mentally challenging/no challenging', 'intellectually stimulating', 'intellectually not stimulating' and alternatively intellectually stimulating/not stimulating'.

Hypermobility. Women were asked at Q1 if they had previously been diagnosed as having hypermobile joints with the response alternatives 'yes' or 'no'. Additionally, they were asked if they had any family member that had been diagnosed as hypermobile and whether they experienced themselves as hypermobile. The response alternatives were 'yes', 'no' and 'do not know'.

Self-rated health (SRH). The women were asked to assess their present health status at Q1, Q2 and Q3. A five category response options was used with the options: 'very good', 'quite good', 'fair', 'quite poor' and 'poor'.

Baseline variables such as pre- and end-pregnancy weight, height, hypermobility, SRH during pregnancy, level of education and work description were obtained from the first questionnaire (Q1). Current weight and SRH at 6 months and 12 months postpartum were obtained from both Q2 and Q3 respectively. BMI was calculated from the self-reported measures at all three measured time points.

Statistical methods

Descriptive statistics was used to investigate sick leave and healthcare utilisation in women with 'recurrent' or 'continuous' PLBP/PGP at approximately 12 months postpartum. The data were analysed through calculation of means and standard deviations (SD) for parametric data. The independent-samples t test was used to test for difference between respondents and non-respondents when possible. Pearson's Chi-square test was used when testing for difference between respondents and non-respondents in regard to categorical data. For data not normally distributed median and interquartile range (IQR) was used.

Statistical significance was set at $p < 0.05$ for all analyses. IBM SPSS Statistics 20 software package was used.

Ethical approval

The study was approved by the Ethics Committee at the Umeå University (Dnr 01–335).

Results

Individuals who responded to Q3 ($N = 176$) were classified into three groups: 'no' pain ($N = 34$, 19.3 %), 'recurrent' pain ($N = 115$, 65.3 %), and 'continuous' pain ($N = 27$, 15.3 %). A detailed description of characteristics of the cohort has been previously presented [1]. Most participants had 2 children (38.1 %) and 36.9 % had one child. The vast majority were married or cohabiting (96.0 %) when responding to Q3. One hundred and fifty-nine (90.3 %) of the women were non-smokers and 170 (96.6 %) had at least achieved a high school education. Six out of 10 women ($N = 107$, 60.8 %) reported physical activity on a regular basis and assessed their health status to be 'quite good' ($N = 84$, 48.0 %) to 'very good' ($N = 27$, 15.4 %). Mean BMI at Q3 was 25.4 (SD 4.6) kg/m^2. Relationship satisfaction was considered stable. No statistically significant differences between the subgroups were found, except for smoking, where the 'continuous' pain group included significant more smokers than the 'recurrent' pain group. Further description of the cohort can be found in Table 1.

Sick leave

The vast majority of women (92.4 %) who responded at Q3 reported no sick leave during the past 6 months. However, Table 2 demonstrates that women with 'continuous' pain at Q3 had been on sick leave to a higher extent at all measure points compared to women reporting 'recurrent' pain at Q3. Additionally, women with 'recurrent' and 'continuous' pain reporting sick leave at Q1, Q2 and Q3 had been so on a full-time basis. Women with 'recurrent' pain reported long-term sick leave of more than 4 weeks to a higher extent compared to the 'no' pain group at Q1 and the 'continuous' pain group demonstrated a higher degree of long-term sick leave at both Q1 and Q2 compared to the 'no' pain group (Fig. 2a, b and c). In addition, women with 'continuous' pain demonstrated more long-term sick leave compared to women with 'recurrent' pain at all three measured time points.

Healthcare utilisation

The majority of women reporting 'recurrent' or 'continuous' pain at Q3 had not sought any healthcare services during the past 6 months ($N = 91$, 64.1 %). However, 59.3 % ($N = 16$) women with 'continuous' pain did report that they had sought healthcare services the past 6 months compared to 30.4 % ($N = 35$) of women with 'recurrent' pain at Q3.

The most sought healthcare service was physical therapy followed by medical doctor (MD) consultation, acupuncture, chiropractic and naprapathic treatment for both groups of women reporting pain at Q3. Other types of treatments that were reported consisted of stretch exercises, ultrasound treatment, Reiki healing, osteopathic treatment, exercise programs and massage therapy (including consultation with a midwife) (Fig. 3).

No treatment alternative was perceived as being more successful than any of the alternatives listed i.e. having a good perceived effect on symptoms.

Discussion
Sick leave

The first objective of this study was to investigate the prevalence, pattern and degree of sick leave in women reporting persistent PLBP/PGP at 12 months postpartum. The findings revealed that most women had no sick leave during the past 6 months before responding to Q3 despite the majority of the women still reported 'recurrent' or 'continuous' pain. Nevertheless, women with 'continuous' pain at Q3 had been on sick leave to a higher extent and demonstrated more long-term sick

Table 1 Descriptive information of the study group

	No pain[a] N = 34	Recurrent pain[b] N = 115	Continuous pain[c] N = 27	Total N = 176
BMI at Q3, mean (SD)	26.23 (4.3)	25.40 (4.8)	24.22 (3.7)	25.37 (4.6)
Pre-pregnancy Q1 (SD)	26.30 (4.9)	25.13 (4.7)	24.33 (4.2)	25.24 (4.7)
< 18.50, n (%)	1 (2.9)	4 (3.5)	-	5 (2.9)
18.50–24.99, n (%)	13 (38.2)	60 (53.1)	16 (59.3)	89 (51.1)
≥ 25.00, n (%)	15 (44.1)	33 (29.2)	8 (29.6)	56 (32.2)
≥ 30.00, n (%)	5 (14.7)	16 (14.2)	3 (11.1)	24 (13.8)
End-pregnancy Q1 (SD)	32.12 (5.3)	30.38 (4.8)	30.15 (4.5)	30.68 (4.9)
Underweight, n (%)	-	-	-	-
Normal range, n (%)	3 (8.8)	14 (12.4)	2 (7.4)	19 (10.9)
Overweight, n (%)	7 (20.6)	41 (36.3)	12 (44.4)	60 (34.5)
Obesity, n (%)	24 (70.6)	58 (51.3)	13 (48.1)	95 (54.6)
At 6 month post-partum Q2 (SD)	26.57 (4.7)	25.37 (4.49)	24.98 (3.9)	25.54 (4.4)
< 18.50 (underweight), n (%)	1 (3.0)	3 (2.8)	-	4 (2.4)
18.50–24.99 (normal range), n (%)	11 (33.3)	56 (51.4)	15 (55.6)	82 (48.5)
≥ 25.00 (overweight), n (%)	16 (48.5)	35 (32.1)	8 (29.6)	59 (34.9)
≥ 30.00 (obesity), n (%)	5 (15.2)	15 (13.8)	4 (14.8)	24 (14.2)
At 14 months post-partum Q3 (SD)	26.23 (4.3)	25.40 (4.8)	24.22 (3.7)	25.37 (4.5)
< 18.50 (underweight), n (%)	1 (3.1)	2 (1.8)	-	3 (1.8)
18.50–24.99 (normal range), n (%)	10 (31.3)	58 (52.3)	19 (70.4)	87 (51.2)
≥ 25.00 (overweight), n (%)	16 (50.0)	34 (30.6)	6 (22.2)	56 (32.9)
≥ 30.00 (obesity), n (%)	5 (15.6)	17 (15.3)	2 (7.4)	24 (14.1)
Employment status Q1				
Gainfully employed	24 (70.6)	77 (68.1)	19 (70.4)	120 (69.0)
Student	4 (11.8)	10 (8.8)	1 (3.7)	15 (8.6)
Maternity leave	3 (8.8)	11 (9.7)	3 (11.1)	17 (9.8)
Unemployed	1 (2.9)	3 (2.7)	-	4 (2.3)
On sick-leave	2 (5.9)	12 (10.6)	4 (14.8)	18 (10.3)
Work description Q1				
Mainly sitting	8 (23.5)	16 (14.0)	6 (33.3)	30 (17.2)
Physical active	18 (52.9)	58 (50.9)	10 (38.5)	89 (49.4)
Alternate sitting/physically active	8 (23.5)	40 (35.1)	10 (38.5)	58 (33.3)
Physically challenging	8 (24.2)	38 (33.9)	8 (33.3)	54 (32.0)
Physically easy	13 (39.4)	33 (29.5)	6 (25.0)	52 (30.8)
Alternate physically challenging/easy	12 (36.4)	41 (36.6)	10 (41.7)	63 (37.3)
Mentally challenging	5 (16.7)	35 (32.1)	8 (32.0)	48 (29.3)
Mentally not challenging	11 (36.7)	17 (15.6)	4 (16.0)	32 (19.5)
Alternate mentally challenging/not challenging	14 (46.7)	57 (52.3)	13 (52.0)	84 (51.2)
Intellectually stimulating	14 (42.4)	56 (50.5)	8 (33.3)	78 (46.4)
Intellectually not stimulating	5 (15.2)	10 (9.0)	4 (16.7)	19 (11.3)
Alternate intellectually stimulating/not stimulating	14 (42.4)	45 (40.5)	12 (50.0)	71 (42.3)
Hypermobility diagnosis Q1				
Yes	7 (20.6)	23 (20.5)	9 (33.3)	39 (22.5)
No	27 (79.4)	89 (79.5)	18 (66.7)	134 (77.5)

Table 1 Descriptive information of the study group *(Continued)*

Number of visits to healthcare providers the past 6 months at Q3, median (IQR)				
Acupuncture	-	4 (4–4)	1 (1–1)	2.5 (1–2.5)
Chiropractic	-	5 (2–5)	1 (0–1)	2 (1–6)
Medical doctor	-	1 (1–1.25)	2 (1–2.5)	1 (1–2)
Naprapathy	-	3 (1–3)	5.5 (3–5.5)	3 (2–6.5)
Physiotherapy	-	3 (1–5.25)	7 (1–12)	3 (1–7.5)
Other (including visits to midwife)	-	2 (1–2)	1 (1–1)	1 (1–2.5)

Numbers in parenthesis are percentage unless otherwise specified
[a]'No pain' denotes respondents reporting remission of LBP/PGP at Q3
[b]'Recurrent pain' denotes respondents reporting recurrent LBP/PGP at approximately 14 months post-partum at Q3
[c]'Continuous pain' denotes respondents reporting continuous LBP/PGP at approximately 14 months post-partum at Q3

leave at all measure points compared to women reporting 'recurrent' pain at Q3.

This cohort had complete baseline information on all subjects and is to the best of the authors' knowledge the first study that has investigated long-term prevalence, pattern and degree of sick leave among women reporting PLBP/PGP during pregnancy. Studies on LBP in the general population show previously reported sick leave and episodes of LBP are predictors of poor outcome and thus persistence of symptoms and delayed recovery rate

Table 2 Sick leave and degree of sick leave due to PLBP/PGP at Q1, Q2 and Q3 with 95 % confidence intervals. Test for difference between respondents and non-respondents (Pearson's Chi test)

	No pain[a]		Recurrent pain[b]		Continuous pain[c]		Non-respondents	
	Number of subjects	95 % CI[e]	Number of subjects	95 % CI[e]	Number of subjects	95 % CI[e]	Number of subjects	p-value[d]
	34		115		27		24	
Sick leave Q1, N (%)								
Yes	16 (72.7)	1.07–1.47	61 (67.8)	1.22–1.42	22 (84.6)	1.01–1.30	10 (58.8)	0.271
No	6 (27.3)		29 (32.2)		4 (15.4)		7 (41.2)	
Sick leave Q2, N (%)								
Yes	2 (5.9)	1.86–2.02	5 (4.4)	1.92–1.99	6 (22.2)	1.61–1.95	1 (4.2)	0.554
No	32 (94.1)		108 (94.7)		21 (77.8)		23 (95.8)	
Sick leave Q3, N (%)								
Yes	-	-	6 (5.3)	1.91–1.99	5 (18.5)	1.66–1.97	-	-
No	3 (8.8)		108 (94.7)		22 (81.5)		-	
Degree of sick leave Q1, N (%)								
Full-time	8 (47.1)	1.29–2.01	50 (73.5)	1.20–1.51	19 (82.6)	1.00–1.61	10 (90.9)	0.276
Part-time	7 (41.2)		12 (17.6)		1 (4.3)		-	
Both full- and part-time sick leave	2 (11.8)		6 (8.8)		3 (13.0)		1 (9.1)	
Degree of sick leave Q2, N (%)								
Full-time	2 (100)	-	4 (80.0)	0.64–1.76	6 (100)	-	1 (100.0)	0.773
Part-time	-		1 (20.0)		-			
Degree of sick leave Q3, N (%)								
Full-time	-	-	4 (66.7)	0.79–1.88	3 (60.0)	0.72–2.08	-	-
Part-time	-		2 (33.3)		2 (40.0)		-	

[a]'No pain' denotes respondents reporting remission of LBP/PGP at Q3
[b]'Recurrent pain' denotes respondents reporting recurrent LBP/PGP at approximately 14 months after pregnancy at Q3
[c]'Continuous pain' denotes respondents reporting continuous LBP/PGP at approximately 14 months after pregnancy at Q3
[d]Respondents vs.non- respondents at Q3
[e]95 % confidence interval (CI) regarding sick leave yes/no and degree of sick leave at Q1, Q2 and Q3
Significance test p < 0.05

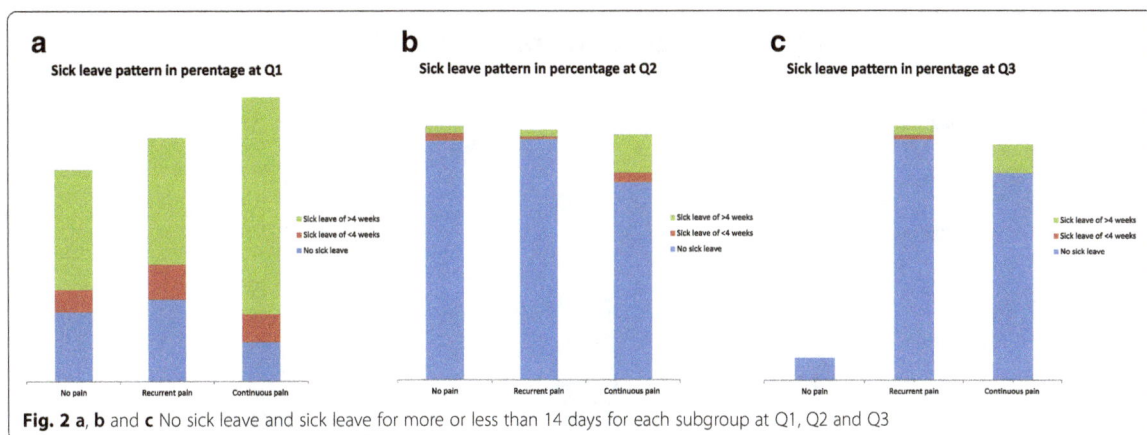

Fig. 2 a, **b** and **c** No sick leave and sick leave for more or less than 14 days for each subgroup at Q1, Q2 and Q3

[8, 26–28]. Thus, there may be reason to believe that sick leave due to persistent PLBP/PGP during and shortly after pregnancy is a risk factor to consider in terms of long-term problems postpartum. Other potential risk factors known to influence poor outcome/persistency of symptoms in regard both LBP and PGP are, but not limited to, age, marital status, duration of symptoms, psychological stress, low levels of physical activity, heavy physical work, high BMI, hypermobility, level of education and reduced SRH [1, 8, 11, 23, 28–33].

It is well established that thoughts, feelings and beliefs of an individual have significant impact on LBP [34]. In addition, individual coping strategies are considered important contributors to future disability in regard to LBP and psychosocial factors appear to exacerbate the clinical component of pain [34, 35]. The presence of emotional distress during pregnancy is shown to be associated with poor outcome [36] and catastrophizing and disability during pregnancy have been shown to increase the risk of postpartum lumbopelvic pain [37].

Albeit the questionnaire used in this study did not include any psychosocial factors with the exception of relationship satisfaction and family situation, reduced SRH has shown to negatively influence the recovery of LBP [29]. In addition, we have demonstrated in a previous paper that women with persistent PLBP/PGP postpartum and 'continuous' pain reported less favourable health status compared to women with 'recurrent' pain [1]. Thus, previous sick leave and poorer SRH could contribute to why women reporting 'continuous' pain at Q1 also reported a higher degree of long-term sick leave at Q2 and Q3.

Healthcare utilisation
Somewhat surprisingly this study shows that women with persistent PLBP/PGP at Q3 had not sought any healthcare service during the past 6 months (Fig. 4). In a previous study, we demonstrated that women with 'continuous' pain did report statistically higher pain intensity compared to women with 'recurrent' pain [1]. However,

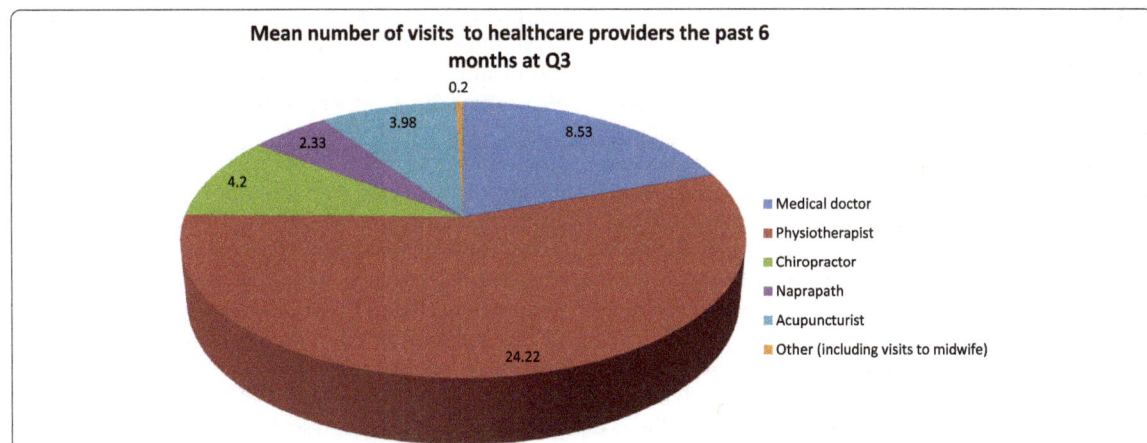

Fig. 3 Number of visits to healthcare providers the past 6 months at Q3

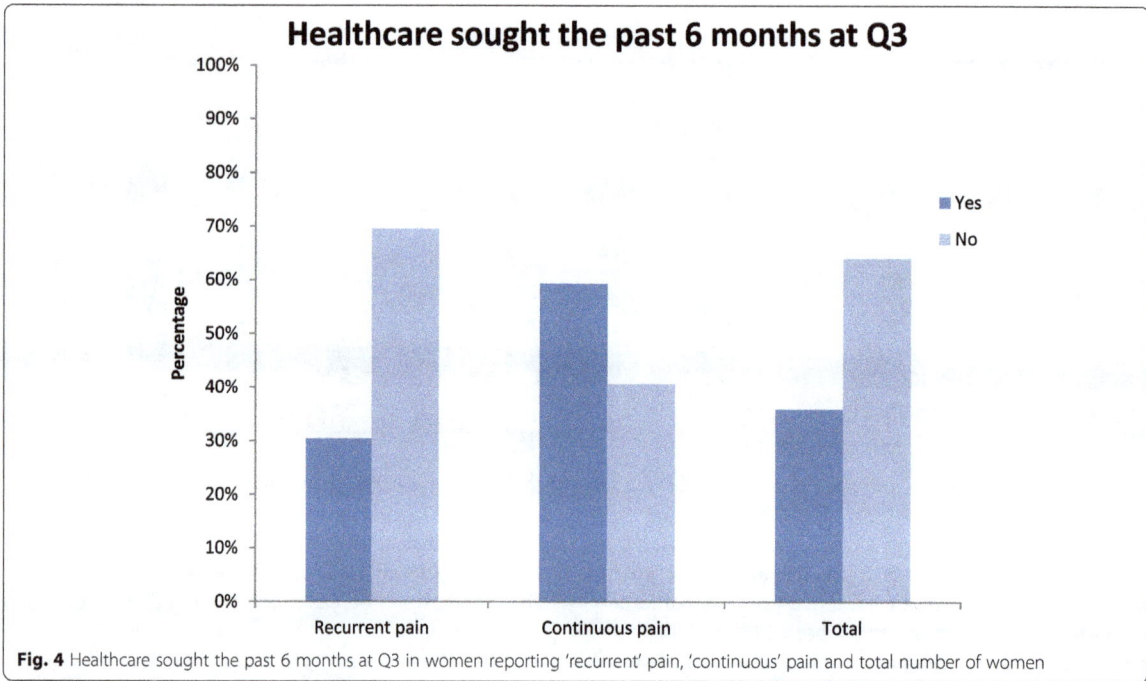

Fig. 4 Healthcare sought the past 6 months at Q3 in women reporting 'recurrent' pain, 'continuous' pain and total number of women

the most important reason for seeking healthcare in the general LBP population has shown to be high levels of disability and not pain itself [38], which could partly explain why most women with persistent PLBP/PGP do not seek care. Most participants may still be on parental leave hence not affecting their work performance or prevent them from taking care of their infant. Another reason could be that there are no effective treatments for this condition today [39–41] and many women with persistent PLBP/PGP postpartum may feel brushed aside by healthcare professionals due to lack of information regarding persistent PLBP/PGP and/or believing themselves that symptoms will subside with time [42, 43]. However, those who seek healthcare appear to suffer from more severe back pain with more functional limitation and demonstrate poorer health-related-quality-of-life scores compared to non-healthcare seekers [44], which can also be a possible explanation to our findings. In a study of the same cohort, we have demonstrated that women with 'continuous' pain have a higher likelihood of poorer SRH compared to women with 'recurrent' pain [1]. These prior findings could therefore explain why women with 'continuous' pain sought care to a higher extent compared to women with 'recurrent' pain at Q3 (Fig. 4).

In this study physiotherapy was the most common sought therapy the past 6 months at Q2 and Q3 among women with 'recurrent' and 'continuous' pain. Physiotherapy in Sweden is well integrated in the public healthcare system and referral from MD is most often

not necessary. In addition, there is a reduced patient's fee, subsidized by the county council, when visiting a public or private practicing physiotherapist. However, a systemic review from 2003, investigating the effectiveness of physiotherapy in women with PLBP/PGP, is inconclusive regarding its effectiveness [45]. The majority of women in this study did report at Q3 that physiotherapy had 'some effect' on their symptoms. However, data is lacking in regard to what kind of treatment was received during the physiotherapy visits.

Stuge et al. [22] examine the long-term effect of physiotherapy with core-stabilizing exercises compared to physiotherapy without core-stabilizing exercises (control group) in women with persistent PGP postpartum. Their study shows a significant difference between the treatment group and the control group where low levels of pain and disability are maintained in the treatment group 2 years postpartum [22]. However, their control group show a significant improvement in functional status from 1 to 2 years after delivery. Conversely, a review article by Ferreira et al. [46] conclude that more high quality randomized clinical trials are needed as evidence regarding effectiveness of physiotherapy in regard to pregnancy related LBP and/or PGP is inconclusive.

Consultation with a medical doctor was the next most commonly sought health service and was also somewhat expected, as MDs are the only health professionals licensed in Sweden to prescribe analgesics (with the exception of dentists and veterinarians). Other aspects that could have affected the number of visits to the MD are that a person on sick leave for more than 1 week needs a sick leave certificate issued by a MD and every fourth person in Sweden believes that a referral issued by a MD is necessary to see a physiotherapist [47]. The majority of women did not find that analgesics had a good effect on their symptoms. Moreover, it is difficult to determine the the effect a specific painkiller had on reported symptoms, as no information was available in respect to what kind of painkillers were used. For instance, recent research shows that paracetamol does not have any effect on LBP symptoms [48, 49]. In addition, paracetamol does not show any effect on pain, disability, function, global system change, sleep quality or quality of life, casting doubt concerning the universal endorsement of the use of paracetamol for LBP [48, 49]; therefore, there are reasons to believe that the same is true for PLBP/PGP.

Acupuncture treatment was reported to have 'some' to 'good' effect on symptoms in women with 'recurrent' and 'continuous' pain at both Q2 and Q3. A study by Elden et al. [50] show that acupuncture has some improvement on performing daily activities; however, acupuncture has no effect on PGP symptoms or the degree of sick leave compared to sham treatment. Unfortunately, information was lacking in regard to the perceived effect of chiropractic and naprapathy on symptoms. To the best of the authors' knowledge, there is a lack of evidence in regard the effectiveness of spinal manipulative therapy (SMT) in women with persistent PLBP/PGP postpartum [39]. Nevertheless, there are some studies that indicate that SMT may decrease pain symptoms as well as having a positive effect on function in women experiencing PLBP/PGP during pregnancy [20, 41, 51]. Other treatment consisted of several different treatments (i.e. stretch exercises, ultrasound treatment, Reiki healing, osteopathic treatment, exercise programs and massage therapy) making it impossible to say what kind of treatment had a good perceived effect on symptoms.

In concurrence with this study, a recently published study demonstrate that individuals with self-reported musculoskeletal pain during the past two weeks show a statistically significant increase in utilisation of general healthcare services [18]. In addition, individuals with primary pain sites from the neck and low back are more likely to seek care from a physiotherapist or chiropractor [18].

Methodological considerations
There are some methodological considerations that need to be addressed in this study. This study commenced in 2002 and at that time no international definition of PGP was available [4]. Instead, pain drawings were used to indicate the location of pain in the pelvic/lumbar area [23]. As a result of the introduction of international definitions and that pain sites of PGP often correlate with common pain location of LBP, some of the cases in our study might be misclassified. However, the lifetime prevalence of LBP is considered stable [52], while pelvic girdle pain increase during pregnancy [33]. In addition, we have previously demonstrated that most women indicated a 'mixed pain location' (back and front of the lumbopelvic area), indicating a strong likelihood that the pain drawings in this study are mostly related to PGP [1]. There also appear to be an increased risk of persistent PGP in women experiencing both LBP and PGP during pregnancy [2, 53]. Thus, a misclassification of noncases would result in an underestimation of associations.

In this study, sick leave was self-reported and could thus be considered a limitation. However, self-reported sick leave is shown to have good agreement with recorded information on number of sick-days, thus retrospectively collected self-reported numbers of sick-days can be useful when registered data are not available [54]. There is also a risk that sick leave was underreported in this study. According to the Swedish Parental Leave Act [55], both mothers and fathers can be on parental leave until the child is 18 months old making it plausible that many women might still have been on parental leave at Q3, thus not bothering to report sick leave to the Swedish Social Insurance Agency as long as their problems did not affect their ability to take care of their infant.

Conclusion
In summary, the main findings in this cohort study was that the majority of women did neither report sick leave nor sought any healthcare services during the past 6 months at Q3 despite reporting 'recurrent' or 'continuous' pain. However, women with more pronounced problems ('continuous' pain) did report a higher prevalence and degree of sick leave and healthcare seeking behaviour compared to women with less pronounced problems ('recurrent' pain). Women with more pronounced problems might constitute a specific subgroup of patients with persistent PGP where the long-term outcome is less favourable. More research is needed in regard to sick leave and healthcare utilisation due to persistent PGP postpartum, powered to determine associations between previously reported poor prognostic factors and sick leave postpartum as well as care-seeking behaviour.

Clinicians need to be attentive that PLBP/PGP may not be transient for some women; instead some will become chronic in nature. Consequently, pregnant women may need to be screened early in pregnancy as well after childbirth facilitating early and customized treatment intervention for PLBP/PGP, consequently reducing individual suffering and societal cost as well as decreasing the risk of transition into chronicity. More clinical research is needed to evaluate the possible effective treatments for this condition both during pregnancy and postpartum.

Competing interests
The authors declare that they have no competing interests.

Authors' contributions
All authors have read and approved the final manuscript. CB was involved in analysis and interpretation of the data, drafting and revising of the manuscript and has given final approval. MP was involved in the interpretation of data and revision of the manuscript and gave final approval. IM was involved in study design, data collection, interpretation of data and revision of the manuscript, and gave final approval.

Acknowledgements
The authors wish to thank all women who shared their obstetric history and experiences with us. Special thanks to all the midwives, at the two Departments of Obstetrics and Gynecology, who contributed greatly to the initial performance of this study. We also thank all other that have been of assistance in this study. Last but not least, we wish to thank the project assistant for excellent work. This study was made possible through grants from the County Council of Västerbotten and Umeå University.

Author details
[1]Department of Clinical Sciences, Obstetrics and Gynecology, Umeå University, Umeå, Sweden. [2]Department of Nursing, Umeå University, Umeå, Sweden.

References
1. Bergstrom C, Persson M, Mogren I. Pregnancy-related low back pain and pelvic girdle pain approximately 14 months after pregnancy - pain status, self-rated health and family situation. BMC Pregnancy Childbirth. 2014;14:48.
2. Gutke A, Ostgaard HC, Oberg B. Predicting persistent pregnancy-related low back pain. Spine (Phila Pa 1976). 2008;33:E386–93.
3. Noren L, Ostgaard S, Johansson G, Ostgaard HC. Lumbar back and posterior pelvic pain during pregnancy: a 3-year follow-up. Eur Spine J. 2002;11:267–71.
4. Vleeming A, Albert HB, Ostgaard HC, Sturesson B, Stuge B. European guidelines for the diagnosis and treatment of pelvic girdle pain. Eur Spine J. 2008;17:794–819.
5. Kanakaris NK, Roberts CS, Giannoudis PV. Pregnancy-related pelvic girdle pain: an update. BMC Med. 2011;9:15.
6. Wu WH, Meijer OG, Uegaki K, Mens JM, van Dieen JH, Wuisman PI, et al. Pregnancy-related pelvic girdle pain (PPP), I: Terminology, clinical presentation, and prevalence. Eur Spine J. 2004;13:575–89.
7. Gutke A, Josefsson A, Oberg B. Pelvic girdle pain and lumbar pain in relation to postpartum depressive symptoms. Spine (Phila Pa 1976). 2007;32:1430–6.
8. Albert HB, Godskesen M, Korsholm L, Westergaard JG. Risk factors in developing pregnancy-related pelvic girdle pain. Acta Obstet Gynecol Scand. 2006;85:539–44.
9. Juhl M, Andersen PK, Olsen J, Andersen AM. Psychosocial and physical work environment, and risk of pelvic pain in pregnancy. A study within the Danish national birth cohort. J Epidemiol Community Health. 2005;59:580–5.
10. Mogren I. Perceived health, sick leave, psychosocial situation, and sexual life in women with low-back pain and pelvic pain during pregnancy. Acta Obstet Gynecol Scand. 2006;85:647–56.
11. Mogren IM. BMI, pain and hyper-mobility are determinants of long-term outcome for women with low back pain and pelvic pain during pregnancy. Eur Spine J. 2006;15:1093–102.
12. Mogren IM. Physical activity and persistent low back pain and pelvic pain post partum. BMC Public Health. 2008;8:417.
13. Robinson HS, Mengshoel AM, Bjelland EK, Vollestad NK. Pelvic girdle pain, clinical tests and disability in late pregnancy. Man Ther. 2010;15:280–5.
14. Vos T, Flaxman AD, Naghavi M, Lozano R, Michaud C, Ezzati M, et al. Years lived with disability (YLDs) for 1160 sequelae of 289 diseases and injuries 1990–2010: a systematic analysis for the Global Burden of Disease Study 2010. Lancet. 2012;380:2163–96.
15. SBU. Metoder för behandling av långvarig smärta. En systematisk litteraturöversikt. Stockholm: Statens beredning för medicinsk utvärdering (SBU); 2006. SBU-rapport nr 177/1. ISBN 91-85413-08-9.
16. Eriksen J, Sjogren P, Ekholm O, Rasmussen NK. Health care utilisation among individuals reporting long-term pain: an epidemiological study based on Danish National Health Surveys. Eur J Pain (Lond Engl). 2004;8:517–23.
17. Hojsted J, Alban A, Hagild K, Eriksen J. Utilisation of health care system by chronic pain patients who applied for disability pensions. Pain. 1999;82:275–82.
18. Hartvigsen J, Davidsen M, Sogaard K, Roos EM, Hestbaek L. Self-reported musculoskeletal pain predicts long-term increase in general health care use: a population-based cohort study with 20-year follow-up. Scand J Public Health. 2014;42:698–704.
19. Albert H, Godskesen M, Westergaard J. Prognosis in four syndromes of pregnancy-related pelvic pain. Acta Obstet Gynecol Scand. 2001;80:505–10.
20. Sadr S, Pourkiani-Allah-Abad N, Stuber KJ. The treatment experience of patients with low back pain during pregnancy and their chiropractors: a qualitative study. Chiropr Man Therap. 2012;20:32.
21. Ostgaard HC, Zetherstrom G, Roos-Hansson E. Back pain in relation to pregnancy: a 6-year follow-up. Spine (Phila Pa 1976). 1997;22:2945–50.
22. Stuge B, Veierod MB, Laerum E, Vollestad N. The efficacy of a treatment program focusing on specific stabilizing exercises for pelvic girdle pain after pregnancy: a two-year follow-up of a randomized clinical trial. Spine (Phila Pa 1976). 2004;29:E197–203.
23. Mogren IM, Pohjanen AI. Low back pain and pelvic pain during pregnancy: prevalence and risk factors. Spine (Phila Pa 1976). 2005;30:983–91.
24. Hartvigsen J, Nielsen J, Kyvik KO, Fejer R, Vach W, Iachine I, et al. Heritability of spinal pain and consequences of spinal pain: A comprehensive genetic epidemiologic analysis using a population-based sample of 15,328 twins ages 20–71 years. Arthritis Rheum. 2009;61:1343–51.
25. Linton SJ, Boersma K. Early identification of patients at risk of developing a persistent back problem: the predictive validity of the Orebro Musculoskeletal Pain Questionnaire. Clin J Pain. 2003;19:80–6.
26. Leboeuf-Yde C, Gronstvedt A, Borge JA, Lothe J, Magnesen E, Nilsson O, et al. The nordic back pain subpopulation program: demographic and clinical predictors for outcome in patients receiving chiropractic treatment for persistent low back pain. J Manipulative Physiol Ther. 2004;27:493–502.
27. Hestbaek L, Leboeuf-Yde C, Manniche C. Low back pain: what is the long-term course? A review of studies of general patient populations. Eur Spine J. 2003;12:149–65.
28. Costa Lda C, Maher CG, McAuley JH, Hancock MJ, Herbert RD, Refshauge KM, et al. Prognosis for patients with chronic low back pain: inception cohort study. BMJ. 2009;339:b3829.
29. Thomas E, Silman AJ, Croft PR, Papageorgiou AC, Jayson MI, Macfarlane GJ. Predicting who develops chronic low back pain in primary care: a prospective study. BMJ. 1999;318:1662–7.
30. George C. The six-month incidence of clinically significant low back pain in the Saskatchewan adult population. Spine (Phila Pa 1976). 2002;27:1778–82.
31. Larsen EC, Wilken-Jensen C, Hansen A, Jensen DV, Johansen S, Minck H, et al. Symptom-giving pelvic girdle relaxation in pregnancy. I: Prevalence and risk factors. Acta Obstet Gynecol Scand. 1999;78:105–10.
32. Ostgaard HC, Andersson GB. Previous back pain and risk of developing back pain in a future pregnancy. Spine (Phila Pa 1976). 1991;16:432–6.
33. Ostgaard HC, Andersson GB, Karlsson K. Prevalence of back pain in pregnancy. Spine (Phila Pa 1976). 1991;16:549–52.
34. Linton SJ. A review of psychological risk factors in back and neck pain. Spine. 2000;25:1148–56.
35. Pincus T, Burton AK, Vogel S, Field AP. A systematic review of psychological factors as predictors of chronicity/disability in prospective cohorts of low back pain. Spine. 2002;27:E109–20.
36. Bjelland EK, Stuge B, Engdahl B, Eberhard-Gran M. The effect of emotional distress on persistent pelvic girdle pain after delivery: a longitudinal population study. BJOG. 2013;120:32–40.
37. Olsson CB, Nilsson-Wikmar L, Grooten WJ. Determinants for lumbopelvic pain 6 months postpartum. Disabil Rehabil. 2012;34:416–22.
38. Ferreira ML, Machado G, Latimer J, Maher C, Ferreira PH, Smeets RJ. Factors defining care-seeking in low back pain–a meta-analysis of population based surveys. Eur J Pain (Lond Engl). 2010;14:747. e1-7.
39. Close C, Sinclair M, Liddle SD, Madden E, McCullough JE, Hughes C. A systematic review investigating the effectiveness of Complementary and Alternative Medicine (CAM) for the management of low back and/or pelvic pain (LBPP) in pregnancy. J Adv Nurs. 2014;70:1702–16.
40. Liddle SD, Pennick V. Interventions for preventing and treating low-back and pelvic pain during pregnancy. Cochrane Database Syst Rev. 2015;9: CD001139.

41. Stuber KJ, Smith DL. Chiropractic treatment of pregnancy-related low back pain: a systematic review of the evidence. J Manipulative Physiol Ther. 2008; 31:447–54.

42. Wuytack F, Curtis E, Begley C. The health-seeking behaviours of first-time mothers with persistent pelvic girdle pain after childbirth in Ireland: A descriptive qualitative study. Midwifery. 2015;31:1104–9.

43. Wuytack F, Curtis E, Begley C. Experiences of First-Time Mothers With Persistent Pelvic Girdle Pain After Childbirth: Descriptive Qualitative Study. Phys Ther. 2015;95:1354–64.

44. Cote P, Cassidy JD, Carroll L. The treatment of neck and low back pain: who seeks care? who goes where? Med Care. 2001;39:956–67.

45. Stuge B, Hilde G, Vollestad N. Physical therapy for pregnancy-related low back and pelvic pain: a systematic review. Acta Obstet Gynecol Scand. 2003; 82:983–90.

46. Ferreira CW, Alburquerque-Sendi NF. Effectiveness of physical therapy for pregnancy-related low back and/or pelvic pain after delivery: a systematic review. Physiother Theory Pract. 2013;29:419–31.

47. Fysioterapeuterna. Ny undersökning: Varannan svensk saknar kunskap om remissfriheten (In Swedish). 2011. http://www.fysioterapeuterna.se/Om-forbundet/nyheter/2011/2011/Nyundersokning-Varannan-svensk-saknar-kunskap-om-remissfriheten-/. Accessed January 16 2016.

48. Machado GC, Maher CG, Ferreira PH, Pinheiro MB, Lin CW, Day RO, et al. Efficacy and safety of paracetamol for spinal pain and osteoarthritis: systematic review and meta-analysis of randomised placebo controlled trials. BMJ. 2015;350:h1225.

49. Williams CM, Maher CG, Latimer J, McLachlan AJ, Hancock MJ, Day RO, et al. Efficacy of paracetamol for acute low-back pain: a double-blind, randomised controlled trial. Lancet. 2014;384:1586–96.

50. Elden H, Ladfors L, Olsen MF, Ostgaard HC, Hagberg H. Effects of acupuncture and stabilising exercises as adjunct to standard treatment in pregnant women with pelvic girdle pain: randomised single blind controlled trial. BMJ. 2005;330:761.

51. Peterson CD, Haas M, Gregory WT. A pilot randomized controlled trial comparing the efficacy of exercise, spinal manipulation, and neuro emotional technique for the treatment of pregnancy-related low back pain. Chiropr Man Therap. 2012;20:18.

52. Leboeuf-Yde C, Nielsen J, Kyvik KO, Fejer R, Hartvigsen J. Pain in the lumbar, thoracic or cervical regions: do age and gender matter? A population-based study of 34,902 Danish twins 20–71 years of age. BMC Musculoskelet Disord. 2009;10:39.

53. Gausel AM, Kjaermann I, Malmqvist S, Dalen I, Larsen JP, Okland I. Pelvic girdle pain 3–6 months after delivery in an unselected cohort of Norwegian women. Eur Spine J. 2015.

54. Voss M, Stark S, Alfredsson L, Vingard E, Josephson M. Comparisons of self-reported and register data on sickness absence among public employees in Sweden. Occup Environ Med. 2008;65:61–7.

55. Försäkringskassan. https://www.forsakringskassan.se/wps/wcm/connect/76573377-cea7-4eda-8e7d-f93bb6f62d0a/4070-foraldrapenning-1512.pdf?MOD=AJPERES. Accessed January 16 2016.

11

The role of information search in seeking alternative treatment for back pain: a qualitative analysis

Hoda McClymont[1*], Jeff Gow[2,3] and Chad Perry[1]

Abstract

Background: Health consumers have moved away from a reliance on medical practitioner advice to more independent decision processes and so their information search processes have subsequently widened. This study examined how persons with back pain searched for alternative treatment types and service providers. That is, what information do they seek and how; what sources do they use and why; and by what means do they search for it?

Methods: 12 persons with back pain were interviewed. The method used was convergent interviewing. This involved a series of semi-structured questions to obtain open-ended answers. The interviewer analysed the responses and refined the questions after each interview, to converge on the dominant factors influencing decisions about treatment patterns.

Results: Persons with back pain mainly search their memories and use word of mouth (their doctor and friends) for information about potential treatments and service providers. Their search is generally limited due to personal, provider-related and information-supply reasons. However, they did want in-depth information about the alternative treatments and providers in an attempt to establish apriori their efficacy in treating their specific back problems. They searched different sources depending on the type of information they required.

Conclusions: The findings differ from previous studies about the types of information health consumers require when searching for information about alternative or mainstream healthcare services. The results have identified for the first time that limited information availability was only one of three categories of reasons identified about why persons with back pain do not search for more information particularly from external non-personal sources.

Keywords: Back pain, Information search, Search effort, Complementary and alternative treatments, Australia

Background

Health consumers are moving away from a heavy reliance on medical practitioner advice to more independent decision processes [1,2]. In countries such as Australia, the United Kingdom and the United States shared decision making and patient self-management are key components of health policy [3]. There are five steps to the consumer health decision making process: need recognition; information search; evaluation of alternatives; purchase decision and post-purchase behavior [4]. In this paper a qualitative examination of the second step, information search, in managing chronic back pain is undertaken.

Information search is particularly relevant to consumers with chronic diseases where doctors cannot recommend one best treatment that will solve the problem [2,5]. One such chronic condition is back pain caused by musculoskeletal disease. Traditionally, information about solutions to back pain and the available treatments has been provided by mainstream health providers such as physiotherapists and, in more serious cases, by surgeons. However, more recent trends indicate that an increasing number of persons with back pain are turning to alternative or complementary treatments such as chiropractic treatments, homeopathy, naturopathy, Bowen therapy, kinesiology and reflexology [5]. This change in treatment direction combined with the multitude of treatment solutions necessitates factual and effective information in order to guide consumer's choices.

* Correspondence: hoda@usq.edu.au
[1]School of Management and Enterprise, University of Southern Queensland, 4350 Toowoomba, QLD, Australia
Full list of author information is available at the end of the article

This area of research is particularly important because back pain is a significant problem affecting people globally [6]. In industrialised countries, more than 80 per cent of people will experience back pain sometime in their life and up to half of the workforce will suffer at least one episode of back pain each year resulting in work absences, lower productivity and increased costs to businesses [6]. For example, half of all working Americans experience back pain each year and it is one of the most common reasons for missing work [7]. In the United Kingdom, there are approximately three million persons with back pain and of the 131 million working days lost to sickness, 34.4 million are due to musculoskeletal conditions such as back pain, neck pain and limb problems [8]. In turn, musculoskeletal disorders are the leading cause of disability in Australia; they accounted for more disability than any other medical condition with 14% (2.8 million people) experiencing back pain and disc disorders [9].

Despite this significance of back pain problems and a trend towards alternative information sources and treatment options, little is known about the information search processes used by persons with back pain to select appropriate treatment types and service providers in particular. This gap is important because persons with back pain search behavior are the *start* of any treatment chain. Other research has addressed search behavior by patients and/or patients' families searching for information about areas like hospitals, physicians and healers [10-12], aged care homes [11], mental health services [13] and cancer [14,15]. Recent research has covered search behavior on the internet for health related issues that did not include back pain [16,17]. But persons with back pain overall information search behavior has not been researched [18] and so requires some qualitative investigation to uncover.

This study aims to extend previous research on information search in healthcare by using the convergent interviewing methodology to investigate how persons with back pain apply three essential elements of the search process to acquire information about treatment types and service providers: what sources do they use and why; what information content do they seek and how; and how do they search for it?

The next section briefly reviews literature on information search in the health care context. Then data collection and analysis methods of convergent interviewing used in this research are described. Analysis of the research data to develop schemas of information search behaviour by persons with back pain, and their implications, follow.

Prior theory - information search

This research extends prior theory to back pain situations and so that theory needs to be established first. Accessing the right information efficiently reduces uncertainty and anxiety [2] and guides the decision making of health consumers. To undertake this information search, a typical consumer has to decide on three key issues that became the three research questions about back pain that drove the data collection and analysis phases of this research: where to search for it [19], what information content to look for [20], and how much search effort to expend when looking for information [21].

Information sources

Firstly, consider sources of information. The literature on information search identifies two main sources: internal and external sources. Internal search comprises searching one's memory to access information about solutions to an existing problem [19,22,23]. This information is basically stored knowledge and experiences gathered over time [24]. Thus prior knowledge is a key to undertaking any effective search for it provides the basis for evaluating new information in later, external search. Furthermore, prior knowledge has been shown to influence both the amount and type of information sought. However, this influence appears to be context specific [25] with certain contexts leading to more information search with greater knowledge while others lead to less information search with greater knowledge [26]. Despite its contextual nature, no studies were found on the use of internal information search within a health care context. Thus, the question arises about how much consumers with back pain rely on their memories (internal sources) for treatment type and service provider information and how does this internal search impact the amount and type of external information search?

In turn, if internal information is deficient, external information sources are usually used. External information search constitutes seeking information from the outside environment [24]. In contrast to the scant research about internal sources, some research findings are available about external information sources used to make health treatment and service provider selections [10,27-29]. For example, [30] suggested that information about mainstream health care services is effectively distributed through external sources such as pamphlets, health professionals and formal educational programs. However, other studies indicate that information search by patients does not rely on these sources and instead uses more "personal" external sources; for example, information about general health matters could be sought from family members, friends, work colleagues and doctors [1,31]. For back pain, studies show booklets and physical-related cues might be effective but other sources like video are not [32,33]. Other external sources about back pain are online [34,35]. But are these *all* the sources for back pain information? This was the first research question.

Information content

The second issue raised in the information search literature is the nature of the content of the information patients look for or indeed avoid looking for [12,36]. The information content sought by health consumers is context specific [20]. For example, [37] found that women going through menopause searched for information to work out which symptoms were 'normal' for their age group; which symptoms they experienced were related to menopause; to get information to prepare for their visit to the doctor, and to later confirm the doctor's diagnosis and expand their knowledge of issues raised by the doctor. As another example, parents of children often have concerns and require specific information to combat misconceptions, and address their doubts about the safety/efficacy of treatments [38]. A final example relates to female cancer patients' whereby women search for information topics relating to therapies available, how to manage a recurrence of cancer if a treatment stops working, types of surgery that can be undertaken for the cancer and pain issues [39]. What context-specific information do persons with back pain seek? This was the second research question.

Search effort

The third element of information search behavior is the search effort expended by consumers. While the search effort construct [40,41] is well recognized and accepted in the marketing literature, there does not appear to be an accepted way to measure it. For example [42], measured this construct using two items: the amount of time and the amount of effort used to locate information [43] also measured search effort for home shoppers using the single item of the number of advertisements referred to in catalogues [21] defined search effort based on the number of sources consulted and the amount of effort required to gather and comprehend information. In health care research [44], measured internet search effort based on a single scale of measuring the extent of agreement/disagreement with the statement: "it took a lot of effort to get the information you needed". Other health care research investigating information search behaviours appear to ignore this issue totally [45]. In brief, search effort has been measured using time, number of sources, effort level or a combination thereof. But what defines search effort by persons with back pain? This was the third and final research question.

Methods

Qualitative research methods are appropriate for the investigation of how and/or why a social phenomenon occurs, and are therefore appropriate for this study's research problems [46,47]. That is, "the aim of qualitative research is to develop concepts that can help us understand social phenomena in natural settings, giving emphasis on the meanings, experiences and views of the participants" [48], p.11. The qualitative method of convergent interviewing was selected. It involved a series of long, initially rather unstructured interviews [49-51]. The interviewer analysed the data and refined the interview questions after each interview, to converge on the emerging issues in the topic area. In brief, flexible exploration of this complex and sensitive topic was possible through the convergent interviewing technique.

This convergent interviewing methodology is *justified* for this research in four ways [50]. Firstly, it converges quickly on important issues. The required number of interviewees in convergent interviewing should be less than traditional interviewing's because any points of convergence or divergence among interviewees are examined after each interview to develop the questions and probes for the next interview; that is, the methodology is a thorough one. Moreover, this efficiency is important when interviewees are time-limited, like many of the busy interviewees in this research project. Secondly, convergent interviewing has a mechanism for knowing when to stop collecting data – the "stability" described below. Finally, it sets a sound stage for further research methodologies such as case research.

However, there are limitations related to convergent interviewing as a research methodology. Firstly, convergent interviews are time consuming and require many consecutive interviews with many different people [46]. But the analysis after each interview allowed a convergence on key issues, and the use of the prior theory permitted a focus on important issues. Secondly, there is a risk of bias because the researcher, as the interviewer, is a participant in the data collection process. This risk was mitigated by the researcher's understanding and experience of the methodology and her use of appropriate interview techniques [52]. Moreover, the methodology's analysis after each interview reduces bias that may exist in traditional interviewing's one-off data analysis process that starts after the final interview. Indeed, the methodology could perhaps be called 'convergent and divergent interviewing' because explanations for any differences of opinion are probed for in each interview. Next, convergent interviewing is an exploratory technique and therefore should be used in conjunction with later research, and this limitation is acknowledged in the 'further research' section below. Finally the lack of interviewee validation could result in misinterpretation of the results by the researcher, but asking interviewees to decide the validity of the social-scientific rendering of interpretations of the interviews would be unreasonable because of their lack of discipline-specific knowledge [53].

Interviews were conducted with adult persons with back pain who had sought either one or more types of treatment for their problem. Study participants were recruited in Australia through notices in physiotherapy practices, government offices and one university. The twelve interviewees were purposively selected to ensure gender, age and educational balance in the sample, as shown in Table 1.

A key question is, "How many interviews should have been conducted?" The answer to this question about convergent interviewing revolves around the concept of "stabilty" or "saturation" when no new information or patterns in the data emerge from the interviews [54]. This stabilty depends on the skill of the interviewer, the type of research problem, the cases themselves, and the depth of data analysis [55], p.245 summarises this difficulty of deciding how many interviews are needed: "The validity, meaningfulness and insights generated from qualitative inquiry have more to do with the information-richness of the cases selected and the observational/analytical capabilities of the researcher than with sample size." The interviewer was an experienced qualitative researcher who had previous interviewing experience and who had a working knowledge of the subject matter.

Estimates of the required number of interviews vary. That minimum can be about six [54,55], 10 [56] or 15 [57]. The maximum can be about 50 [56,58]. Stability is often reached after only five or so convergent interviews [50]. The final convergent interview occurs when interview data analysis of that interview shows there is stability through a consistent pattern of agreements and disagreements in the last two interviews [46,50,51]. In this study, this stability appeared after the eleventh interview. To ensure that stability had been reached, an additional interview was conducted but no new information emerged.

At each interview, the researcher clarified a number of administrative issues including ethical clearance and whether the interview could be taped. The opening question was broad [46] and then detail-oriented probes, elaboration probes, and clarification probes were used within the interview [59]. Incidentally, "back pain" is defined in

this report in general terms: "a pain in the lumbar, lumbo-sacral, or cervical regions of the back, varying in sharpness and intensity. Causes may include muscle strain or pressure on the root of a nerve" [60]. Each interview ran for approximately 60 minutes and was taped and then transcribed before analysis. Each interview was transcribed within a day of the interview and the transcript was triangulated with the notes taken by the researcher during the interview. The interviewer undertook preliminary analysis of each of the interview transcripts and accessed literature about issues that emerged as a result of the interview in order to better understand the subject matter. These steps allowed the researcher to modify the interviewer's guide as necessary (in line with the convergent interviewing methodology) to obtain more detailed and relevant information in the following interviews.

Data reduction was undertaken to condense data to assist in the development of a conceptual framework. Thus, transcripts were coded into themes and sub-themes according to the issues identified during the literature review. The three themes were information sources, information content and search effort although each of these were further divided into sub-themes such as internal information sources, external personal sources and external non-personal sources under the information sources theme. Where new and contrary information was found in the data, these were coded to new categories and discussed later. Next, the data from the various coded themes and sub-themes were linked together to find regularities and make sense of the data [61]. These regularities were tallied in a table next to each theme or sub-themes and the interviewee number and quote recorded alongside them.

In order to validate findings and their interpretations, one researcher undertook the analysis and discussed the findings with the other researchers. Next, the analysis was put aside for some time and then returned to by the researcher and re-analysed. This action resulted in some minor errors in the initial interpretations. These were rectified by revisiting the interview transcripts to clarify what the interviewees had said and assessing the logic with which ideas were categorized into a theme or sub-theme based on prior literature and data reduction techniques.

Ethical approval was obtained from the University of Southern Queensland's Human Research Ethics Committee (Ethical Approval number: H05REA495).

Results and discussion

Research question 1: what sources of information do persons with back pain use, and why?

Persons with back pain use a variety of internal, external personal (subjective) and external non-personal (objective) information sources during decision making, as summarized in Table 2, where the relative importance of each item is estimated.

Table 1 Sample characteristics of convergent interview interviewees (n = 12)

	Frequency		Frequency
Gender		**Highest education level**	
Females	5	Secondary	5
Males	7	Post secondary	2
		Tertiary	5
Age			
Less than 25 years		**Occupation**	
25 – less than 40 years	2	Professional	6
40 – less than 60 years	3	Semi-professional	2
	7	Trades	1
		Student	2
		Disability pension	1

Table 2 Information sources used to select treatment types/service providers

Information sources	Interviewees	No. of interviewees using each source	Rank of frequency of sources used
Internal source – memory of past knowledge and experiences	1, 2, 3, 4, 5, 7, 8, 9, 10, 11, 12	6	2
External personal sources			
Word of mouth – friends	1, 2, 4, 5, 7, 9, 11	7	1
Doctor/other therapists' referrals	1, 4, 5, 7, 9, 11	6	2
Word of mouth – family	1, 5, 8, 9	4	3
Word of mouth – work colleagues	1, 2, 6, 12	4	3
Speaking with a provider prior to appointment	2, 10	2	5
Word of mouth - other (for example, teacher, receptionist at my doctor's practice)	3, 10	2	5
External non-personal sources			
Yellow/white pages	1, 2, 3, 8	4	3
Promotional sign at provider's office	2, 3, 11	3	4
Internet	5, 7	2	5
Books	5	1	6
Radio talk back show	7	1	6

One of the two most important sources of information is *internal*. Almost all interviewees (11 of 12 interviewees) stated using internal sources in one or more of their decision making situations for back pain treatment selection This frequent use of internal information sources (including past knowledge and/or personal experiences) reflects other consumer research about services that require experience to evaluate [4] and indicates that persons with back pain tend to rely on their own memories. But how comprehensive and accurate is their internal information?

In order to ascertain how accurate and comprehensive interviewee's knowledge and experiences were, they were asked to explain why they chose the treatment type that they had. The majority (66%, or interviewees 2, 3, 4, 5, 7, 8, 9, 12) of interviewees explained that they had made their choices based on their perceptions of their back problem, their perception of what each treatment type could offer and thus which would be most suitable for their problem. For example, interviewee 9 said:

'I thought my muscles were tight from sitting at the computer every day at work so the masseuse would relax my muscles. I didn't think I had a medical problem to be sorted out by a chiropractor or physiotherapist'.

Misconceptions and biases about chiropractors and physiotherapists

An interesting finding was that most interviewees had misconceptions of the nature of their problem and workings of chiropractic and physiotherapy treatments even though these treatments were the ones most used by interviewees. Some misconceptions were:

- That they perceived their bones were 'out' of their spine' and that they needed to be 'put back in'

Chiropractors manipulate the bones and put them in so they loosen the muscles but they don't retighten them. Physiotherapists don't actually put the bones in but they make the muscles work so that the bones go in by themselves. I know this from my suppositions mainly and from talking to physiotherapists (Interviewee 3).

But, I knew chiropractors put bones back into place and so in my first accident when I popped a vertebra out I knew a chiropractor would put the bones back into place ... I picked [Bowen Therapy] because I thought that chiropractors put people's bones into place but I also knew that muscles keep your bones in place and so there is no point getting your bones put into place if they (your muscles) are not working right. So I wanted to go to Bowen therapy (Interviewee 5).

I chose a chiropractor because I knew it was something structural – something was 'out' and it had to be put back in. And my perception is the physiotherapists work more with muscles and give massage and exercise things. But I felt like something had gone out so I just felt like I needed to have it pushed back in (Interviewee 9).

- That physiotherapists have nothing to do with treating pain and muscle spasm:

When people think of physiotherapists, they don't think of them as people who could help heal muscle spasm and pain. And people think of chiropractors as aligning the back which has little to do with muscle pain and spasm (Interviewee 2).

- That physiotherapists and chiropractors only deal with injuries and rehabilitation

I liked the notion that chiropractors could deal with the manipulation ....like the operation of a chiropractic move. Like, they are realigning what you have. So if your back is causing you grief due to the tension that you may be carrying around then they can realign the neck and fix your headache. Whereas other treatments, I am not sure how they work but I don't like the idea of taking a tablet for a headache. I would rather deal with the cause. I always associate physiotherapists with sports injury and rehabilitation (for example, people who have their arm in a cast and they build the muscle up.' (Interviewee 10).

- That chiropractors are only helpful for non-specific back pain

Chiropractors are good for general back pain which I initially had. The treatments allowed me to wake up in the mornings without feeling stiff. They straightened my back which was crooked and I will go back for my general back pain to them but not for the spondylolisthesis. *I try to stretch my treatments to 4–5 weeks now* (Interviewee 7).

- That physiotherapists are better than chiropractors or vice versa

'I thought of seeing a chiropractor but what I had learnt about physiotherapists and chiropractors was the physiotherapists were better' (Interviewee 4).

Knowledge and experience void relating to alternative treatments

Unlike the multitude of opinions provided about physiotherapy and chiropractic care, some interviewees appeared not to know as much or express strong opinions about other treatment types (interviewees 5, 6, 7, 10, 11). Therefore, they relied mainly on their emotions and memories of vicarious learning and recommendations made by others to select a treatment type. For example, interviewee 7 chose an acupuncturist because of desperation rather than because of his knowledge of the treatment: *'I chose this type of treatment out of desperation and the lack of success with physiotherapists and chiropractors. Also, I was curious about this type of treatment and wondered what*

benefits it could have.' Interviewee 10 chose chiropractors because she did not like needles despite the fact that acupuncture needles do not function in the same way that injections do: *' I always associate physiotherapists with sports injury and rehabilitation (for example, people who have their arm in a cast and they build the muscle up. And, I don't like acupuncture because I don't like needles'.* Interviewee 5 said: *'I found out about Reiki from mum and her books'.* Respondent 1 used memories of vicarious learning to select a treatment type: *'I didn't really know anything about physiotherapists and chiropractors other than they help with pain. But I knew that my sister had had luck with a chiropractor and so I just chose to go to them'* (Interviewee 1).

However, once interviewees had had back problems for some time and had experienced a treatment, they used various criteria to decide on the treatment type and provider. Therefore, their criteria for selection included their past knowledge as well as their present experience with which to construct their decision.

Biased attitudes towards non-mainstream treatments

Some interviewees revealed biases against non-mainstream treatments. For example, interviewee 11 was biased against non-mainstream treatments because of his rural upbringing: *'The others (acupuncture, osteopath or any treatment outside of physiotherapy and chiropractors) are voodoo. ... well I come from a rural background and family members and people I associate with said to go to a physiotherapist. You wouldn't go to a chiropractor because they could injure you, crack your bones. As far as any alternative things like acupuncture – they are extreme'.*

Similarly, interviewee 4 showed bias toward alternative treatments like chiropractic care based on his experience:

I thought of seeing a chiropractor but what I had learnt about physiotherapists and chiropractors, was the physiotherapists were better. I knew a chiropractor as a friend when I told him my symptoms, he said that I am better off with a physiotherapist who works with musculoskeletal issues rather than spinal issues (which is what a chiropractor does).

External sources

Persons with back pain also rely on *external* personal sources to provide credence about the treatment and service they seek. Two external personal sources are word of mouth by friends, and referrals by doctors and other therapists. Other external personal sources used include word of mouth by family and work colleagues, speaking with a provider prior to booking an appointment, and speaking with others such as teachers and receptionists.

External non-personal sources are not used as much as external personal sources, because they do not have the credence of personal sources [4], as discussed below. These external non-personal sources include the telephone directory, advertising signage outside the provider's office, the internet, books and talk-back shows.

No interviewee relied solely on an internal source, even if they have past experience and knowledge to fall back on – all those using an internal source also used an external personal source, and some of them used an external non-personal source as well. Clearly, for back pain services, credence is required as well as experience [4].

Effectiveness of external personal sources

One question that remains unanswered in the literature is how effective are external personal sources in achieving positive treatment outcomes? To investigate this issue, a summary of all incidents in which interviewees outlined information sources used to select a treatment type and subsequent treatment outcomes was developed (refer Table 3).

Table 3 summarises 26 incidents where interviewees had selected a treatment provider based on word of mouth. Of the 26 incidents, only 12 (46.2%) had positive outcomes. A positive outcome is defined as adequate relief of symptoms for an acceptable period of time as judged by the respondent. The other 14 incidents were 11 (42.3%) who had no symptom relief (a negative outcome) and another 3 (11.5%) who had some symptom relief but were not fully satisfied (a somewhat positive outcome). In brief, we propose that although word of mouth is heavily relied on for decisions about which treatment type and provider to use, it might not be the most effective source to use. Further research is warranted to establish the validity of this finding and to identify any other factors which may be contributing to this outcome.

In brief, the findings of the internal and external information sources indicated that persons with back pain have and obtain little if any accurate information about the nature of their problem and what different treatments can and should be used for. As a result, interviewees' final choice of treatment type is based more on trial and error. This finding is supported by a cancer study in which its noted that many patients do not know how to access credible information and make informed decisions about cancer [62].

One poorly resolved issue in the literature relates to the reasons for the limited use of some information sources and this research makes a contribution about this issue. In particular, why are not more external non-personal sources used? Three categories of reasons for *not* searching more extensively for external information about treatment types or service providers emerged in the interviews. First, many interviewees provided *personal* reasons for not searching for information such as:

- A lack of interest as noted by interviewee 11:

I don't look for much information about what my problems are or treatments because usually you are so busy and flat out that you, sort of, are very reactive in everything you do....

- Not wanting to self- diagnose:

Nowadays I suppose you could look on the internet but I don't reckon I would do that probably because I would rather be led by an expert rather than have a look at a whole lot of stuff and start deciding... (Interviewee 12).

- Being able to self-diagnose as stated by interviewee 9: 'No I didn't look for any other information because being a nurse, you self-diagnose a lot.'

The second category of reasons for limiting search of external non-personal sources can be labeled provider-related. Two reasons were offered:

- Loyalty to the treatment provider. For example, interviewee 3 said that her loyalty stopped her from searching for information: "He [the physiotherapist] was the one I went to 25 years ago after my high jump accident, I had success with him and I was ... loyal."

- The provider provided sufficient information about their treatment relative to other providers.

I didn't look for any other information because on my first consultation with the chiropractor, they took me through what chiropractic care is and how it differs from a doctor, physiotherapist or acupuncturist. So I felt they gave me enough information (Interviewee 10).

Finally, *information-supply reasons* for limited use of external sources included reasons such as patients not knowing what information to look for, where to look for information, or the information not being readily available. For example, interviewees 7 and 12 both believed that information was not readily available. Interviewee 7, who suffers from spondylolisthesis, a rare spinal pressure produced by the forward dislocation of one vertebra over the one beneath it, said that he had only looked for information about this problem on the Internet because it is a very specific condition and information could not be found through general sources such as general interest magazines. Interviewee 2 also found it difficult to find information readily and said:

It was difficult to find information about back pain. The Yellow Pages [telephone directory] just had names

Table 3 External personal sources used to select treatment types/service providers

Interviewee	External source	1st ever treatment	2nd treatment	3rd treatment	Treatment outcome
1	WOM – family		Pain subsided from chiropractor		Positive
1	WOM - friend			Pain subsided from physiotherapy	Positive
2	WOM - colleague		Pain subsided from masseuse		Positive
3	WOM – teacher		Paid subsided from chiropractor		Positive
4	GP - referral	Pain relief but problem progressively worsened with physiotherapy			Negative
4	GP - referral		Some pain relief but got problem got progressively worse with physiotherapy		Negative
4	GP - referral			Some pain relief but got problem got progressively worse with physiotherapy	Negative
5	WOM – friends	Inadequate length of pain relief from chiropractor			Negative
5	WOM – family		No pain relief with colour therapy		Negative
5	WOM – family			Inadequate length of pain relief	Negative
6	WOM - colleague	Unhappy with chiropractor's behaviour			Negative
6	WOM – friends		Inadequate length of pain relief from acupuncture		Somewhat positive
6	WOM – friends			Inadequate length of pain relief from acupuncture	Somewhat positive
7	GP and WOM – friends	Not totally pain free with physiotherapy			Somewhat positive
7	WOM – friends		In adequate relief of symptoms with chiropractor		Negative
7	WOM - friend			No pain relief from acupuncture	Negative
8	WOM - mum	Adequate pain relief with chiropractor			Positive
8	WOM and marketing sources		Adequate pain relief with chiropractor		Positive
9	WOM friends/others	Adequate pain relief with chiropractor			Positive
10	Chiropractor's referral		Adequate pain relief		Positive
10	Chiropractor's referral			Adequate pain relief	Positive
11	WOM –friends	Inadequate pain relief			Negative
11	GP referral		Adequate pain relief		Positive
11	WOM – friend and family			Inadequate pain relief	Negative
12	WOM - friend	Adequate pain relief			Positive
12	WOM - friend		Adequate pain relief		Positive

Table 3 External personal sources used to select treatment types/service providers *(Continued)*

All	Total treatment outcomes	**26**
All	Total 'somewhat positive' outcomes*	**3 (11.5%)**
All	Total 'positive' outcomes	**12 (46.2%)**
All	Total negative outcomes	**11 (42.3%)**

*Note: somewhat positive outcomes frequency was excluded from the final calculation because of the outcomes were not satisfactory enough for the patient to remain loyal to the practitioner.

and contact details of physiotherapists and chiropractors but they didn't have a list of people who could assist with back pain."

In turn, interviewee 1 did not know what information to look for or where to look for it: *"I didn't look for information because I didn't know what to look for or where to look for it ... there wasn't any real information in your face."*

In brief, internal and only external *personal* sources of information are most important for persons with back pain. External non-personal information in not as used because of personal, provider or supply related reasons.

Research question 2: what information content is sought by persons with back pain, and how?

Interviewees sought information about two items: their *treatment options*, and their choice of service providers within a selected treatment option. The content sought about treatment options included information about the types of back problems that exist and their symptoms; the types of treatment options that exist and the specific symptoms they address or benefits they have; how each treatment option works and its origins; the efficacy of each treatment option; and self-help tips.

In addition to information sought about treatment options, interviewees wanted information about *service providers* including:

1. Finding service providers within each treatment type and their area of expertise. For example, interviewee 6 said: *"I ended up talking to friends to find out ... which ones [acupuncturists] were good to go to."*
2. Service providers' reputation. For example, interviewee 10 said:

"I went and saw Dr X and he fixed my neck and I went out and my mum was talking to her [the receptionist] about my prescription and how Dr X realigned my neck and she said "I go to a really good chiropractor if you are looking for one" and then she suggested X Chiropractic."

3. Provider's contact details. For example, interviewee 8 said: *"I found out about him through mum ... Then I jumped on the Internet for the White Pages to find his number..."*

4. Proximity to provider. For example, interviewee 1 looked through the Yellow Pages to locate a chiropractor close to where she lived. In turn, interviewee 2 said that he was in pain and walked by the masseuse therapist's shop and decided to go in for a massage. He made this decision because he was in city Y at the time that he experienced this pain and so could not wait to see his masseuse back home in city X.

5. How speedily an appointment could be obtained with the provider. For example, interviewee 11 said: *"And I needed someone that I could get into straight away..."*

6. Accessibility of the provider to discuss matters before making an appointment. For example, interviewee 2 searched for information about a provider by phoning a masseuse therapist, telling him about his problem and asking him what he could do about it.

The relationship between information content and information source

Another issue, not highlighted in the extant literature, emerged from the interview data: there was a link between some information items sought about treatment options and about service providers, and the types of information sources used to locate such information. Figure 1 shows these linkages, with treatment options and service providers on the left and information sources on the right.

To begin, information about *treatment options* was sourced through internal sources (when it was available), and through several external personal and external non-personal sources, as shown in Figure 1. Next, consider the findings about the linkages about *service provider* information and information sources, as also summarized in Figure 1. These linkages had three patterns. First, information about the availability of providers practicing a treatment type and their reputation and expertise was sourced mainly through internal sources (such as past experience) and external personal sources including word of mouth from friends, family, colleagues, doctors and others. Second, very specific information about a service provider such as the contact details, location of practice, speed of obtaining an appointment and access to the provider before an appointment, was sourced mainly from external sources such as the telephone directory, signage outside the practice and through direct contact with the provider prior to

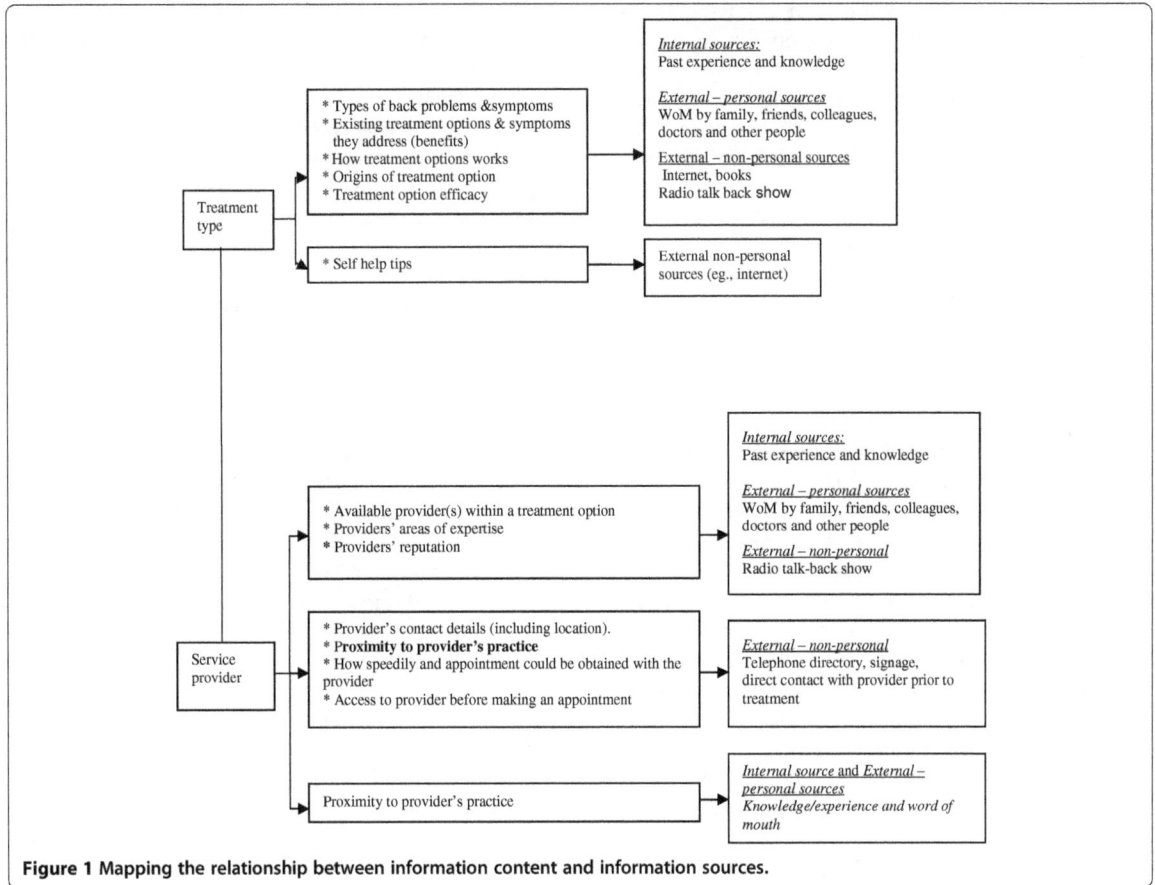

Figure 1 Mapping the relationship between information content and information sources.

treatment bookings. Third, information about the location of a service provider's practice was also sourced through internal sources (that is, past experience and knowledge) and through external personal sources of word of mouth.

In brief, the context-specific items of information sought by persons with back pain were identified for the first time, and the linkages between their sources of information and type of information were identified for the first time for any health care patient.

Research question 3: How do persons with back pain search for information?

The meaning of "search effort" emerged as the number of sources used and whether a patient deliberately or incidentally looked for information prior to making a decision. The term "deliberately" refers to situations where interviewees made a deliberate decision to look for information. By contrast, situations are categorized as "incidentally" when interviewees were exposed to certain information even though they were not deliberately searching for it. This distinction between deliberate and incidental search effort has not been identified before.

First, consider *deliberate* search through the examples provided by interviewees. Naturally, the decision was a deliberate one when the interviewee referred to their memory banks (internal information) to select a suitable treatment type and service provider (for example, interviewees 3, 8 and 9). Similarly, deliberate search was undertaken by interviewees who sought information externally through the Yellow/White Pages, the internet, books, doctors, speaking with service providers before the appointment and, in some cases, speaking with family members (for example, interviewees 1, 2, 4, 5 7, 8 and 10).

Interviewees who deliberately consulted family members about their back problems and sought assistance from them, were dependents living at home. Of the five interviewees (interviewees 1, 3, 5, 8 and 10) who did consult family members, four did so to obtain assistance. For example, the younger, dependent interviewees 3, 5, 8 and 10 had all told their parents about their pain and their parents had then suggested a course of action such as seeing a doctor (interviewees 3, and 10) or seeking treatments from providers such as a reiki healer and a physiotherapist (interviewees 5 and 8). Only interviewee 1 (an adult living independently) did not consult her family for specific back pain assistance, and raised the issue only in conversation with them.

Next, consider *incidental* search. Incidental search occurred when interviewees did not usually deliberately attempt to find information but were exposed to it from external sources such as from colleagues, friends, advertising signs on providers' doors and talkback shows. For example, interviewees 6, 7, 11 and 12 were having a general conversation with a work colleague and the issue of back pain arose as a topic in the conversation. In brief, it became evident from the analysis that search effort is a function of deliberate or incidental search.

Implications

The findings of this research have *implications* for public and private health sectors, and also for marketing management researchers. Persons with back pain rely mainly on internal information and external personal word of mouth by their doctor and friends which does not appear to provide an effective strategy for choosing treatment types and providers. Therefore, the public health system could provide more treatment related information about mainstream *and* complementary and alternative treatments. Furthermore they could provide generic information about how to select a service provider (for example, what steps to take to find a reputable and qualified service provider with the desired area of expertise) through a range of media. As a first option, information can be channeled through GP practices, in preference to the television and radio shows that have been shown to be more effective for the less information savvy, health conscious consumer [28]. However, research indicates that GPs may be unlikely to refer patients to complementary and alternative treatments due to their lack of belief in them [63]. This stance could be due to the fact that many GPs are not familiar with the research advances relating to alternative treatments like chiropractic care and massage. Therefore, an alternative solution is to use social workers who are trained in complementary and alternative treatments [62] and who understand physiology and anatomy. These professionals can assist patients to explore choices, discuss concerns, ask questions to increase understanding and make more informed decisions without judgment or bias.

As well, this information could be channeled through printed pamphlets/booklets in back health professional practices aimed at persons with back pain and their family and friends who are more health conscious and information savvy. Of course, the psychographic and media profiles of all these segments may need to be researched as a precursor to this action.

The findings of this study also have implications for health service providers. Knowledge of the information content required by interviewees can be used to better communicate services so that consumers can make better decisions. Service providers have two options: they can provide information about their service only and/or provide additional information about other competing treatment options available and compare the differences/benefits to their specific treatment offering. Service providers can also target this information through various media. Some of these media include more personal sources like the word of mouth of their own patients (who speak with friends and family) and office staff as well as their websites, pamphlets located in doctor's practices (for more in-depth treatment and service related information), radio advertising, signage and the telephone directory (for contact details and other specific service provider related queries). In order to provide personal ratings of the practice and provider, the websites could host a patient review site where past and present patients can discuss the outcomes of their experiences and even suggest improvements. The website could also provide an appointment availability function whereby patients could book or cancel appointments and find out if appointment slots are available when needed.

Next, the research has implications for market researchers. The convergent interviewing methodology was an efficient and effective way of undertaking inductive research in an under-researched area and so could be used in similar research projects. However, two limitations are evident from this study, each providing grounds for *further research* into this topic. One limitation relates to the sample size, which although adequate for constructing a preliminary model of search behavior, requires statistical generalization (theory testing) through a survey to complement the analytic generalization (theory building) of this research [47]. A final limitation is that we were not able to find any strong deviations in interviewee's answers and this could be because of the sample size. Further *quantitative* research about information search should be undertaken to investigate the presence of deviations in responses and investigate the roles of demographic, psychographic, behavioural and back pain characteristics on response differences.

Conclusions

This study has explored how persons with back pain search for information when trying to choose from a range of treatment options and service providers. Three main issues were researched: where to search for information, what information to search for, and how much effort to expend searching. In terms of where to search for information, persons with back pain rely heavily on their own memories (internal) and external personal sources such as friends and doctors when searching for information about treatment types and service providers. However, more often than not, these perceptions are wrong, biased or too limited to provide a useful guide for decisions.

These findings differ from the findings of previous studies [30] about the types of information health consumers require when searching for information about alternative or mainstream healthcare services. First, internal search was not mentioned in the literature even though it is the source most used and appears to be inaccurate, and interviewees did not rely to any extent on pamphlets. The results have identified for the first time that limited information availability was only one of three categories of reasons identified about why persons with back pain do not search for more information particularly from external non-personal sources.

Next, this study confirms findings from other research [36] that information *content* sought by patients is health context specific. For example, some interviewees required information about self-help techniques for their back problem. Examples of service related information content included the speed with which an appointment with the provider could be obtained, a providers' area of expertise and their reputation. In turn, this research outlined for the first time the exact information items sought by interviewees for both back pain treatment types and service providers, and its linkages to sources. Furthermore, extending previous studies [36], this research showed that the sheer number of treatment options and service providers required interviewees to undertake a more complex search step (combining internal search, and external personal and non-personal search) than in some other health care areas.

Finally, the information sources used by persons with back pain are a function of the information content they seek; this link is a new finding. For example, the use of external non-personal sources such as the telephone directory, contacting the provider directly or using practice signage was reserved for acquiring more detailed service provider information such as the speed of acquiring an appointment; whereas information about the provider's reputation and expertise was obtained from internal and other external personal sources. This situation reflects the information available from each source rather than the information search preferences of these persons with back pain, as evidenced by the reasons given for their low reliance on external non-personal sources.

Competing interests
The authors declare they have no competing interests.

Authors' contributions
HM conceived of the study, conceived the research design, conducted the interviews, undertook data analysis and wrote the first draft of the manuscript and approved the final manuscript. JG assisted in the research design, assisted in the data analysis and wrote additional sections of the second draft of the manuscript as well as writing the final version of the manuscript and approving the final manuscript. CP advised on research design and wrote some sections of the second draft of manuscript and approved the final manuscript.

Acknowledgements
The authors would like to thank the 12 participants who shared their back pain treatment journeys with us.

Author details
[1]School of Management and Enterprise, University of Southern Queensland, 4350 Toowoomba, QLD, Australia. [2]School of Commerce, University of Southern Queensland, Toowoomba, Australia. [3]Research Associate, Health Economics and HIV/AIDS Research Division (HEARD), University of KwaZulu-Natal, Westville Campus, Durban, South Africa.

References
1. Stewart DW, Hickson GB, Pechmann C, Koslow S, Altemeier WA: Information search and decision making in the selection of family health care. *J Health Care Market* 1989, 9(2):29–39.
2. Sepucha KR, Belkora J: **Putting shared decision making to work in breast and prostate cancers: tools for community oncologists.** *Comm Oncol* 2007, 4(11):685–689.
3. Fullwood C, Kennedy A, Rogers A, Eden M, Gardner C, Protheroe J, Reves D: **Patients' experiences of shared decision making in primary care practices in the United Kingdom.** *Med Decis Making* 2013, 33(1):26–36.
4. Kotler P, Keller K: *Marketing Management.* New York: Prentice Hall; 2008.
5. Yen L, Jowsey T, McRae S: **Consultation with complementary and alternative medicine by older Australians: Results from a national survey.** *BMC Complement Altern Med* 2013, 13(73):1–8.
6. Disease Control Priorities Project: *Musculoskeletal Conditions are the Most Common Cause of Chronic Disability;* 2007. Available at: http://www.dcp2.org/file/84/DCPP-Musculoskeletal.pdf (accessed 12 May 2013).
7. American Chiropractic Association: *Back Pain Facts and Statistics;* 2013. Available at: http://www.acatoday.org/level2_css.cfm?T1ID=13&T2ID=68 (accessed 5 September 2013).
8. Office for National Statistics: *31 Million Days Lost to Sickness in 2011 – but it's Falling;* 2012. Available at: ons.gov.uk/ons/rel/mro/news-release/131-million-working-days-lost-to-sickness-in-2011—but-it-s-falling/sanr0512.html, (accessed 21 October 2012).
9. Australian Bureau of Statistics: *Health.* Year Book Australia; 2012. Available at http://www.abs.gov.au/ausstats/abs@.nsf/Lookup/by%20Subject/1301.0~2012~Main%20Features~Health%20status~229. (accessed 21 October 2012).
10. Harris KM: **How do patients choose physicians? Evidence from a national survey of enrolees in employment-related health plans.** *Health Serv Res* 2003, 38(2):711–732.
11. McClymont H: **Search and evaluation behaviours in hospital selection of rural health consumers.** *Asian J Mark* 2005, 11(1):81–91.
12. Kind T, Wheeler K, Robinson B, Cahana M: **Do leading children's hospitals have quality websites? A description of children's hospital web sites.** *J Med Internet Res* 2004, 6(2):e20.
13. Lipscomb T, Root T, Shelley K: **Strategies for seeking mental health services.** *Serv Mark Q* 2004, 25(4):1–12.
14. Kwon N, Kyunghye K: **Who goes to a library for cancer information in the e-health era? A secondary data analysis of the Health Information National Trends Survey (HINTS).** *Lib Info R* 2009, 31(3):192–200.
15. Weber K, Solomon D, Meyer B: **A qualitative study of breast cancer treatment decisions: evidence for five decision making styles.** *Health Commun* 2013, 28(4):408–421.
16. Huh J, DeLorme DE, Reid LN, Kim J: **How Korean and White Americans Evaluate and Use Online Advertising and Non-advertising Sources for Prescription Drug Information.** *Ther Inno Reg Sci* 2013, 47(1):116–124.
17. Park J, Chung E, Yoo WS: **Is the internet a primary source for consumer information search?: Group comparison for channel choices.** *J Retailing & Consumer Services* 2009, 16(2):92–99.
18. Mortimer M, Ahlberg G, MUSIC-Norrtalje Study Group: **To seek or not to seek? Care-seeking behaviour among people with low-back pain.** *Scand J Public Healt* 2003, 31(3):194–203.
19. Moorman C, Diehl K, Brinberg D, Kidwell B: **Subjective knowledge, search, locations and consumer choice.** *J Consum Res* 2004, 31(3):673–680.

20. Wathen NC, Harris RM: I try to take care of it myself. How rural women search for health information. *Qual Health Res* 2007, **17**(5):639–651.

21. Duncan CP, Olshavsky RW: External search: the role of consumer beliefs. *J Marketing Res* 1982, **19**(1):32–43.

22. Rijnsoever FJ, Castaldi C, Dijst MJ: In what sequence are information sources consulted by involved consumers? The case of automobile pre-purchase search. *J Retail Consum Serv* 2012, **19**(3):343–352.

23. Kitamura S: The relationship between use of the internet and traditional information sources: an empirical study in Japan. *SAGE Open* 2013, **3**: doi:10.1177/2158244013489690.

24. Lamb JF, Hair JF, McDaniel C: *Marketing*. Mason: Thompson – South Western; 2009.

25. Rose S, Philip S: Internal psychological versus external market-driven determinants of the amount of consumer information search amongst online shoppers. *J Mark Manag* 2009, **25**(1–2):171–190.

26. Johnson EJ, Russo EJ: Product familiarity and learning new information. *J Consum Res* 1984, **11**(1):542–550.

27. Diviani N, Camerini A, Reinholz D, Galfetti A, Schulz PJ: Health literacy, health empowerment and health information search in the field of MMR vaccination: a cross-sectional study protocol. *BMJ Open* 2012, **19**:2(6).

28. Dutta-Bergman MJ: Primary sources of health information: comparisons in the domain of health attitudes, health cognitions, and health behaviours. *Health Commun* 2004, **16**(3):273–289.

29. Flynn M, Smith M, Freese J: When do older adults turn to the internet for health information? Findings from the Wisconsin longitudinal study. *J Gen Intern Med* 2006, **21**(12):1295–1301.

30. Ansani NT, Bethany MV, Henderson AF, McKaveney TP, Weber RJ, Smither RB: Quality of arthritis information on the Internet. *Am J Health Syst Pharm* 2005, **62**(1):1184–1189.

31. Mahoney C, Heavin C, Sammon D: *A Tool for Analyzing the Information Behavior of Expectant and new Mothers*. Proceedings of the 21st European Conference on Information Systems; 2013. viewed 25 May 2013, < http://www.staff.science.uu.nl/~vlaan107/ecis/files/ECIS2013-0873-paper.pdf.

32. Henrotin YE, Cedraschi C, Duplan B, Bazin T, Duquesnoy B: Information and low back pain management: a systematic review. *Spine* 2006, **31**(11):E326–E334.

33. Little P, Roberts L, Blowers H, Garwood J, Cantrell T, Langridge J, Chapman J: Should we give detailed advice and information booklets to patients with back pain?: a randomized controlled factorial trial of a self-management booklet and doctor advice to take exercise for back pain. *Spine* 2001, **26**(19):2065–2072.

34. Butler L, Foster N: Back pain online: a cross-sectional survey of the quality of web-based information on low back pain. *Spine* 2003, **28**(4):395–401.

35. Li L, Irvin E, Guzmin J, Bombardier C: Surfing for back pain patients: the nature and quality of back pain information on the Internet. *Spine* 2001, **26**(5):545–557.

36. Davey HM, Lim J, Butow PN, Barratt A, Houssami N, Higginson R: Consumer information materials for diagnostic breast tests: women's view on information and their understanding of test results. *Health Expect* 2003, **4**(6):298–311.

37. Genius SK: Constructing "sense" from evolving health information: a qualitative investigation of information seeking and sense making across sources. *J Am Soc Inf Sci Tec* 2012, **63**(8):1553–1566.

38. Kennedy A, LaVail K, Nowak G, Basket M, Landry S: Confidence about vaccines in the United States: understanding parents' perceptions. *Health Affair* 2011, **30**(6):1151–1159.

39. Kim SC, Shah DV, Namkoong K, McTavish FM, Gustafson DH: Predictors of online health information seeking among women with breast cancer: the role of social support perception and emotional well-being. *J Comput-Mediat Comm* 2013, **18**(2):212–232.

40. Webster FE: Modeling of industrial buying behavior. *J Marketing Res* 1965, **2**(4):370–376.

41. Beatty SE, Smith SM: External search effort: an investigation across several product categories. *J Consum Res* 1987, **14**(1):83–95.

42. Bunn MD, Butaney GT, Hoffmann NP: An empirical model of professional buyers' search effort. *J Bus-Bus Mark* 2001, **8**(4):55–84.

43. Sundaram DS, Taylor RD: An investigation of external information search effort: replication in in-home shopping situations. *Advances Consum Res* 1998, **25**:440–445.

44. Geana M, Greiner KA: Health information and the digital divide. *J Manag & Mark Healthcare* 2011, **4**(2):108–112.

45. Enwald HPK, Niemelä RM, Keinänen-Kiukaanniemi S, Leppäluoto J, Jämsä J, Herzig K, Oinas-Kukkonen H, Huotari MA: Human information behaviour and physiological measurements as a basis to tailor health information. An explorative study in a physical activity intervention among prediabetic individuals in Northern Finland. *Health Info Libr J* 2012, **29**(2):131–140.

46. Carson D, Gilmore A, Gronhaug K, Perry C: *Qualitative Research in Marketing*. London: Sage; 2001.

47. Yin RK: *Case Study Research*. 4th edition. London: Sage; 2009.

48. Al-Busaidi Z: Qualitative research and its uses in health care. *Sultan Qaboos University Medical J* 2008, **8**(1):11–19.

49. Driedger SM, Gallois C, Sanders CB, Santesso N: Finding common ground in team-based qualitative research using the convergent interviewing method. *Qual Health Res* 2006, **16**(8):1145–1157.

50. Rao S, Perry C: Convergent interviewing to build a theory in under-researched areas: principles and an example investigation of internet usage in inter-firm relationships. *Qual Mark Res: An International J* 2003, **6**(4):236–247.

51. Rao S, Perry C: Convergent interviewing: a starting methodology for an enterprise research program. In *Innovative Methodologies in Enterprise Research*. Edited by Hine D, Carson D. Northampton: Edward Elgar; 2007.

52. Perry C: *Efficient and Effective Research*. Adelaide: AIB Publications; 2013.

53. Bryman AE: *Member Validation' Accessed: 22 January 2014*. Available at: http://www.referenceworld.com/sage/socialscience/mem_valid.pdf.

54. Guest G, Bunce A, Johnson L: How many interviews are enough? An experiment with data saturation and variability. *Field Method* 2006, **18**(1):59–82.

55. Morse JM: Determining sample size. *Qual Health Res* 2000, **19**(3):3–5.

56. de Ruyter K, Scholl N: Positioning qualitative market research: reflections from theory and practice. *QualMark Res: An International J* 1998, **1**(1):7–14.

57. Betraux D: From the life-history approach to the transformation of sociological Practice. In *Biography and Society: The Life History Approach In The Social Sciences*. Edited by Betraux D. London: Sage; 1981:29–45.

58. Mason M: Sample size and saturation in PhD studies using qualitative interviews. *Forum: Qualitative Science Research* 2010, **11**(3):8.

59. Patton MQ: *Qualitative Evaluation and Research Methods*. 3rd edition. Newbury Park: Sage; 2002.

60. Medical Dictionary: *Medical Definition of Back Pain*; 2013. The Free Dictionary, viewed 28 May 2013, http://medical-dictionary.thefreedictionary.com/back+pain.

61. Miles MB, Huberman AM: *Qualitative Data Analysis (2nd edition)*. Thousand Oaks: Sage; 1994.

62. Runfola J, Levine E, Sherman P: Helping patients make decisions about complementary and alternative treatments: The social work role. *J Psychosoc Oncol* 2006, **24**(1):81–106.

63. Charles C, Gafni A, Whelan T: Self-reported use of shared decision-making among breast cancer specialists and perceived barriers and facilitators to implementing this approach. *Health Expect* 2004, **7**(4):338–348.

12

Attitudes and beliefs of Australian chiropractors' about managing back pain: a cross-sectional study

Stanley I Innes[1*], Peter D Werth[2], Peter J Tuchin[3] and Petra L Graham[4]

Abstract

Background: Chiropractors are frequent providers of care for patients with lower back pain. Biopsychosocial approaches to managing patients are regarded as best practice and are gaining wider acceptance. Recent evidence suggests that practitioners' attitudes and beliefs may also have an important effect on patients' recovery from back pain. Past studies have pooled manual therapists from differing professions. Dissonant findings have been hypothesised as being a result of the chiropractic subpopulation within multi-practitioner participant pools who are hypothesised to focus on biomedical aspects of treatment and minimize biopsychosocial dimensions.
The aim of this study is to determine whether a study population of only chiropractors would demonstrate similar attitudes and beliefs to other manual therapists' biopsychosocial or biomedical approach to the management of their patients.

Methods: A survey of chiropractors in Victoria Australia in September 2010 was undertaken utilising the Pain Attitude and Belief Scale (PABS.PT), a tool which has been developed to determine the orientation (biopsychosocial or biomedical approach) of practitioners to the management of people with low back pain. The survey also obtained demographic data from respondents to determine whether variables such as education, gender or practice related factors influenced their orientation.

Results: The overall response rate was 29% (n = 218). The majority of the sample was male (68%), with a mean age of 44 years. The 6 point Likert scale scores were 34.5 (6.3) for the biomedical factor scale and 31.4 (4.1) for the biopsychosocial scale. Internal consistency of the psychosocial subscale was poor. None of the demographic variables were found to influence the biomedical or psychosocial scales.

Conclusions: Chiropractors in the state of Victoria were found to have similar biomedical and psychosocial orientations in their attitudes and beliefs when compared to other manual therapists' levels of previous studies from differing cultural and educational backgrounds. This study was unable to replicate any of the relationships from past studies with any of the demographic variables. The psychosocial scale internal consistency may be a significant factor in this non-finding. Future research should address the identification of more robust items of the biopsychosocial attitudes of Victorian chiropractors toward treating lower back pain.

Keywords: Low back pain, Chiropractic, Attitudes and beliefs, Biopsychosocial

* Correspondence: s.innes@murdoch.edu.au
[1]Discipline of Chiropractic, Health Professions, Murdoch University, Murdoch, WA 6150, Australia
Full list of author information is available at the end of the article

Background

Low back pain is now the leading cause of disability globally and was estimated to be responsible for 83 million years lived with disability in 2010 [1]. Manual therapists, such as chiropractors, physiotherapists and osteopaths, are a significant consumer choice for the treatment and management of this condition. During 2005, in Victoria Australia, over 3 million people sought care at least once from a chiropractor [2]. While a recent study has documented the type of conditions chiropractors encounter, there has been little research exploring therapists' attitudes and beliefs which may improve patient outcomes and thus reduce levels of associated disability [3].

It is now well established that the problem of persistent low back pain and associated levels of disability are not fully explained by biological factors alone and that best practice care should include more than the musculoskeletal system. There is good evidence that psychological constructs such as pre-existing depression, anxiety, fear-avoidance beliefs, poor coping strategies and poor self-efficacy are significant predictors of greater functional disability and work loss [4]. These constructs appear to play an important role in the transition from the acute setting to persistent pain and disability. Evidence also suggests that social and organisational factors may play a role in these negative outcomes, though the exact mechanism remains unclear [5]. Consequently this investigation sought to expand the understanding of chiropractic interventions by studying these non-mechanical dimensions.

The most dominant current model in understanding these is the biopsychosocial model (BPSM) of health. It describes the influence of the biological, psychological and sociological factors in the manifestation of pain and illness [6]. It may best be considered as a heuristic to better understand these dimensions of care [7]. There are now validated outcome measures stemming from BPSM research that enhances the primary contact practitioner's ability to detect in the early phases this transition into disability [8]. The practitioner is thus able to avoid inappropriate and ineffective passive modalities of care and implement more appropriate interventions [9].

Despite the BPSM recently celebrating its 25th birthday not all manual therapists are cognisant of the impact of the psychological and sociological domains. In response to this various government and insurance agencies have attempted to implement readily applicable assessment frameworks and education programs to improve patient outcomes [10]. Despite these efforts there has been no appreciable diminution of the rates of disability or its financial impost. Psychological and sociological interventions to date have only produced modest changes at best [11]. Subsequently researchers are now beginning to explore other facets of the BPSM.

One line of exploration that researchers have turned their focus toward is that of the attitudes and beliefs of the practitioner [12]. A systematic review of the relationship between practitioners' beliefs and behaviours concluded that there is moderate evidence that practitioners' fear-avoidance beliefs are associated with reported sick leave prescription thus directly influencing patient's behaviour [13]. For example, a practitioner may be overly anxious about the patient exacerbating a lower back injury and may unnecessarily recommend reduced activity, bed rest and time away from work, thus reinforcing pain behaviours. Several studies have now been conducted to explore the possibility of measuring these attitudes and beliefs in various manual therapy groups [14-17].

One instrument used to explore these attitudes is the Pain Attitudes and Beliefs Scale for Physiotherapists (PABS.PT) [16,17]. It was developed in an attempt to identify the extent to which practitioner attitudes and beliefs in two domains; biomedical and/or psychosocial which impact on patients response to lower back pain. While the developers of the PABS.PT state that these domains do not sit on a continuum, several studies have shown a low negative correlation [18-20]. A practitioner who scores highly on the biomedical orientation is thought to have a strong belief that there is a relationship between pain and tissue damage. Those who attain higher scores on the psychosocial dimension are thought to be more likely to believe that lower back pain outcomes are a result of tissue damage and can be influenced by social and psychological factors. Thus it may be possible to identify those practitioners by their high scores on biomedical orientation and low psychosocial orientation who are less likely to follow evidence-based guidelines best quality care and can be assisted with further education interventions to improve the quality of care delivery [18].

The initial version PABS.PT was comprised of 31 items which were extracted from existing psychosocial related questionnaires by an expert physiotherapist panel [16]. Factor analysis revealed two discrete factors: "Biomedical Orientation or factor 1" and "Behavioural Orientation or factor 2" which explained 25% and 8% of the variance respectively. "Biomedical Orientation" demonstrated adequate internal consistency (Cronbach's alpha 0.83) but the "Behavioural Orientation" obtained a Cronbach's alpha of 0.54. Subsequently the authors suggested future research into the items of factor 2 in order to improve its psychometric properties. They recommended the recruitment of practitioners from a variety of professions (orthopaedic surgeons and chiropractors) in order to achieve extreme scores. It was noted that women tended to score higher on both scales than men and men of greater than 42 years of age scored significantly higher on the "Behavioural factor".

Houben et al. [17] continued the psychometric development of the PABS.PT and followed these recommendations by recruiting 295 Dutch physiotherapists, manual therapists and chiropractors. They also selected 5 additional items based on "face value" and added these to the original PABS.PT. These additional items were aimed at enhancing the second factor. Statistical analysis produced a 19 item inventory with 2 factors closely resembling those of Ostelo et al. [16]. Factor 1 (Biomedical Orientation) was best described by 10 items and explained 23.4% (Cronbach's alpha 0.80) of the variance. Factor 2 (BPS orientation) was best described by 9 items and these explained 10% (Cronbach's alpha 0.68) of the variance. No differences were observed on the factors with regard to gender, age or years of work experience. Chiropractors scored significantly lower on factor 2 compared to the other treatment disciplines. Chiropractors also obtained the highest score on the Biomedical factor but this did not reach a level of significance.

Subsequent studies have verified the two factor structure of the PABS.PT [18-21]. These studies have also explored other dimensions and related factors. A significant linear trend of increasing disparity with treatment guidelines as biomedical scores increased and behavioural scores decreased was found in a United Kingdom study who recruited 1012 general practitioners (GPs) and physical therapists [19]. Irish GPs low biomedical scores were more likely to be found in those who were more recently qualified and more likely to follow best practice guidelines, however the authors removed 9 items from the Houben et al. version of the PABS.PT to improve the internal consistency of the questionnaire [18]. Brazilian male physiotherapists and those with less experience were significantly more likely to follow a biomedical approach to the treatment of patients with chronic lower back pain [21]. It should be noted that this Brazilian study summed the short form of the PABS.PT on a 0 = "totally disagree" and 5 = "totally agree" Likert scale as opposed to a "1 through 6" Likert scale standard in prior studies. This Brazilian study, when discussing differences in mean scores on the PABS.PT between previous studies suggested that the high scores could possibly be a result of a group of professionals such as chiropractors who would be expected to have a stronger biomedical orientation.

This suggestion of the chiropractic population possessing different qualities to other health professionals is not without precedent. For example the STarT back screening tool had been developed to help primary care practitioners make care decisions about the likely need LBP patients have for secondary prevention based on modifiable risk factors for poor outcomes [22,23]. It had been validated with physiotherapists and medical practitioners but was unable to be replicated with chiropractors in the UK [24]. The authors suggested several

possibilities for this outcome. First that this was due to patient population differences as these were a self-selecting population who sought chiropractic care privately and as such had a different psychological profile. Other reasons included higher expectations of a positive outcome. They also mused that differences in treatment approaches used by chiropractors could be a factor. Finally they suggested that chiropractors may have consciously or unconsciously addressed the patients' psychological needs. In contrast, a Norwegian study has suggested that psychological factors are not relevant in the prediction of treatment outcomes in chiropractic patients as psychosocial issues constitute a negligible portion of their daily encounters [25].

Other possible explanations for this professional dissonance include the presence of a significant portion who hold unorthodox views [26], a limited research capacity, a lower value placed on scientific knowledge, a short history with decision support systems such as guidelines and a lack of developed coordinated efforts to address low coherence of beliefs and evidence-based practices [27].

Therefore, the primary aim of this study was to further explore chiropractors' attitudes and beliefs in an effort to understand these reported differences. In particular it sought to measure and compare their attitudes and beliefs in regard to biomedical and psychosocial aspects of patient care in a sample of only chiropractors in Victoria, Australia. A secondary aim was to determine if sociodemographic characteristics may be also be associated with their beliefs and attitudes.

Methods

The study consisted of a retrospective survey of chiropractors practising in the state of Victoria Australia in October 2010. Ethical approval was obtained from Human Research Ethics Committee of Macquarie University, New South Wales, Australia (HE25SEP2009-ROO143). All questionnaire responses were completed anonymously, thus written consent was not obtained from individual respondents with completion of the questionnaire indicating consent.

Instruments

The 19 item shortened version PABS.PT was used to evaluate the role of chiropractors' attitudes and beliefs on the development and maintenance of persistent low back pain [17]. Previous studies have produced and validated the presence of 2 discrete scales. The Biomedical scale consists of 10 items which are scored on a 6 point Likert scale (1="totally disagree" to 6 "totally agree") and are summed to produce a score between 0 and 60 points. A high score indicates a belief in the relationship between low back pain and tissue damage. The Psychosocial scale consists of 9 items and is likewise summed to produce a score between 0 and 54. A high score indicates a belief in the influence of psychological, social and biological factors.

A recently published systematic review of the psychometric properties of the PABS.PT found positive results for its construct validity, reliability and responsiveness [20].

Sample

A mailing list of all registered chiropractors in the state of Victoria was obtained from the national chiropractic registration board. Duplicate names, incomplete details and practitioners who were not practising in Victoria and returned mail from practitioners who were no longer practising at the designated address were excluded from the sample. This resulted in a list of 750 eligible practitioners.

Survey dissemination

All 750 practitioners were mailed an invitation letter which consisted of the PABS.PT and 10 demographic questions. The survey was accompanied by a reply paid envelope to return to the authors. Alternatively, practitioners were given the opportunity to complete the survey online via an online survey tool (Survey Monkey™). A reminder was forwarded to practitioners via electronic mail with the assistance of the professional associations.

Statistical methods

Data were analysed with SPSS V21. Descriptive statistics were calculated for the demographic items and Cronbach's alpha was used to examine internal consistency of the questionnaire items.

Median scores on the biomedical and psychosocial factors were calculated and the sample was dichotomised using these values. Logistic regression was then used to determine whether any demographic variables (age in years, gender, number of patients per week, years working chiropractor, whether or not post graduate studies had been undertaken, urban or rural practice location, type of chiropractic national body membership) could explain the dichotomisation (i.e. whether or not the chiropractors have higher odds of the particular domain tendency).

In order to compare this sample to the national population, figures were obtained from the Australian Workforce Data Analysis and Planning, Department of Health [28]. These data were only available in 10 year age ranges.

The mean and standard deviation scores for the biomedical and psychosocial scales were calculated on a "1 to 6" Likert scale and a "0 to 5" Likert scale to allow for comparison to the Magalhães et al., [14,21] study.

A multiple regression analysis was used with the biomedical and psychosocial scale scores as the dependent variables and the demographic factors were entered as independent variables to test for the presence of independent predictors.

Results

The overall response rate to the survey was 29% (n = 218). Demographic data are summarised in Table 1. The average age of the chiropractors in this study was 44 years of age, males constituted the majority of the sample (68%) and had been in practice for an average of 17.5 years. They worked 30 hours per week, consulting 90 patients per week and approximately one third held post graduate degrees.

The average 6 point Likert scale scores were 34.5 (6.3) for the biomedical factor and 31.4 (4.1) for the biopsychosocial scores. The 5 point Likert scale produced biomedical factor scores of 24.7 (6.3) and a biopsychosocial score of 22.4 (4.1) (Table 2).

The biomedical subscale Cronbach's alpha reached an acceptable level of 0.74 and the psychosocial subscale was 0.42.

The biomedical and psychosocial scales were inversely related as shown in several previous studies ($r = -0.27$).

Logistic regression analysis indicated no evidence that any of the demographic variables helped to predict domain tendency ($p > 0.140$, results not presented). Multiple linear regression analysis demonstrated that the chiropractic demographic variables accounted for 12% of the variance of the biomedical factor (F (8, 131) = 1.210, $p = 0.298$, $R^2 = 0.12$) and 20% of the psychosocial factor (F(8,131) = 1.348, $p = 0.226$, $R^2 = 0.20$) (Tables 3 and 4). Only the number of patients for the psychosocial scale approached significance at the 5% level (beta coefficient = 0.175; 95% CI: -.0003 to 2.704; p = 0.05). Sample size adequacy to perform the regression analysis was calculated with GPower 3.1. With a sample size of 218 participants and 8 independent variables, 99.6% power was obtained to detect a low correlation.

Discussion

This study's aim was to determine if chiropractors' attitudes and beliefs regarding the management of patients with back pain were consistent with previous findings where a contemporary biopsychosocial approach or a biomedical approach has been shown to impact on the management of back pain when delivered by first contact practitioners. Anomalous findings in past studies suggested that the chiropractic subpopulation may be a cause of experimental artefact [20,24]. This is the first study to investigate the attitudes and beliefs of chiropractors in isolation.

Table 1 Demographic data of Victorian chiropractic participants and national demographic data (where available)

	(n = 218)	National workforce (4854)
Gender (% female)	69 (31.7)	479 (35.7)
Age in Years: 16-34	18.9%	35.6%
35-44	40.0%	30.4%
45-54	24.0%	18.4%
55-64	14.0%	10.7%
65-74	2.2%	4.3%
75-89	-	0.8%
Practice type (%)		
Group	47.9%	54%
Solo	52.1%	46%
Location (%)		
Metro	67.1%	75%
Rural	32.4%	24%
Remote	0.5%	1%
Postgraduate qualifications	32.7%	n/a
Professional Association (%)		
CAA	122 (56.2)	n/a
COCA	59 (27.2)	n/a
CAA and COCA	15 (6.9)	n/a
Other	8 (3.7)	n/a
None	13 (6.0)	n/a
Average number of years in practice (SD)	17.5 (9.2)	13.1
Average hours per week in practice (SD)	30.3 (11.6)	n/a
Median number of patients per week (range, SD)	90 (0-380)	n/a
Years worked		
0-5	17.3	25.6
6-10	23.7	18.3
11-15	22.5	13.6
16-20	15.6	9.2
21-25	13.3	7.6
26 or more	7.5	14.6
Hours Per Week		
1-10	4.2	9.6
11-15	10.0	7.6
16-20	2.6	9.0
21-25	14.7	10.0
26-30	20.5	16.9
31-35	17.9	14.4
36-40	15.8	15.3

Table 1 Demographic data of Victorian chiropractic participants and national demographic data (where available) *(Continued)*

41-45	5.8	3.9
46-50	5.8	3.2
51-55	1.6	0.9

The chiropractic sample in this study, when compared to the national chiropractic workforce data, had similar proportion of female chiropractors and average hours per week worked. However several differences were noted. The current study had a smaller portion of chiropractors participating in group practice compared to the national figures (48% versus 52%) and were less represented in the younger age groups (16 -34 years) compared to the national figures (18.9% versus 35.6% respectively). Chiropractors in this study tended to have more work experience in the 10 to 20 years range (38% compared to 21%). So this sample may be over represented by "mid-life" chiropractors.

The results of this study showed that the estimated chiropractic population's scores on the two subscales of the 19 item PABS.PT were within the ranges of previous studies. Scores were calculated on a "0-5" Likert scale for comparison to the Brazilian chronic pain physiotherapists in Magalhães et al. [14,21] and were also of a similar magnitude (biomedical = 27.6, psychosocial = 24.3 compared to this study of 24.7 and 22.4 respectively). Calculating means and SD using the "1 – 6" Likert scale, Victorian chiropractors were most similar to the United Kingdom GPs and physiotherapists [19] and least similar to Irish GPs [18]. The findings of this study do not support the hypothesis that chiropractors have an extreme tendency towards biomedical or biopsychosocial orientations as proposed by Magalhães et al. [14,21].

Magalhães et al. [14,21] raise several alternative explanations for the variability in mean subscale scores across the studies, notwithstanding their alternative Likert scale scoring system which significantly reduced scale scores. These include cultural aspects, type of academic training and differences in the curricular training of university programs. Magalhães et al. also suggested that healthcare providers in European countries would produce lower biomedical but higher psychosocial beliefs because the biopsychosocial model originated in this continent.

If the Magalhães et al., study was scored on a "1-6" Likert scale and increased by a similar amount as those of Victorian chiropractors when re scaled, which appears highly likely as standard deviations are similar between studies, then those scores would fall within the midrange of previous studies. This suggests that practitioner responses are similar across culture and educational training.

Magalhães et al. [14,21] suggested that healthcare professionals whose attitudes and beliefs reflect a stronger

Table 2 Means and standard deviations of PABS.PT past studies scores

Study	PABS.PT_{biomedical}		PABS.PT_{biopsychosocial}	
	Score	SD	Score	SD
Innes et al (1-6 Likert scale)	34.5	6.3	31.4	4.1
Houben et al, 2005 [17]	29.5	7.9	35.6	5.6
Bishop et al, 2008 [19]	31.1	7.2	32.5	4.8
Fullen et al, 2011 (10 items version)	38.8	7.7	16.3	3.1
Magalhães et al, 2011 [14,21]	**27.6**	**7.2**	**24.3**	**6.3**
Innes et al (1-5 Likert scale)	**24.7**	**6.3**	**22.4**	**4.1**

biomedical profile are more likely to search for a specific cause of low back pain and prescribe more imaging exams, encourage rest and time off work in an attempt to reduce tissue damage. In contrast to this expectation Victorian chiropractors have been shown to largely adhere to evidence-based guidelines for X-ray referrals [29]. This further suggests that the chiropractic population is not biased toward a biomedical or psychosocial orientation.

The most significantly disparate score is that of the Irish GP's psychosocial scale, which was 16.3 (SD = 3.1) [18]. The authors removed 9 items which excludes the possibility of comparisons. This is unfortunate as the study of Queally et al. (2008) suggested that training in musculoskeletal medicine in Ireland was inadequate and required urgent attention and data from the PABS.PT may have been useful in identifying educational competency gaps [30].

The biomedical orientation scale internal consistency in this study was found to replicate levels of previous studies. Other studies have reported less favourable internal consistency levels in the psychosocial scale. This study obtained the lowest Cronbach's alpha to date (0.44). The original study of Ostelo et al. [16] achieved a

level of 0.54, which was strengthened by the items added by Houben et al. [17] and achieved a level of 0.68. The items in the psychosocial scale do not appear to capture the psychosocial orientation in Victorian chiropractors. There is a need for the identification of alternative items to more robustly quantify this dimension in the PABST.PT.

While several demographic variables have been found to influence the biomedical orientation in other studies (gender, age, number of years in practice) this study was not able to identify any such relationships. The number of patients treated per week approached significance at the 5% level in relation to the psychosocial scale. This unexpected finding suggests that the practitioner who sees larger numbers of patients per week is more likely to believe that psychosocial factors play a role in patients' lower back pain. The poor Cronbach's alpha result for the psychosocial scale may also be a possible explanation for this trend and casts uncertainty over this finding.

This study did not replicate past studies which have identified relationships with the biomedical scale and GPs and physiotherapists in early and late working life stages. This study's population was biased toward those

Table 3 Multiple regression analysis of PABS.PT psychosocial (dependent variable) with sociodemographic variables

Coefficients

Model	Unstandardized coefficients		Standardized coefficients	t	Sig.	95.0% confidence interval for B	
	B	Std. error	Beta			Lower bound	Upper bound
1 (Constant)	34.765	2.335		14.891	.000	30.146	39.383
Patients	1.351	.684	.175	1.974	.050	−003	2.704
Years_Prac	.051	.077	.120	.656	.513	−102	.204
Age	−095	.072	−.249	−1.320	.189	−236	.047
PostGrad	−092	.711	−011	−.129	.897	−1.499	1.315
Location	−801	.703	−101	−1.139	.257	−2.193	.591
PracType	−749	.692	−097	−1.082	.281	−2.118	.620
ChiroAssoc	−244	.772	−028	−317	.752	−1.772	1.283
Gender	.104	.775	.013	.134	.894	−1.430	1.637

Table 4 Multiple regression analysis of PABS.PT biomedical (dependent variable) with sociodemographic variables

Coefficients

Model	Unstandardized coefficients		Standardized coefficients	t	Sig.	95.0% confidence interval for B	
	B	Std. error	Beta			Lower bound	Upper bound
1(Constant)	35.346	3.831		9.226	.000	27.768	42.924
Patients	−1.917	1.115	−153	−1.719	.088	−4.122	.289
Years_Prac	−031	.127	−045	−244	.808	−283	.221
Age	.019	.118	.031	.162	.871	−214	.252
PostGrad	−1.475	1.154	−108	−1.278	.203	−3.757	.807
Location	−1.442	1.144	−112	−1.261	.210	−3.705	.820
PracType	1.482	1.131	.118	1.311	.192	−755	3.719
ChiroAssoc	1.296	1.263	.092	1.026	.307	−1.202	3.795
Gender	.288	1.254	.022	.229	.819	−2.193	2.769

chiropractors in "mid-life" and a targeted study seeking to recruit larger numbers from those age groups may be required to reveal if this pattern exists in Victorian chiropractors.

The results of this study and previous studies have not found any relationship to the PABS.PT psychosocial sub-scale and demographic variables. The lower scores for internal consistency may be a possible explanation. Future studies exploring alternative items may overcome this concern and add to the potential utility of the PABS.PT.

Limitations of this study

This study was limited by its low response rate. Comparison to the national workforce data suggests that this studies sample approximated it, aside from the younger age groups. Nonetheless non-responders may be aligned to those of high biomedical and low psychosocial patterns but only a larger sample would clarify this possibility.

When compared to the national chiropractic data this sample was underrepresented by younger aged practitioners with fewer years in practice. This will be the "longest practicing" portion of the population who this study focused on and will subsequently have the potential to deliver suboptimal care for many years. A baseline measure would allow an insight into the changes in attitudes across their working lifespan and to determine if future generations of manual therapists are improving in their ability to deliver best practice guideline based care.

This poor internal consistency of the psychosocial scale suggests that the survey items are not capturing this dimension in the chiropractic population. The development of alternative items remains an objective for future research.

A strength of this study was the single professional practitioner base of participants. It enabled a comparison to previous studies comprised of various populations. Chiropractic practitioners do not appear to differ significantly from other health care providers. Thus the PABS.PT, in particular the biomedical scale may offer some utility in identifying non guideline based chiropractitioners.

Conclusions

Practitioner attitudes and beliefs have been shown to be associated with clinical outcomes for patients with low back pain [12]. This study is the first to explore chiropractors' attitudes and beliefs in isolation to determine whether their attitudes and beliefs are consistent with previous studies of mixed practitioner populations and differing cultural backgrounds. Past studies have suggested that chiropractors may hold extreme views which bias toward a biomedical emphasis. The results of this study suggest that the sample of Victorian chiropractors demonstrated similar levels to that of other health professions from differing cultures and educational backgrounds as measured on the PABS.PT. Future research is needed to identify items to improve the internal consistency of the psychosocial scale. Once achieved a larger study may be conducted to explore if the non-findings of age, gender and years in practice are robust.

Competing interests
The authors declare that they have no competing interests.

Authors' contributions
All authors read and approved the final manuscript. PW was responsible for the study design and securing the funding for the project. PT obtained ethics approval and contributed to the development of the questionnaire. PG and SI undertook the data analysis and interpretation. SI was responsible for reviewing and redrafting the final manuscript. PW developed the initial draft of the manuscript and all contributed to the final version.

Acknowledgements
The project was funded by the Chiropractors Registration Board of Victoria.

The views expressed herein do not necessarily reflect the views of the Chiropractors Registration Board of Victoria.

Author details
[1]Discipline of Chiropractic, Health Professions, Murdoch University, Murdoch, WA 6150, Australia. [2]Private Practice, Australian Injury Management Consulting, 117 Hall Road, Carrum Downs, VIC 3201, Australia. [3]Department of Chiropractic, Faculty of Science, Macquarie University, Sydney, NSW 2109, Australia. [4]Department of Statistics, Faculty of Science, Macquarie University, Sydney, NSW 2109, Australia.

References

1. Murray CJ, Vos T, Lozano R, Naghavi M, Flaxman AD, Michaud C, et al. Disability-adjusted life years (DALYs) for 291 diseases and injuries in 21 regions, 1990–2010: a systematic analysis for the Global Burden of Disease Study 2010. Lancet. 2012;380:2197–223.
2. Xue CC, Zhang AL, Lin V, Da Costa C, Story DF. Complementary and alternative medicine use in Australia: A national population based study. J Alt Comp Med. 2007;13:643–50.
3. French SD, Charity MJ, Forsdike K, Gunn JM, Polus BI, Walker BF, et al. Chiropractic and Observational Analysis Study (COAST). Providing an understanding of current chiropractic practice. MJA. 2013;10:687–91.
4. Pincus T, Kent P, Bronfort G, Loisel P, Pransky G, Hartvigsen J. 25 Years with the Biopsychosocial model of Low Back Pain – Is it time to celebrate? Spine. 2013;38(24):2118–23.
5. Antao L, Shaw L, Ollson K, Reen K, To F, Bossers A, et al. Chronic pain in episodic illness and its influence on work occupations: a scoping review. Work. 2013;44(1):11–36. doi:10.3233/WOR-2012-01559.
6. Engel G. The need for a new medical model: a challenge for biomedicine. Science. 1977;196(4286):129–36.
7. Gatchel R, Turk D. Criticisms of biopsychosocial model in spine care: creating then attacking a straw person. Spine. 2008;33(25):2831–6.
8. Forster N, Thomas E, Bishop A, Dunn KM, Main CJ. Distinctiveness of psychological obstacles to recovery in low back pain patients in primary care. Pan. 2010;148(3):389–406.
9. Kamper SJ, Apeldoorn AT, Chiarotto A, Smeets RJ, Ostelo RW, Guzman J, van Tulder MW. Multidisciplinary biopsychosocial rehabilitation for chronic low back pain. Cochrane Database Syst Rev. 2014 Sep 2;9:CD000963. [Epub ahead of print].
10. The New Zealand Acute Low Back Pain Guide (1999 review) and Assessing Yellow Flags in Acute Low Back Pain: Risk Factors for Long-term Disability and Work Loss (1997).
11. Ramond-Roquin A, Bouton C, Gobin-Tempereau AS, Airagnes G, Richard I, Roquelaure Y, et al. Interventions focusing on psychosocial risks for patients with chronic low back pain in primary care – a systematic review. Fam Pract. 2014;31(4):379–88.
12. Pincus T, Vogel S, Santos S. The attitudes and beliefs of clinicians do they affect patients outcomes? In: Hasenbring MI, Turk DC, editors. From acute to chronic back pain: risk factors mechanisms and clinical implications. New York: Oxford University Press; 2012. p. 405–18.
13. Darlow B, Fullen BM, Dean S, Hurley DA, Baxter GD, Dowell A. The association between health care professional attitudes and beliefs and the attitudes and beliefs clinical management and outcomes of patients with low back pain: A systematic review. Eur J Pain. 2012;16(1):12–21.
14. Magalhães MO, Costa LO, Ferreira ML, Machado LA. Clinimetric testing of two instruments that measure attitudes and beliefs of health care providers about chronic low back pain. Rev Bras Fisioter. 2011;15(3):249–56.
15. Vonk F, Pool JJ, Ostelo RW, Verhagen AP. Physiotherapists' treatment approach towards neck pain and the influence of a behavioural graded activity training: an exploratory study. Man Ther. 2009;14(2):131–7.
16. Ostelo RW, Stomp-van den Berg SG, Vlaeyen JW, Wolters PM, de Vet HC. Health care provider's attitudes and beliefs towards chronic low back pain: the development of a questionnaire. Man Ther. 2003;8(4):214–22.
17. Houben RM, Ostelo RW, Vlaeyen JW, Wolters PM, Peters M. Stomp-van den Berg SG. Health care providers orientations towards common low back pain predicted harmfulness of physical activities and recommendations regarding return to normal activities. Eur J Pain. 2005;9(2):173–83.
18. Fullen BM, Baxter GD, Daly LE, Hurley DA. General Practitioners attitudes and beliefs regarding the management of chronic low back pain in Ireland. Clin J Pain. 2011;27(6):180–9.
19. Bishop A, Forster NE, Thomas E, Hay EM. How does the self-reported clinical management of patients with low back pain relate to the attitudes and beliefs of health care practitioners? Pain. 2008;135(1-2):187–95.
20. Mutsaers JH, Peters R, Pool-Goudzwaard AL, Koes BW, Verhagen AP. Psychometric properties of the Pain Attitudes and Beliefs Scale for Physiotherapists: a systematic review. Man Ther. 2012;17(3):213–8. doi:10.1016/j.math.2011.12.010. Epub 2012 Jan 23.
21. Magalhães MO, Costa LO, Ferreira ML, Machado LA. Attitudes and beliefs of Brazilian physical therapists about chronic low back pain; A cross sectional study. Rev Bras Fisioter S&o Carlos. 2011;16(3):248–53.
22. Hay EM, Dunn KM, Hill JC, Lewis M, Mason EE, Konstantinou K, et al. A randomised clinical trial of subgrouping and targeted treatment for low back pain compared with best current care. The STarT Back Trial Study Protocol. BMC Musculoskelet Disord. 2008;9:58.
23. Hill JC, Dunn KM, Lewis M, Mullis R, Main CJ, Foster NE, et al. A primary care back pain screening tool: Identifying patient subgroups for initial treatment. Arthritis Rheum. 2008;59:632–64.
24. Field J, Newell D. Relationship between STarT Back Screening Tool and prognosis for low back pain patients receiving spinal manipulative therapy. Chiropractic & Manual Therapies. 2012;20:17. 12 June 2012.
25. Leboeuf-Yde C, Rosenbaum A, Axén I, Lövgren PW, Jørgensen K, Halasz L, et al. The Nordic Subpopulation Research Programme: prediction of treatment outcome in patients with low back pain treated by chiropractors - does the psychological profile matter? Chiropractic & Osteopathy. 2009;17:14. doi:10.1186/1746-1340-17-14.
26. McGregor M, Puhl AA, Reinhart C, Injeyan HS, Soave D. Differentiating intraprofessional attitudes toward paradigms in health care delivery among chiropractic factions: results from a randomly sampled survey. BMC Complement Altern Med. 2014;14:51. doi:10.1186/1472-6882-14-51.
27. Kawchuk G, Bruno P, Busse JW, Bussières A, Erwin M, Passmore S, et al. Knowledge Transfer within the Canadian Chiropractic Community. Part 1: Understanding Evidence-Practice Gaps. J Can Chiropr Assoc. 2013;57(2):111–5.
28. Workforce Data Analysis and Planning, within the Department of Health. [http://www.hwa.gov.au/resources/health-workforce-data] Viewed October 22 2014.
29. Walker BF, Stomski NJ, Hebert JJ, French SD. A survey of Australian chiropractors' attitudes and beliefs about evidence-based practice and their use of research literature and clinical practice guidelines. Chiropr Man Therap. 2013;21(1):44.
30. Queally JM, Kiely PD, Shelly MJ, O'Daly BJ, O'Byrne JM, Masterson EL. Deficiencies in the education of musculoskeletal medicine in Ireland. Ir J Med Sci. 2008;177(2):99–105. doi:10.1007/s11845-008-0153-z. Epub 2008 Apr 15.

13

Bladder metastasis presenting as neck, arm and thorax pain: a case report

Clinton J. Daniels[1,2,3*], Pamela J. Wakefield[1,2] and Glenn A. Bub[1,2]

Abstract

Background: A case of metastatic carcinoma secondary to urothelial carcinoma presenting as musculoskeletal pain is reported. A brief review of urothelial and metastatic carcinoma including clinical presentation, diagnostic testing, treatment and chiropractic considerations is discussed.

Case presentation: This patient presented in November 2014 with progressive neck, thorax and upper extremity pain. Computed tomography revealed a destructive soft tissue mass in the cervical spine and additional lytic lesion of the 1st rib. Prompt referral was made for surgical consultation and medical management.

Conclusion: Distant metastasis is rare, but can present as a musculoskeletal complaint. History of carcinoma should alert the treating chiropractic physician to potential for serious disease processes.

Keywords: Chiropractic, Neck pain, Transitional cell carcinoma, Bladder cancer, Metastasis, Case report

Background

Urothelial carcinoma (UC), also known as transitional cell carcinoma (TCC), accounts for more than 90 % of all bladder cancers and commonly metastasizes to the pelvic lymph nodes, lungs, liver, bones and adrenals or brain [1, 2]. The spread of bladder cancer is mainly done via the lymphatic system with the most frequent location being pelvic lymph nodes. Bladder cancer is the most common malignant disease of the urinary tract with a higher incidence in older age and more prevalent in men than women [3]. There is a higher prevalence in white persons; however, delayed diagnosis has lead to higher mortality rates in black persons [4]. More than 80 % of skeletal metastases are from carcinomas of the lung, breast and prostate with bladder tumors responsible for just 4 % of all bone metastases [5, 6]. Although uncommon, studies confirm that bone is the preferred site of metastasis (35 %) of UC outside of the pelvis, with the spine being most common site (40 percent of bone metastases) [7]. The cervical spine is only affected in 8 to 20 % of metastatic spine disease cases [8, 9]. The most

serious complication of UC is distant metastasis—with higher stage cancer and lymph involvement worsening prognosis and cancer survival rate [10]. The 5-year cancer-specific survival rate of UC is estimated to be 78 % [10, 11].

Neck pain accounts for 24 % of all disorders seen by chiropractors [12]. Although infrequently encountered, malignancy and infiltrative processes are a potential pathological source of neck pain [13]. Cancer is among the most common life threatening conditions presenting to chiropractic treatment facilities, with 58.9 % of chiropractors self-reporting identification of previously undiagnosed carcinomas [14]. A recent systematic review identified more than 60 published cases of diverse cancers recognized by chiropractic physicians [15]. The objective of this case report is to describe a patient presenting for chiropractic care with neck, arm and thorax pain due to metastatic disease secondary to urothelial carcinoma and provide brief review including clinical presentation, diagnosis, and treatment.

Case presentation

History

An 81-year-old white male presented to the Saint Louis Veterans Health Affairs chiropractic clinic in November 2014 with a referral for low back pain and he described additional complaints of neck pain, upper thoracic pain,

* Correspondence: Clinton.daniels@logan.edu
[1]Chiropractic Clinic, VA St. Louis Healthcare System, 1 Jefferson Barracks Rd, Saint Louis, MO, USA
[2]Logan University, College of Chiropractic, 1851 Schoettler Rd, Chesterfield, MO, USA
Full list of author information is available at the end of the article

radiating numbness, tingling and pain into the left arm, and pain that radiated into his left lateral and anterior chest wall. Coughing and sneezing significantly increased his pain in all areas of complaint and he denied chest pain and shortness of breath. Relevant medical history included concurrent care for high-grade papillary transitional cell carcinoma (TCC) of the bladder, and presence of a pacemaker. He was a 50-year non-smoker, but with a 30-pack year history of cigarette use.

His bladder cancer was diagnosed approximately one year prior after he presented with gross hematuria. Cystoscopy confirmed the presence of an 8 mm papillary tumor near the right ureteral opening and trigone, and a second cystoscopy identified a 5 mm mass on the left lateral bladder wall. Two prior biopsy and transurethral resections of bladder tumor (TURBT) procedures had been performed. Pathology report revealed high-grade transitional cell carcinoma that invaded subepithelial connective tissue, but was negative for muscular infiltration. Upon presenting for chiropractic care he was in the process of completing a second round of Bacillus Calmette-Guérin (BCG) immunotherapy.

Diagnosis and management

Cervical radiographs taken one week prior to presentation were read as moderate degenerative changes of the cervical spine with moderate carotid bulb atherosclerosis (Fig. 1). Physical examination revealed tenderness to touch of cervical paraspinal muscles and left upper trapezius, and diminished light touch of the left upper extremity. Left anterior chest wall pain was reproduced with manual over pressure of the left lower cervical spine. The provider could not clearly identify the cause of the upper back, chest and arm pain and did not provide any treatment to the cervical region. MRI was

contraindicated due to the presence of an implanted pacemaker. Computed tomography was obtained; multiplanar multidetector CT images revealed a large destructive soft tissue mass along the leftward aspect of C6-T1 with frank osseous destruction of the vertebral bodies and transverse processes (Fig. 2). An additional lytic lesion was identified within the first right rib (Fig. 3). The patient was sent to the emergency department for stabilization and consultation with an orthopedic surgeon. He selected non-operative management and was stabilized with a Miami-J cervical collar. The patient expired 4-weeks following the discovery of these lesions on the CT scan.

Discussion

Metastatic disease of the cervical spine can present with a variety of clinical signs and symptoms; including mechanical, nonmechanical, and referred pain due to pathologic fracture and/or neurologic dysfunction from cord or nerve root compression. Localized nonmechanical pain is the most common complaint, and is often described as not being related to any activities, progressively worsening, and exacerbated in the evening [16]. For patients with a history of carcinoma and a new onset of nonmechanical pain it is imperative to rule out the presence of metastatic disease [17–19]. Our patient's history of UC, cigarette use, and new onset of neck pain was a red flag for potential pathologic processes.

There is a clear correlation between smoking and the risk of developing bladder carcinomas [20]. Cigarette smoking is credited as responsible for more than 50 % of cases within the developed world [21], and a four to seven times greater risk than nonsmokers [22, 23]. An additional 5 to 10 % of cases can be linked to occupational exposures, such as aromatic amines used in

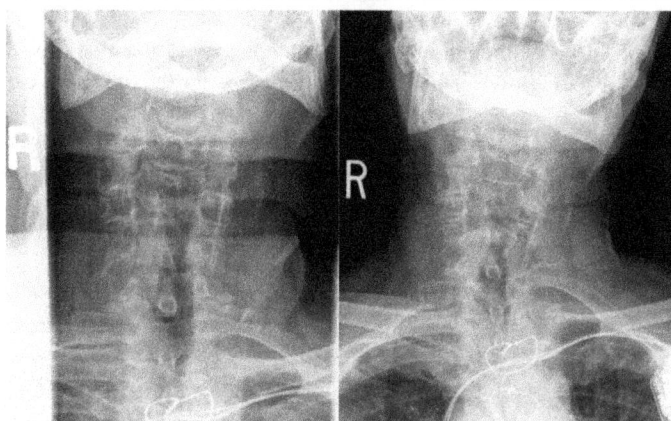

Fig. 1 AP cervical radiograph taken in 2010 (*Left*) AP cervical radiograph demonstrating missing left C6 pedicle and articular pillar taken in 2014 (*Right*)

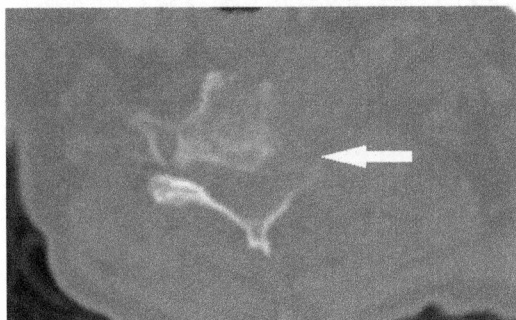

Fig. 2 Axial CT demonstrating destructive mass C6 left vertebral body and transverse process

manufacturing of chemical dyes and pharmaceuticals, and in gas treatment plants [24, 25]. While our patient was a long-term non-smoker his prior smoking may still have been contributory to disease development.

The most common symptom of patients with urothelial carcinomas is painless hematuria. Gross blood throughout urination is suggestive of bladder cancer [20]. Our patient sought medical care in the presence of hematuria and this ultimately lead to his cancer diagnosis. Early stage, local bladder disease, or carcinoma in situ, most commonly presents with urinary frequency, urgency and other signs of bladder irritation [20]. If the lesion is located near the urethra or bladder neck then the patient may experience obstructive symptoms. Signs of obstruction include decreased force or intermittent stream, sensation of incomplete voiding and straining. Pain may be present in the flanks with advanced stages of disease caused by urethral obstruction. Physical pain may also present in abdomen, pelvis, buttock or at distant bone sites [20, 26].

Practitioners should begin investigation of patients with urinary symptoms with a thorough history of cigarette smoking and occupational exposures. Physical examination does not provide much insight for early bladder cancer, however, palpable masses of the kidney

and pelvis may be detectable in later stages [20]. Urinalysis with urine microscopy and a urine culture is first line screening to rule out infection and hematuria. If bladder cancer is suspected, then urine cytology and cystoscopy would be indicated. Urine cytology is a noninvasive test that consists of sending urine sample to a laboratory for pathologist assessment to identify and monitor for high-grade tumors. Cytology interpretation is user dependent [27] with a sensitivity for carcinoma in situ of 28 to 100 % [28] and specificity exceeding 90 % [29]. Cystoscopy is an office procedure performed under local anesthesia, and is the mainstay of diagnosis and surveillance [20]. This involves insertion of a hollow tube with a lens (cystoscope) into the urethra and advanced towards the bladder. The cystoscope provides information on tumor location, appearance, and size. Bladder wash cytology is very sensitive for carcinoma in situ and obviates the need for random bladder biopsies. Patients with symptoms of bladder cancer should be evaluated with cystoscopy and bladder wash cytology [30].

Patients with a known history of cancer presenting with persistent neck pain (including mechanical and nonmechanical) should be evaluated for pathologic processes [16]. A history of nocturnal pain further escalates the suspicion of a neoplastic process [16]. Early diagnosis can be aided with basic neurologic screening for spasticity, hyperreflexia, Hoffman sign, and abnormal plantar reflexes [31]. In our case, the patient presented with vague mechanical symptoms and neurological symptoms that quickly progressed between visits—although pathologic reflexes remained absent. Evaluation for metastatic disease includes common laboratory tests such as complete blood count, blood chemistry tests, liver function tests, chest radiography, and CT or MRI [32]. Follow-up bone scan may be performed if in the presence of symptoms indicating potential bone metastasis or elevated alkaline phosphatase levels [20].

Men have a higher incidence of spinal metastases than women, and individuals in the fourth and sixth decade are most likely to be affected [33]. The main mechanisms by which a lesion can metastasize to the spine are dependent on the primary neoplasm and include: direct extension or invasion, hematogenous metastasis, and cerebrospinal fluid (CSF) seeding [16]. Direct extension occurs through primary lesions becoming locally aggressive and extending to involve bony spine. Hematogenous seeding is facilitated by the vast arterial supply of the vertebra and via the valveless venous drainage plexi such as Batson's plexus. Seeding of a primary lesion through the CSF occurs much less frequently and is most often caused by surgical manipulation of cerebral lesions [34]. Post-mortem biopsy was not performed on this patient, therefore it is not possible to definitively state that his cervical metastasis was a direct result of his urinary carcinoma.

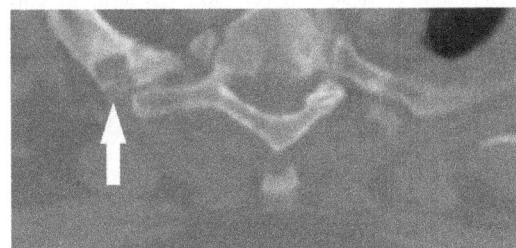

Fig. 3 Lytic lesion in right 1st thoracic rib

Management of metastatic disease of cervical spine requires a multidisciplinary approach. In general, nonsurgical management of metastatic spine is recommended when tumor involvement has not resulted in spinal instability, neurological involvement, and pain nonresponsive to medical management [35]. Nonoperative management consists of radiotherapy, chemotherapy, hormonal therapy, and high-dose steroid therapy [16]. Radiotherapy is specifically aimed to reduce tumor size and response to therapy varies widely depending on tumor type. To reduce localized intramedually edema, acutely presenting symptoms of cervical epidural spinal cord compression by a neoplasm can be managed with corticosteroids such as Dexamethosone [16]. Chemotherapy may be utilized as an adjuvant therapy to treat the primary tumor(s), as it has no direct effect on spinal instability [16]. Although not a primary method of treatment, bisphosphonate use in the setting of metastatic cervical spine disease is advocated to reduce the incidence of skeletal-related events such as pathologic vertebral fractures and cord compression [16]. Surgery is generally palliative and indicated in cases of neurologic dysfunction, spinal instability, and intractable pain (Table 1). In cases of metastatic tumor the most common surgical intervention is anterior cervical corpectomy with fusion. Laminectomy with fusion is used less frequently as most lesions are located anteriorly. However, posterior decompression and stabilization may be the best treatment option at the craniocervical junction [16]. Detailed discussion of each individual therapy is beyond the scope of this paper and can be found elsewhere [8, 36, 37] (Table 2).

The effectiveness of these treatment modalities and the patient survival rate depends on the histological tumor type, tumor stage, therapeutic control of the primary tumor, and spread of the tumor [36]. Indications for treatment are guided not simply by neurocompression, but also by quality of life factors—such as pain and loss of

Table 2 Treatment rationale for non-operative procedures

Treatment	Purpose/Goal
Corticosteroid (i.e., Dexamethosone)	Reduce intramedullary edema and subsequent pressure
Chemotherapy/Hormone Therapy	Treat or manage primary tumor
Irradiation	Reduce tumor size
Bisphosphonates	Prevent and/or reduce likelihood of skeletal-related events

mobility. The oncology clinical decision process is further hampered, as a surgical option is often inappropriate due to possible comorbidities.

One of three cancer patients experience pain either directly related to their lesion or as an adverse result of cancer treatment—for instance radiation related fibrosis and joint contracture or chemotherapy-induced neuropathy [38]. Chiropractic care with high-velocity manipulation is widely considered an absolute contraindication [39]. Potential diminished bone strength and integrity from malignancy puts the patient at risk of skeletal-related events with forceful treatments. Low force treatment techniques such as mechanical-assisted manipulation methods [40], myofascial release, stretching and gentle exercise may be appropriate on a case by case basis as an adjuvant for pain management [39]. While prudent use of chiropractic services in cancer patients may offer effective strategies for reducing the pain and suffering, we do not believe that any chiropractic care was appropriate for our patient's chief complaint.

Consent

Written informed consent could not be obtained. The Saint Louis Veterans Health Affairs privacy officer and Research Development Committee provided approval for publication of this report and associated images. A written approval is available for review by the Editor-in-Chief of this journal.

Conclusions

This case describes the presentation of metastatic urothelial carcinoma as a source of neck, arm and thorax pain. Development of urothelial carcinoma is strongly correlated with smoking and occupational exposures. Although distant metastasis is rare, it can present as musculoskeletal pain and it is not uncommon for previously undiagnosed cases to present to chiropractic physicians.

Competing interests
The authors declare they have no competing interests.

Authors' contributions
CJD performed the literature review, and prepared the manuscript. PJW assisted in preparation of the manuscript. GAB cared for the patient and provided editorial review. All authors' read and approved the final manuscript.

Table 1 Indications for neurosurgery in the presence of malignancy [35]

Surgical Indications

• Pain due to mechanical compression of pain producing structures or clear instability

• Symptomatic mechanical compression of neurostructures (neurological deficit)

• Rapidly progressing neurological deficit due to mechanical compression

• Unknown primary tumor with clearly defined metastatic involvement of the spine

• Radioresistant tumor

• Neurological deterioration or increasing pain during or after radiotherapy (should be avoided by a careful evaluation of the tumor potential before irradiation is decided)

Authors' note

The views expressed in this article are those of the authors and do not reflect the official policy or position of the Department of Veterans Affairs. This material is the result of work supported with resources and the use of facilities at VA St. Louis Health Care System.

Author details

[1]Chiropractic Clinic, VA St. Louis Healthcare System, 1 Jefferson Barracks Rd, Saint Louis, MO, USA. [2]Logan University, College of Chiropractic, 1851 Schoettler Rd, Chesterfield, MO, USA. [3]811 Rowell St., Steilacoom, WA 98388, USA.

References

1. Rozanski TA, Grossman HB. Recent developments in the pathophysiology of bladder cancer. Am J Roentgenol. 1994;163:789–92.
2. Weizer AZ, Shariat SF, Haddad JL, Escudier S, Lerner SP. Metastatic Transitional Cell Carcinoma of the Urinary Bladder to the Shoulder Girdle. Rev Urol. 2002;4(2):97–9.
3. Shinagare AB, Nikhil HR, Jagannathan JP, Fennessy FM, Taplin ME, Van den Abbeele AD. Metastatic pattern of bladder cancer: Correlation with the characteristics of the primary tumor. Genitourin Imaging. 2011;196:117–22.
4. Jemal A, Murray T, Ward E, et al. Cancer statistics, 2005 [published correction appears in CA Cancer J Clin 2005;55(4):259]. CA Cancer J Clin. 2005;55(1):10–30.
5. Coleman RE. Skeletal complications of malignancy. Cancer Suppl. 1997;80:1588–94.
6. Semino MA, Cabria RO, Garcia EC, Banez ET, Alonso A, Rodriguez FV. Distal bone metastases from carcinoma transitional cell bladder. Arch Esp Urol. 2002;55(1):69–70.
7. Sengelov L, Kamby C, Maase H. Pattern of metastases in relation to characteristics of primary tumor and treatment in patients with disseminated urothelial carcinoma. J Urol. 1996;155:111–4.
8. Fehlings MG, David KS, Vialle L, et al. Decision making in the surgical treatment of cervical spine metastases. Spine (Phila Pa 1976). 2009;34 Suppl 22:S108–17.
9. Talbot JN, Paycha F, Balogova S. Diagnosis of bone metastasis: recent comparative studies of imaging modalities. Q J Nucl Med Mol Imaging. 2011;55:374–410.
10. Ehdaie B, Shariat SF, Savage C, Coleman J, Dalbagni G. Postoperative nomogram for disease recurrence and cancer-specific death for upper tract urothelial carcinoma: comparison to American Joint Committee on Cancer staging classification. Urol J. 2014;11(2):1435–41.
11. Pollack A, Zagars GK, Cole CJ, et al. The relationship of local control to distant metastasis in muscle invasive bladder cancer. J Urol. 1995;154:2059–63.
12. Coulter ID, Hurwitz EL, Adams AH, Genovese BJ, Hays R, Shekelle PG. Patients using chiropractors in North America: Who are they, and why are they in chiropractic care? Spine (Phila Pa 1976). 2002;27(3):291–7.
13. Teichtahl AJ, McColl G. An approach to neck pain for the family physician. Aust Fam Physician. 2013;42(11):774–7.
14. Daniel DM, Ndetan H, Rupert RL, Martinez D. Self-reported recognition of undiagnosed life threatening conditions in chiropractic practice: a random survey. Chiropr Man Ther. 2012;20:21.
15. Alcantara J, Alcantara JD, Alcantara J. The chiropractic care of patients with cancer: A systematic review of the literature. Integr Cancer Ther. 2012;11(4):304–12.
16. Molina CA, Gokaslan ZL, Sciubba DM. Diagnosis and management of metastatic cervical spine tumors. Orthop Clin N Am. 2012;43:75–87.
17. Sciubba DM, Petteys RJ, Dekutoski MB, et al. Diagnosis and management of metastatic spine disease. J Neurosurg Spine. 2010;13(1):94–108.
18. Sundaresan N, Krol G, DiGiacinto G, Metastatic tumors of the spine. Tumors of the Spine. In: Sundaresan N, Schmidek H, Schiller A, editors. Diagnosis and Clinical Managemen. Philadelphia: WB Saunders; 1990.
19. Sundaresan N, Boriani S, Rothman A, et al. Tumors of the osseous spine. J Neurooncol. 2004;69(1–3):273–90.
20. Sharma S, Ksheersagar P, Sharma P. Diagnosis and treatment of bladder cancer. Am Fam Physician. 2009;80(7):717–23.
21. Jankovic S, Radosavljevic V. Risk factors for bladder cancer. Tumori. 2007;93(1):4–12.
22. Morrison AS. Advances in the etiology of urothelial cancer. Urol Clin North Am. 1984;11(4):557–66.
23. Burch JD, Rohan TE, Howe GR, et al. Risk of bladder cancer by source and type of tobacco exposure: a case–control study. Int J Cancer. 1989;44(4):622–8.
24. Quilty PM, Kerr GR. Bladder cancer following low or high dose pelvic irradiation. Clin Radiol. 1987;38(6):583–5.
25. Lin J, Spitz MR, Dinney CP, Etzel CJ, Grossman HB, Wu X. Bladder cancer risk as modified by family history and smoking. Cancer. 2006;107(4):705–11.
26. Murphy DR, Morris NJ. Transitional cell carcinoma of the ureter in a patient with buttock pain: A case report. Arch Phys Med Rehabil. 2008;89:150–2.
27. Raitanen M-P, Aine R, Rintala E, et al. Finn Bladder Group. Differences between local and review urinary cytology and diagnosis of bladder cancer. An interobserver multicenter analysis. Eur Urol. 2002;41(3):284–9.
28. Tetu B. Diagnosis of urothelial carcinoma from urine. Mod Pathol. 2009;22 Suppl 2:S53–9.
29. Lokeshwar VB, Habuchi T, Grossman HB, et al. Bladder tumour markers beyond cytology: international consensus panel on bladder tumour markers. Urology. 2005;66(6 Suppl 1):35–63.
30. Mohr DN, Offord KP, Owen RA, Melton III LJ. Asymptomatic microhematuria and urologic disease. A population-based study. JAMA. 1986;256(2):224–9.
31. Sciubba DM, Gokaslan ZL. Diagnosis and management of metastatic spine disease. Surg Oncol. 2006;15(3):141–51.
32. Greene FL, Page DL, Fleming ID, editors. Urinary bladder, AJCC Cancer Staging Manual. 6th ed. New York: Springer-Verlag; 2002. p. 335–40.
33. Molina CA, Gokaslan ZL, Sciubba DM. Spinal tumors. In: Norden AD, Reardon AD, Wen PC, editors. Primary Central Nervous System Tumors: Pathogenesis and Therapy. New York, NY: Humana Press. 2011;529.
34. Arguello F, Baggs RB, Duerst RE, et al. Pathogenesis of vertebral metastasis and epidural spinal cord compression. Cancer. 1990;65(1):98–106.
35. Mazel C, Balabaud L, Bennis S, et al. Cervical and thoracic spine tumor management: surgical indications, techniques, and outcomes. Orthop Clin North Am. 2009;40(1):75–92. vi–vii.
36. Eur AM, Spine J. Spinal metastasis in the elderly. Eur Spine J. 2003;12 Suppl 2:S202–13.
37. Mesfin A, Buchowski JM, Gokaslan ZL, Bird JE. Management of metastatic cervical spine tumors. J Am Acad Orthop Surg. 2015;23(1):38–46.
38. Evans RC, Rosner AL. Alternatives in cancer pain treatment: The application of chiropractic care. Semin Oncol Nurs. 2005;21(3):184–9.
39. Schneider J, Gilford S. The chiropractor's role in pain management for oncology patients. J Manipulative Physiol Ther. 2001;24(1):52–7.
40. Schneider M, Haas M, Glick R, Stevans J, Landsittel D. Comparison of spinal manipulation methods and usual medical care for acute and subacute low back pain: A randomized clinical trial. Spine (Phila Pa 1976). 2015;40(4):209–17.

Chiropractic identity, role and future: a survey of North American chiropractic students

Jordan A Gliedt[1,2*], Cheryl Hawk[2], Michelle Anderson[2], Kashif Ahmad[3], Dinah Bunn[3], Jerrilyn Cambron[4], Brian Gleberzon[5], John Hart[6], Anupama Kizhakkeveettil[7], Stephen M Perle[8], Michael Ramcharan[9], Stephanie Sullivan[10] and Liang Zhang[11]

Abstract

Background: The literature pertaining to chiropractic students' opinions with respect to the desired future status of the chiropractic physician is limited and is an appropriate topic worthy of study. A previous pilot study was performed at a single chiropractic college. This current study is an expansion of this pilot project to collect data from chiropractic students enrolled in colleges throughout North America.

Objective: The purpose of this study is to investigate North American chiropractic students' opinions concerning professional identity, role and future.

Methods: A 23-item cross-sectional electronic questionnaire was developed. A total of 7,455 chiropractic students from 12 North American English-speaking chiropractic colleges were invited to complete the survey. Survey items encompassed demographics, evidence-based practice, chiropractic identity and setting, and scope of practice. Data were collected and descriptive statistical analysis was performed.

Results: A total of 1,247 (16.7% response rate) questionnaires were electronically submitted. Most respondents agreed (34.8%) or strongly agreed (52.2%) that it is important for chiropractors to be educated in evidence-based practice. A majority agreed (35.6%) or strongly agreed (25.8%) the emphasis of chiropractic intervention is to eliminate vertebral subluxations/vertebral subluxation complexes. A large number of respondents (55.2%) were not in favor of expanding the scope of the chiropractic profession to include prescribing medications with appropriate advanced training. Most respondents estimated that chiropractors should be considered mainstream health care practitioners (69.1%). Several respondents (46.8%) think that chiropractic research should focus on the physiological mechanisms of chiropractic adjustments.

Conclusion: The chiropractic students in this study showed a preference for participating in mainstream health care, report an exposure to evidence-based practice, and desire to hold to traditional chiropractic theories and practices. The majority of students would like to see an emphasis on correction of vertebral subluxation, while a larger percent found it is important to learn about evidence-based practice. These two key points may seem contradictory, suggesting cognitive dissonance. Or perhaps some students want to hold on to traditional theory (e.g., subluxation-centered practice) while recognizing the need for further research to fully explore these theories. Further research on this topic is needed.

Keywords: Chiropractic, Cross-sectional survey

* Correspondence: jordan.gliedt@gmail.com
[1]Private Practice, 725 S. Dobson Rd, Suite 100, Chandler, AZ 85224, USA
[2]Logan University College of Chiropractic, 1851 Schoettler Rd, Chesterfield, MO 63017, USA
Full list of author information is available at the end of the article

Introduction

The last thirty years in health care have brought about many changes in thoughts and practice ideologies. One of these recent trends is an emphasis on cost-effective treatments and interprofessional collaboration [1-3]. Additional changes in health care over this time have included an increase in medical specialization and sub-specialization, the concept and implementation of evidence-based practice, and a greater acceptance of complementary and alternative medicine (CAM) therapies in mainstream medicine. Amid all of these transformations and shifts in the health care arena, a primary spine care specialist role has not been established. The current state of spinal care has been classified as a "supermarket approach" consisting of multiple practitioners including primary care providers, chiropractic physicians, acupuncturists, physical therapists, physiatrists, orthopedic surgeons, neurosurgeons, massage therapists, and naturopathic physicians with multiple treatment philosophies, high salesmanship and little interprofessional communication [4]. Chiropractic physicians possess many attributes that would be required of a primary spine care practitioner, and with specific modifications in education and practice, chiropractors may be in a position to make a relatively lateral transition to occupy this role [4]. As factions of the chiropractic profession are establishing a pathway for chiropractors to assume an evidence-based primary spine care practitioner role integrated in mainstream health care, it has been asserted this may not be the route many field providers desire to pursue [5]. Although most professions may have internal factions with conflicting viewpoints, such factions within chiropractic are particularly contentious [6]. According to McGregor et al., progressing toward a collaborative focus will demand a more visible appreciation of the professional strata that exist, and the mutual goals that exist between them [1]. Because chiropractic students represent the future of the profession, examining their views on professional identity might provide insight into the future of the profession. However, to date, there has been little research done among this population, with only one related specifically to this topic; this study, in fact, served as the pilot study for the current project [7]. The aim of this investigation was to survey chiropractic students' opinions about chiropractic identity, role and future. Results may yield an insight into future practitioners' perspective about the future of the profession, thus aiding in chiropractic's progression. This study may further act as a catalyst for future studies directed to current practicing chiropractors.

Methods

Survey development

A 23-item survey instrument (Additional file 1) was developed by the lead investigators at Logan University, based on the pilot survey previously used by the principal investigator among chiropractic college students at one university [7]. The survey instrument was reviewed by all remaining investigators and feedback was provided about the content, with subsequent revisions made. Survey items encompassed demographics, evidence-based practice, chiropractic identity and setting, and scope of practice. The first 8 survey items collected demographic information that included participants' current chiropractic institution in which they are enrolled, age, sex, current enrollment status, education and degrees achieved prior to enrollment, and student chiropractic organization affiliations. The enrollment status question was constructed to standardize the various institutions' use of semesters, trimesters, and quarters into 1st, 2nd or 3rd year. The remaining 15 survey items (9–23) explored participants' opinions concerning evidence-based practice, chiropractic identity and setting, and scope of practice. Of the final 15 items, 11 were constructed in 5-point Likert scale with the following ratings: 1 = Strongly Agree; 2 = Agree; 3 = Neutral; 4 = Disagree; 5 = Strongly Disagree.

Sample population

Initially, the research directors of all 19 accredited North American chiropractic colleges were invited by email to participate by administering the survey at their institution and contributing to the analysis and reporting of results. Of these 19 institutions, 12 participated (63%), each with at least one designated on-site representative to administer the survey. The participating institutions were:

- Canadian Memorial Chiropractic College
- Logan University
- National University of Health Sciences
- Northwestern Health Sciences University
- Palmer College of Chiropractic – Davenport campus
- Palmer College of Chiropractic – Florida campus
- Palmer College of Chiropractic – West campus
- Sherman College of Chiropractic
- Southern California University of Health Sciences
- Texas Chiropractic College
- University of Bridgeport

Eligibility criteria

Students enrolled in an accredited Doctor of Chiropractic (DC) degree program at the time of survey administration at a participating institution were eligible. Students enrolled in a bachelor, master or non-chiropractic doctoral degree program without concurrently being enrolled in a DC program, or those enrolled part-time in a DC program, were ineligible.

Survey administration

An anonymous cross-sectional survey to identify chiropractic students' opinions regarding chiropractic identity, role and future was administered among 12 North American English-speaking chiropractic colleges. The lead institution's (Logan University) Institutional Review Board (IRB) approved this study and all participating colleges that required IRB submission of the project obtained approval from their respective institutions. A notice of participant consent was included at the beginning of the electronic survey. Participation in this study was voluntary and no compensation was provided to students for participating in this study. The electronic survey was conducted through Survey Monkey. Logan University's Survey Monkey Platinum account ensured HIPAA compliance at the highest level to all survey participants. Survey Monkey is electronic survey administrations system in which questions appear on the screen and scroll to the next item after being answered. Respondents were able to return to questions and change their responses at any time until they submitted the questionnaire; at that time it was no longer accessible by that respondent. We used a setting which only allows one survey response per IP address, in order to avoid duplication. Responses were then downloaded into an Excel file.

The study's program coordinator uploaded the survey instrument into Survey Monkey. A representative at each participating institution disseminated student recruitment invitations and the survey instrument to all eligible chiropractic students via email between November 2013 and April 2014. However, specific survey recruitment varied depending upon policies and procedures in place at each institution. Due to logistical difficulties and also to avoid duplicate responses, reminders were not sent to the students.

Data analysis

Results were downloaded from Survey Monkey directly into SPSS (v.22). Descriptive statistics were computed. Frequencies were computed for all variables, including those items with Likert scale categories (strongly agree, agree, neutral, disagree, strongly disagree and missing). Responses were compared for each item, stratified by year in program. Using a Chi square test, an alpha level of .05 was used to indicate statistically significant differences among responses by year in program.

Results

A total of 1,247 surveys were completed. Among the 12 institutions participating, response rates varied from 38.0% to 6.1%, with a mean response of 16.72. Table 1 details the response rates by institution.

Table 1 Response rates by institution

Institution	n distributed	n completed	Response rate (%)
1	677	257	38.0
5	434	99	22.8
3	485	104	21.4
10	744	137	18.4
2	602	106	17.6
6	310	49	15.8
9	234	36	15.4
8	1830	263	14.4
12	920	93	10.1
4	148	14	9.5
7	725	53	7.3
11	346	21	6.1
Total	**7455**	**1247**	**16.7**

Respondent demographics are reported in Table 2. The majority of respondents were between the ages of 18–25 years (50.9%) and male (53.6%). However, when comparing the sample by year in program, the proportion of men was less for earlier years in the program (50.3% for year 1, 53.2% for year 2, and 58.6% for year 3). Most respondents (83.4%) reported obtaining a bachelor's degree prior to enrollment in chiropractic college, with few respondents indicating further education beyond a bachelor's degree. The majority of respondents (62.1%) reported belonging to neither Student International Chiropractic Association (SICA) nor Student American Chiropractic Association (SACA). Respondents' current status in the Doctor of Chiropractic (DC) program were well represented throughout each year of enrollment with 394 respondents (31.6%) reporting a status of 1st year, 400 (32.1%) as 2nd year, and 446 (35.8%) as 3rd year. A significant number of 3rd year respondents (86.0%) reported having completed a course in evidence-based practice in their chiropractic curriculum.

Responses to statements regarding evidence-based practice, identity and settings, and scope of practice are outlined in Table 3. Most respondents agreed (34.8%) or strongly agreed (52.2%) that it is important for chiropractors to be educated in evidence-based practice. Approximately half (51.9%) of the respondents strongly agreed (21.6%) or agreed (30.3%) that contemporary and evolving scientific evidence is more important than traditional chiropractic theory. Nearly half (45.8%) of respondents strongly agreed (17.4%) or agreed (28.4%) that it is important for chiropractors to hold strongly to traditional chiropractic theories and practices. Many respondents strongly agreed (39.5%) or agreed (29.7%) that it is important for the progression of the chiropractic profession to include clinical chiropractic training internships

Table 2 Respondent demographics

Sex	n	%
Male	668	53.6
Female	565	45.3
Missing	14	1.1
Age		
18-25 years	635	50.9
26-35 years	489	39.2
36-45 years	91	7.3
46-55 years	20	1.6
55 years and older	7	.6
Missing	5	.4
Highest level of education prior to enrollment		
Associate degree	110	8.8
Bachelor degree	1040	83.4
MA/MS/MPH degree	63	5.1
Doctoral degree (Ph.D, EdD, etc.)	16	1.3
Missing	18	1.4
Professional degrees prior to enrollment		
MD/DO from USA	4	.3
MD/DO from other country	6	.5
Other health professional degree (RN, PT, etc.)	111	8.9
Other professional degree (JD, etc.)	59	4.7
None	1036	83.1
Missing	31	2.5
Membership in chiropractic organizations		
Student International Chiropractic Association	94	7.5
Student American Chiropractic Association	326	26.1
Both	45	3.6
Neither	775	62.1
Missing	7	.6
Current enrollment status in DC program		
1st year	394	31.6
2nd year	400	32.1
3rd year	446	35.8
Missing	7	.6
Total	1247	100.0
Report having completed a course in evidence-based practice in chiropractic program	782	63.5
Year 1	137	35.0
Year 2	265	66.4
Year 3	380	86.0

and post-graduate residencies in integrative medical settings. A majority agreed (35.6%) or strongly agreed (25.8%) the emphasis of chiropractic intervention is to eliminate vertebral subluxations/vertebral subluxation complexes; however very few respondents strongly agreed (6.5%) or agreed (6.6%) that chiropractic intervention should consist of chiropractic adjustment only. A large number of respondents (55.2%) were not in favor of expanding the scope of the chiropractic profession to include prescribing medications with appropriate advanced training.

Table 4 shows additional responses relating to identity and setting, and scope of practice. Most respondents deemed that chiropractors should be considered mainstream health care practitioners (69.1%). The largest proportion of respondents (46.9%) deemed the most important chiropractic practice paradigm is one that focuses on primary spine/musculoskeletal care; 25.5% thought it should be primary care; and 15.4% that it should focus on subluxation correction only. The highest proportion of participants (46.8%) reported that chiropractic researchers should focus future efforts primarily on physiological mechanisms of chiropractic adjustments.

Responses were additionally analyzed by year of respondents' current DC program status. Table 5 illustrates respondents' responses to statements about practice and identity, by topic and year in DC program. Items included in Table 5 were only those in which there was a statistically significant difference among years in program. Nearly all respondents agreed that chiropractic providers should maintain portal of entry status (84.7% 1st year, 90.1% 2nd year, and 90.1% 3rd year). Respondents tended to disagree with the idea of expansion of chiropractic scope to include prescribing medications more so in 2nd (61.6%) and 3rd (60.2%) year respondents compared to 1st year (53.5%). Respondents in their 3rd year (18.7%) agreed that chiropractic intervention should consist of chiropractic adjustment only more so than 1st (11.3%) and 2nd (10.9%) year respondents, although most respondents disagreed with this statement regardless of year in DC program.

Table 6 shows respondents' opinions by year in DC program. Items included in Table 6 were those in which there was a statistically significant difference among years in program. A greater percentage of respondents viewed primary spine/musculoskeletal care as the most important practice paradigm for the chiropractic profession in 3rd year (54.2%) respondents compared to 1st (48.7%) and 2nd (45.7%) year respondents. Interestingly, students in favor of a subluxation correction only focus paradigm tended to increase in 3rd year (21.0%) respondents compared to 1st (15.6%) and 2 year (12.0%) respondents. Respondents tended to view physiological mechanisms of chiropractic adjustments as the most important focus for chiropractic researchers less as they progressed in the DC program (54.7% 1st year, 49.1% 2nd year, and 46.4% 3rd year). Additionally, respondents in favor of outcomes/cost-effectiveness of chiropractic care as a primary chiropractic research focus increased

Table 3 Respondents' agreement with statements about practice and identity

	SA (%)	A (%)	N (%)	D (%)	SD (%)	M (%)
Evidence based practice						
It is important for chiropractors to be educated in evidence based practice.	52.2	34.8	6.0	1.3	0.2	5.5
It is appropriate to allow for updating and enrichment of chiropractic theories based on current scientific advancements.	47.8	39.1	5.0	2.1	.8	5.3
Contemporary and evolving scientific evidence is more important than traditional chiropractic theory	21.6	30.3	25.2	13.6	3.8	5.6
It is important for chiropractors to hold strongly to traditional chiropractic theories and practices.	17.4	28.4	23.5	19.0	6.2	5.5
Identity and setting						
Chiropractic providers should maintain portal of entry (direct access) status.	57.2	26.2	9.1	1.3	.5	5.7
Inclusion of clinical chiropractic training internships and post-graduate residencies in integrative medical settings is important to the progression of the chiropractic profession.	39.5	29.7	12.7	7.2	5.5	5.5
Scope of practice						
Emphasis of chiropractic intervention is to eliminate vertebral subluxations/vertebral subluxation complexes.	25.8	35.6	15.2	10.3	6.9	6.1
The primary purpose of the chiropractic examination is to detect vertebral subluxations.	20.7	23.9	15.8	22.0	12.0	5.6
The chiropractic profession should expand its scope of practice to include prescribing of medication, with appropriate advanced training	12.9	13.2	13.2	18.8	36.4	5.5
It is appropriate for the chiropractic profession to distinguish and promote two separate subgroups of broad scope (providing manual and other non-drug procedures) and limited scope (providing subluxation correction only).	10.3	20.7	26.6	21.6	15.6	5.3
Chiropractic intervention should consist of chiropractic adjustment only.	6.5	6.6	8.9	34.2	38.5	5.4

SA = Strongly Agree; A = Agree; N = Neutral; D = Disagree; SD = Strongly Disagree; M = Missing.

by percentage as respondents progressed in the DC program (23.8% 1st year, 32.3% 2nd year, and 32.7% 3rd year).

By the third year of chiropractic education, most (86.0%) students reported taking a class in evidence-based practice. A majority of respondents expressed an appreciation for education in evidence-based practice (87.0%), the importance of contemporary scientific evidence (51.9%), and the appropriateness of enriching chiropractic theories based on current scientific advancements (86.9%). Comparison of respondents based on year in DC program showed little variance in issues related to opinions on evidence-based practice.

Discussion

This study suggests that North American chiropractic students appreciate evidence-based practice, have a desire to participate in mainstream health care, be considered mainstream practitioners, concentrate in musculoskeletal/primary spine care, and are not in favor of expanding the chiropractic scope of practice to include prescribing medications. Results of this study also suggest that chiropractic students desire to hold onto aspects of traditional chiropractic theories and practices such as emphasizing subluxation/vertebral subluxation complex as part of the evaluation and treatment of patients. However, a majority of the students also expressed the desire for researching physiological mechanisms of chiropractic adjustments.

This may indicate a trend that future chiropractors want to maintain traditional principles while pursuing a more scientific understanding of those principles. According to the Institute for Alternative Futures (IAF) Chiropractic 2025 report, general recommendations were set out for the chiropractic community to pursue including: 1. Integrate chiropractic into health care systems and integrative care models, 2. Increase research, including why chiropractic adjustments produce cost-effective outcomes, why they often show positive non-musculoskeletal effects, and how they influence gene expression and self-healing, 3. Continue to strive for high standards of practice, including promoting the use of evidence-based guidelines [8]. Results of this survey suggest that chiropractic students' ideologies mirror these aforementioned recommendations of IAF which might suggest positive strides toward continued chiropractic acceptance and growth.

The opinions and perceptions of these students may indicate future implications for the chiropractic profession. According to IAF, chiropractic has remained largely secluded from integrated health care delivery systems. [8] It is expected that 30-85% of health care will be comprised of these integrated systems. [8] Inclusion in these models, which students in this study supported, may yield greater public acceptance and utilization of chiropractic services [8]. This may additionally require modifications and shifts in traditional emphasis in chiropractic

Table 4 Respondents' opinions, by topic

Doctors of chiropractic should be considered	n	%
Complementary/alternative health practitioners	312	25.0
Mainstream health care practitioners	862	69.1
Missing	73	5.9

The most important practice paradigm for the chiropractic profession is	n	%
Subluxation correction only focus	192	15.4
Primary spine/musculoskeletal care physician	585	46.9
General/Primary care physician	318	25.5
Other	81	6.5
Missing	71	5.7

The most important setting for chiropractic health care is	n	%
Integrated settings with other health care disciplines including allopathic medicine	354	28.4
Integrated settings with alternative medicine practitioners only	51	4.1
Alone or with other DC's, without integration with any other health care disciplines	102	8.2
Any/all of the above	670	53.7
Missing	70	5.6

Chiropractic researchers should focus future efforts primarily on	n	%
Physiological mechanisms of chiropractic adjustments	584	46.8
Outcomes/cost-effectiveness of chiropractic care	349	28.0
Outcomes/cost-effectiveness of integrative care models	240	19.2
Missing	74	5.9

Table 5 Respondents' agreement with statements about practice and identity, by topic and year in program*

	A (%)	N (%)	D (%)
Identity and setting			
Chiropractic providers should maintain portal of entry (direct access) status.			
Year 1	84.7	14.0	1.3
Year 2	90.1	8.3	1.6
Year 3	90.1	7.3	2.6
Inclusion of clinical chiropractic training internships and post-graduate residencies in integrative medical settings is important to the progression of the chiropractic profession.			
Year 1	74.3	17.9	7.8
Year 2	73.0	13.1	13.9
Year 3	72.5	9.4	18.1
Scope of practice			
Emphasis of chiropractic intervention is to eliminate vertebral subluxations/vertebral subluxation complexes.			
Year 1	67.6	17.8	14.6
Year 2	67.2	17.1	15.7
Year 3	61.8	14.2	23.9
The chiropractic profession should expand its scope of practice to include prescribing of medication, with appropriate advanced training.			
Year 1	33.1	13.4	53.5
Year 2	22.7	15.7	61.6
Year 3	26.9	12.9	60.2
It is appropriate for the chiropractic profession to distinguish and promote two separate subgroups of broad scope (providing manual and other non-drug procedures) and limited scope (providing subluxation correction only).			
Year 1	37.8	29.5	32.7
Year 2	28.4	28.1	43.5
Year 3	32.1	26.9	41.0
Chiropractic intervention should consist of chiropractic adjustment only.			
Year 1	11.3	11.0	77.7
Year 2	10.9	6.4	82.7
Year 3	18.7	10.5	70.7

NOTE—all the above differed significantly.
*Items are only included if the differences among year in program responses were significant at the $p < .05$ level (Chi square test).
A = agree; N = neutral; D = disagree.

curriculum such as increased exposure to integrative settings, emphasis in primary spine care management in an integrative setting, accelerating research, and emphasis on evidence-based guidelines.

The majority of students (61.4%) would like to see an emphasis on correction of vertebral subluxation in chiropractic practice. In addition, a larger percent (87.0%) said it is important to learn about evidence-based practice. These two key points may seem contradictory, suggesting cognitive dissonance. Or perhaps some students want to hold on to traditional theory (e.g., subluxation-centered practice) while recognizing the need for further research to fully explore these theories, as suggested by the data that showed 86.9% of the sample said that it is appropriate to update chiropractic theories based on scientific advancements. More research on this topic is needed.

As health care continues to evolve and take strides toward the establishment of collaborative multidisciplinary teams and a shift from fee-for-service reimbursements to bundled payments, risk sharing, and/or capitation [8], chiropractors must decide their identity and role in relation to this new model of health care. The chiropractic profession has been handcuffed with internal discord [9,10] and multiple strata within the profession exist. Current chiropractic students will play a role in contributing to choosing the path the profession chooses to pursue in this time of health care reorganization and this study shows the current climate of North American chiropractic students' ideologies in relation to professional identity and role. Future studies should focus on assessing practicing chiropractic physicians, and this study can provide a springboard for future investigations.

Table 6 Respondents' opinions by year in program*

	Yr 1 (%)	Yr 2 (%)	Yr 3 (%)	Total (%)
Doctors of chiropractic should be considered				
Complementary/alternative health practitioners	25.3	23.0	30.8	26.6
Mainstream health care practitioners	74.7	77.0	69.2	73.4
The most important practice paradigm for the chiropractic profession is				
Subluxation correction only focus	15.6	12.0	21.0	16.4
Primary spine/musculoskeletal care physician	48.7	45.7	54.2	49.7
General/Primary care physician	29.6	34.3	18.4	27.0
Other	6.2	8.0	6.4	6.8
The most important setting for chiropractic health care is				
Integrated settings with other health care disciplines including allopathic medicine	25.5	34.2	30.5	30.1
Integrated settings with alternative medicine practitioners only	5.6	2.4	5.0	4.3
Alone or with other DC's, without integration with any other health care disciplines	7.8	6.1	11.8	8.7
Any/all of the above	61.1	57.3	52.7	56.9
Chiropractic researchers should focus future efforts primarily on				
Physiological mechanisms of chiropractic adjustments	54.7	49.1	46.4	49.9
Outcomes/cost-effectiveness of chiropractic care	23.8	32.3	32.7	29.8
Outcomes/cost-effectiveness of integrative care models	21.4	18.7	20.9	20.4

NOTE—all the above differed significantly.
*Items are only included if the differences among year in program responses were significant at the $p < .05$ level (Chi square test).

Limitations

This study, much like other studies of similar nature, had limitations. The low response rate (16.7%) was the greatest limitation; a 2008 study reported online surveys to have an average response rate of 33% [11]. There is consequently likely to be a response bias. Repetitive survey distributions or reminders may have provided an increase in response rate. The survey may not have been representative due to response bias; we were only able to assess response bias in terms of gender and SACA membership. Nearly half of respondents (45.3% of total respondents and 49.7% of 1st year respondents) of this study were female. This represents a higher percentage of females in the chiropractic profession than previously reported [12]. In 2009 only 22.4% of the chiropractic profession was made up of females, unlike the typical chiropractic patient which is estimated to be approximately 60% female, compared to 48.8% of female medical graduates that year [12]. This high proportion of women students might suggest that women were overrepresented in our sample.

Approximately one fourth (26.1%) of respondents reported membership in Student American Chiropractic Association (SACA). Recent reporting of enrollment in United States (US) based chiropractic colleges has been described as 9,946 students in 2010 [8]. As of June 2014, SACA membership is 3,429 students (Hall LC, ACA Director of Membership Operations/SACA Liaison, personal communication Jun 3, 2014), representing approximately

35% of US based chiropractic students, which is comparable to the results of this study. This provides evidence of the representativeness of our sample in terms of SACA membership.

A substantial proportion of respondents reported a "neutral" stance for multiple survey items. As with all surveys constructed with a middle response option, potential sources of response error exist. [13] A vast majority of respondents reported having a course in evidence-based practice; however responses to this survey item, along with responses to all items of the survey instrument, may be incomplete due to the bias of the sample available to this study.

Our sample in this study may not be representative of all North American chiropractic colleges in terms of approach to chiropractic philosophy, although this study did include colleges with diverse philosophical approaches [8].

Results of this study represent only a subset of North American students at a particular time in history. Particularly given that there were only 63% of North American chiropractic colleges that participated in this study, and there are more chiropractic colleges located outside of North America, results of this study may not be representative of chiropractic students as a whole.

Conclusion

Results of this study indicate that North American chiropractic students show a preference for participation in integrative health care, have been exposed to evidence-based practice concepts, and appreciate a practice paradigm focusing on musculoskeletal/primary spine care. However students indicate a desire to hold strongly to traditional chiropractic theories and practices, including emphasis in vertebral subluxation/vertebral subluxation complex. Students in our study display certain ideologies that are in alignment with recommendations for the accelerated progression of chiropractic's future.

Additional file

Additional file 1: Survey instrument.

Competing interests
The authors declare that they have no competing interests.

Authors' contributions
JG contributed to concept and design of the study, and assisted in drafting the manuscript. CH contributed to design of the study, collection of data, interpretation of the data, and assisted in drafting the manuscript. MA contributed to collection of data, and interpretation of the data. KA contributed to collection of data and assisted in review of the manuscript. DB contributed to collection of data and assisted in review of the manuscript. JC contributed to collection of data and assisted in review of the manuscript. BG contributed to collection of data and assisted in review of the manuscript. JH contributed to collection of data and assisted in review of the manuscript. AK contributed to collection of data and assisted in review of the manuscript. SP contributed to collection of data and assisted in review of the manuscript. MR contributed to collection of data and assisted in review of the manuscript. SS contributed to collection of data and assisted in review of the manuscript/ LZ contributed to collection of data and assisted in review of the manuscript. All authors read and approved the final manuscript.

Acknowledgements
We would like to thank all those who participated in assisting the authors in this study; David Beavers, MEd, DC, MPH, Logan University; Daniel Haun, DC, Logan University; and Atanas Ignatov, PhD, Logan University for participating in survey administration and data collection.

Author details
[1]Private Practice, 725 S. Dobson Rd, Suite 100, Chandler, AZ 85224, USA. [2]Logan University College of Chiropractic, 1851 Schoettler Rd, Chesterfield, MO 63017, USA. [3]Northwestern University of Health Sciences, 2501 W. 84th St, Bloomington, MN 55431, USA. [4]National University of Health Sciences, 200 E. Roosevelt Rd, Lombard, IL 60148, USA. [5]Canadian Memorial College of Chiropractic, 6100 Leslie St, Toronto, Ontario, Canada. [6]Sherman College of Chiropractic, 2020 Springfield Rd, Boiling Springs, SC 29316, USA. [7]Southern California University of Health Sciences, 16200 E. Amber Valley Dr., Whittier, CA 90604, USA. [8]University of Bridgeport, Bridgeport, CT 06604, USA. [9]Texas Chiropractic College, 5912 Spencer Highway, Pasadena, TX 77505, USA. [10]Life University, 1269 Barclay Circle, Marietta, GA 30060, USA. [11]Palmer College of Chiropractic - Florida, 4777 City Center Parkway, Port Orange, FL 32129, USA.

References
1. McGregor M, Puhl AA, Reinhart C, Injeyan HS, Soave D. Differentiating intraprofessional attitudes toward paradigms in health care delivery among chiropractic factions: results from a randomly sampled survey. BMC Complement Altern Med. 2014;14:51.
2. Gaboury I, Bujold M, Boon H, Moher D. Interprofessional collaboration within Canadian integrative healthcare clinics: key components. Soc Sci Med. 2009;69(5):707–15.
3. Kreitzer MJ, Kligler B, Meeker WC. Health professions education and integrative healthcare. Explor. 2009;5(4):212–27.
4. Murphy DR, Justice BD, Paskowski IC, Perle SM, Schneider MJ. The establishment of a primary spine care practitioner and its benefits to health care reform in the united states. Chiropr Man Ther. 2011;19(1):17.
5. Villanueva-Russell Y. Caught in the crosshairs: identity and cultural authority within chiropractic. Soc Sci Med. 2011;72(11):1826–37.
6. McGregor-Triano M: Jurisdictional Control of Conservative Spine Care: Chiropractic Versus Medicine. The University of Texas at Dallas: University of Texas at Dallas; 2006.
7. Gliedt JA, Briggs S, Williams JS, Smith DP, Blampied J. Background, expectations and beliefs of a chiropractic student population: a cross-sectional survey. J Chiropr Educ. 2012;26(2):146–60.
8. Institute for Alternative Futures. Chiropractic 2025: Divergent Futures. Alexandria, VA: Institute for Alternative Futures; 2013.
9. Gliedt JA: Finding a common ground in chiropractic: the key to progression. *Top Integr Health Care* 2011, 2(4).
10. Kaptchuck TJ, Eisenberg DM. Chiropractic: origins, controversies, and contributions. Arch Intern Med. 1998;158(20):2215–24.
11. Nulty D. The adequacy of response rates to online and paper surveys: what can be done? Assess Eval High Educ. 2008;33(3):301–14.
12. Johnson CD, Green BN. Diversity in the chiropractic profession: preparing for 2050. J Chiropr Educ. 2012;26(1):1–13.
13. Sturgis P, Roberts C, Smith P. Middle alternatives revisited: how the neither/nor response acts as a way of saying "i don't know"? Sociol Methods Res. 2014;43(1):15–38.

15

The use of diagnostic coding in chiropractic practice

Cecilie D Testern[1], Lise Hestbæk[1] and Simon D French[2,3*]

Abstract

Background: Diagnostic coding has several potential benefits, including improving the feasibility of data collection for research and clinical audits and providing a common language to improve interdisciplinary collaboration. The primary aim of this study was to determine the views and perspectives of chiropractors about diagnostic coding and explore the use of it in a chiropractic setting. A secondary aim was to compare the diagnostic coding undertaken by chiropractors and an independent coder.

Method: A codin exercise based on the International Classification of Primary Care version 2, PLUS extension (ICPC-2 PLUS) provided the 14 chiropractors with some experience in diagnostic coding, followed by an interview on the topic. The interviews were analysed thematically. The participating chiropractors and an independent coder applied ICPC-2 PLUS terms to the diagnoses of 10 patients. Then the level of agreement between the chiropractors and the coder was determined and Cohen's Kappa was used to determine the agreement beyond that expected by chance.

Results: From the interviews the three emerging themes were: *1) Advantages and disadvantages of using a clinical coding system in chiropractic practice, 2) ICPC-2 PLUS terminology issues for chiropractic practice* and *3) Implementation of a coding system into chiropractic practice.* The participating chiropractors did not uniformly support or condemn the idea of using diagnostic coding. However there was a strong agreement that the terminology in ICPC-2 PLUS would not be applicable or desirable for all practice types. In the coding exercise the chiropractors in total coded 202 diagnoses for 135 patients. The overall percentage agreement between the chiropractors and the coder was 52% (17% expected by chance) with a Kappa score of 0.4 (95% CI 0.3-0.7). Agreement was lower for more detailed coding (percentage agreement 35%; Kappa score of 0.3 (95% CI 0.2-0.5)).

Conclusion: It appears that implementation of diagnostic coding would be possible in the majority of the chiropractic practices that participated in this study. However for those chiropractors who do not focus on symptoms in their approach to clinical care, it could be challenging to use the ICPC-2 PLUS coding system, since ICPC-2 PLUS is a symptom-based classification.

Keywords: Diagnostic coding, Chiropractors

Background

Diagnostic coding in chiropractic practice has several potential benefits. These benefits include improving the feasibility of data collection for research and clinical audits, improving the clinical applicability of research, and providing a common clinical language to help improve interdisciplinary collaboration. Diagnostic coding allows for systematic classification of clinical information in clinical practice and assists with the conduct of clinical audits and data collection for research purposes. Use of the same classification system by different clinical groups creates a common language between different healthcare professions and sectors and could enhance interdisciplinary collaboration. This could lead to better communication, improved continuity of care as well as simplifying the process of referring patients [1].

* Correspondence: Simon.french@queensu.ca
[2]General Practice and Primary Health Care Academic Centre, University of Melbourne, Melbourne, VIC, Australia
[3]School of Rehabilitation Therapy, Faculty of Health Sciences, Queen's University, Kingston, Ontario, Canada
Full list of author information is available at the end of the article

The International Classification of Primary Care (ICPC) is an example of a diagnostic coding system that could be relevant for chiropractic practice [2]. The ICPC consists of 17 chapters based on body systems following the principle that localisation has precedence over aetiology. A second version of the diagnostic code system, International Classification of Primary Care, Version 2 (ICPC-2), was published in 1998. Originally ICPC was designed for paper based data collection and analysis, but it has spread to electronic clinical and research systems. ICPC has gradually received increasing recognition and use, especially in Europe and Australia [2].

Diagnostic coding is not commonly undertaken in chiropractic practice, and the choice of an appropriate coding system is important as the profession moves towards this. A study in Danish general medical practice showed that the ICPC has a good reliability and validity at the chapter level for musculoskeletal conditions [3]. Thus, it would appear that ICPC is a good choice for diagnostic coding in chiropractic practice since most conditions treated are musculoskeletal [4]. Additionally, the ICPC-2 is already integrated in several healthcare systems [3], as well as into the International Classification of Disease (ICD-10), a coding system used in hospital settings [2].

ICPC-2 classifies clinical information using three character codes called a *rubric* [5]. The first character, a letter, represents a chapter or a body system (such as Musculoskeletal, Cardiovascular or Neurological), and the two additional characters, a number, represent a concept within this body system (a symptom/complaint, problem/diagnosis or process of care). To allow for greater detail and specificity, the ICPC-2 PLUS terminology was developed. ICPC-2 PLUS is a clinical terminology (*terms*) classified to the ICPC-2. ICPC-2 PLUS has been developed for the Bettering the Evaluation And Care of Health (BEACH) research project, which is an ongoing Australian national study of general medical practice activity [6]. ICPC-2 PLUS is also used in Australia in age-sex disease registers, morbidity registers and electronic health records in primary care.

New ICPC-2 PLUS codes are created by aligning a *term* with the description of the specific problem/diagnosis, or type of care, with the most appropriate ICPC-2 *rubric*. For each of the ICPC-2 PLUS *terms* a three digit code is assigned. This provides ICPC-2 PLUS with a six-character identifier as oppose to the three digits identifier for ICPC-2. As such, the final three digits of the six character ICPC-2 PLUS code identify the specific *term* within the *rubric*. For example, the three character ICPC-2 code L01 represents 'Neck Symptom or Complaint'. In ICPC-2 PLUS there are 11 neck-related *terms* in the L01 rubric to describe patient problems. For example 'Pain;neck' is represented in ICPC-2 PLUS as L01 004 and the 'Cervicalgia' as L01 006 [2].

Knowledge of who receives chiropractic care and what care they receive is important to understand contemporary chiropractic practice [3]. The Chiropractic Observation and Analysis STudy (COAST) [4] was a cross sectional observational study that described the clinical practice of chiropractors in Victoria, Australia. COAST explored why people seek chiropractic care, what diagnoses chiropractors make and what treatment chiropractors provide. The research method used in COAST was based on the BEACH study methods [6]. In coding the chiropractic clinical information, some new *terms* were required to describe chiropractic clinical practice. In developing the chiropractic specific ICPC-2 PLUS (Chiro), researchers followed the BEACH coding rules [7].

The long-term aim of this area of work is to implement diagnostic coding into chiropractic clinical practice. We are not aware of any previous research exploring the use of diagnostic coding in the chiropractic profession. This project explored chiropractors' attitudes towards diagnostic coding to provide important information about how coding will be received in this setting. Specifically, the primary purpose was to investigate the views among practising chiropractors in relation to feasibility, applicability and future perspectives of diagnostic coding in chiropractic clinical practice. A secondary aim was to compare the diagnostic coding undertaken by chiropractors to that undertaken by an independent coder.

Method
Summary
This study consisted of quantitative and qualitative components. Each of the chiropractors took part in a coding exercise and this exercise then formed the basis for the subsequent interview. The coding exercise primarily provided the chiropractors with some experience in diagnostic coding for them to describe in the interview. The coding exercise also provided the opportunity to compare the diagnostic coding undertaken by chiropractors to diagnostic coding undertaken by an independent coder. We aimed to determine how accurate the coding process was by determining if an independent coder used the same codes, (in this case *terms*) that chiropractors used, considering the chiropractors had more information available to them. The interviews were analysed qualitatively and the coding exercise was analysed quantitatively.

Participants and recruitment
Chiropractors approached for this study had all participated in the COAST project in 2011 [4] and were currently in clinical practice in Victoria. Chiropractors had

already received training in completing the COAST encounter forms and they were familiar with the background for the study. Fifty-two chiropractors participated in COAST and they were all approached for this study. The chiropractors received an invitation pack in the post, including an invitation letter for the study, a Plain Language Statement describing what participation in the study consisted of, and a consent form. Chiropractors opted into the study by returning a signed consent form via post or fax/email.

After two weeks the chiropractors who had not responded to the invitation letter were sent a follow up letter. After two additional weeks, non-responders were contacted by telephone until 15 chiropractors agreed to participate.

Patients were invited to participate in the study when they attended the practices of participating chiropractors during the recording period. Patients were approached if they were 18 years or older and had spinal pain (neck or back pain). Patients received a Plain Language Statement with information about the study and the chiropractors were trained to obtain verbal consent from patients wishing to participate.

Sample size

The number of chiropractors chosen (15) was by convenience. This number of interviews was feasible to complete considering resources and time available. Further, we are not aware of any similar studies conducted in this setting so this preliminary data would provide important information that can be used for future, larger studies.

For the quantitative analysis, we assumed the agreement on the choice of codes between the coder and the chiropractors would be around 50% with an intra-cluster correlation of 0.1. Therefore a sufficient sample size to provide a 95% confidence interval with a margin of error of 11% was 150 encounters or 10 patients per chiropractor.

Data collection and analysis

First, the 15 chiropractor participants were asked to complete encounter forms for 10 consecutive patients with neck or back pain. The encounter form used for the data collection was a slightly modified version of the encounter form used in COAST and included patient demographics, up to three reasons for encounter, relevant health information, presenting pain, diagnosis and care given (see Additional file 1 for a copy of the form).

After the chiropractor had completed their patient data collection, face-to-face semi-structured interviews were conducted between the chiropractor and the first author (CT). During the interviews the first author presented the chiropractors with a short introduction to

ICPC-2 PLUS. Chiropractors were then asked to choose the ICPC-2 PLUS *terms* most relevant for the diagnoses of the patients. In order to make the coding decision, the chiropractors were asked to use their memory of the patient encounter, the patient's clinical file and the encounter recording form they had completed at the time of the consultation. The chiropractor could document up to three diagnoses for each patient encounter and therefore also choose up to three ICPC-2 PLUS *terms* per patient encounter.

To make the coding exercise feasible and relevant to back and neck pain problems/diagnoses, the chiropractor was provided with a shortened list of ICPC-2 PLUS *terms* to choose from. The list only included *terms* relevant to neck and back pain from the ICPC-2 PLUS musculoskeletal chapter (254 *terms*).

The face-to-face interview consisted of open-ended questions about the chiropractors' perspective and views on the use of diagnostic coding in chiropractic practice. The questions enquired about the chiropractors' views on diagnostic coding, the potential role of a diagnostic coding system in chiropractic practice, the chiropractors' views on using the ICPC-2 PLUS *terms* in chiropractic practice, and finally the facilitators and barriers the chiropractors faced when trying to use ICPC-2 PLUS. All interviews were audio recorded and transcribed verbatim.

The patient encounter forms completed by the chiropractors, together with the chiropractors' choice of ICPC-2-PLUS *terms*, were collected at the end of the interviews. An independent hospital trained coder examined the encounter forms and assigned relevant ICPC-2 PLUS *terms* to the diagnosis recorded by the chiropractor on the forms. The coder used the "Demonstrator" function on the ICPC-2 PLUS website to select the appropriate *terms* for the diagnosis provided by the chiropractors [8]. The Demonstrator is an online search tool that allows access to all of the ICPC-2 PLUS *terms*. This coder searched an extensive keyword list with keywords linking the ICPC-2 PLUS six-character codes. When selecting a keyword, the coder was presented with all the available associated *terms*. The coder then selected the *term* that most closely reflected the chiropractors' exact wording of the diagnosis written on the encounter forms. The only information available about the patient for the coder was the information on the encounter forms, as is the case for the BEACH and COAST studies. Encounters were excluded from agreement analysis where the ICPC-2 PLUS *term* chosen by the coder was not included on the list provided to the chiropractors.

For the qualitative analysis, all interviews were examined by the first author (CT) by reading through and listening to each of the transcripts/audio files and labeling paragraphs with descriptive and interpretive codes as suggested by King [9]. After the first read through commonly repeating patterns were identified for each transcript. The same process was performed by the third author (SF) for the interview transcripts of three chiropractors, each with a different type of clinical practice. Descriptive and interpretive codes were then compared between the first and third author for the three interview transcripts, and divergent views between the two authors were resolved through discussion. The first author then re-examined the remaining 11 transcripts in light of this discussion.

For each of the interviews the repeating patterns were merged to define broader themes [10]. The interview were then finally analysed by looking for common themes across all of the 14 interviews, as well as areas of differences in the views and perspectives of the participants [11].

For the quantitative analysis of the coding exercise, the agreement between the independent coder and the chiropractors for their choices of ICPC-2 PLUS *terms* was determined at two levels: ICPC-2 *Rubric level*, three-character code; and also ICPC-2 PLUS *term level*, six-character code. The analysis was undertaken at two levels to determine whether more specific coding at the *term level* resulted in lower agreement. The overall percentage agreement was calculated, as well as the percentage agreement for each practitioner. Cohen's Kappa was used to determine the agreement beyond that expected by chance, using the statistical software Stata. Kappa was derived by comparing whether each chiropractor and the coder agreed (or not) on the choice of codes, and a mean Kappa value with 95% confidence intervals was determined. The guidelines of Landis and Koch [12] were used for interpreting the Kappa values. Finally, the time taken for the chiropractors to make a choice about a diagnostic code was determined from the audio recordings.

Ethics approval
The project received full approval from the Human Ethics Subcommittee at the University of Melbourne on 20th of June 2012 (ID1237727) as a Minimal Risk Project following the ethical guidelines described by the Australian National Health and Medical Research Council, NHMRC [13]. All participants (chiropractors and patients) gave informed consent to participate.

Results
Fourteen chiropractors completed the study and their demographic characteristics are described in Table 1. One chiropractor did not have the encounter forms available at the time of the coding exercise and was therefore not included in the study. Most of the chiropractors were males practising in metropolitan

Table 1 Characteristics of participating chiropractors

Chiropractor characteristics (N = 14)

Chiropractor characteristics	Average	Range
Age in years	46	30-57
Years in practice	19	5-32
	No.	**%**
Gender		
Female	1	7
Male	13	93
Location		
Metropolitan*	10	72
Rural	4	28
Graduated in Australia	13	92
Holds Postgraduate qualification	5	35
Involved in Teaching	3	20
Membership:		
CAA	6	42
COCA	5	35
Other **	6	42
Computer use in clinic:		
Do not have computer in practice	2	14
Clinical records paperless	1	7
Clinical records partially paperless	5	35
Clinical records paper only	7	50

*Determined from Australian Standard Geographical Classification - Remoteness Area (ASGC-RA).
**Other includes: The Australasian College of Chiropractors, Gonstead Chiropractic group, Australian Spinal Research Foundation, CAA sports. CAA = Chiropractors' Association of Australia; COCA = Chiropractic and Osteopathic College of Australasia.

Melbourne. All participated in the COAST project, but typically did not have any other experience participating in research.

The characteristics of the 135 participating patients are described in Table 2. The majority of the patients were between 46 and 70 years of age. There were more female than male patients but the difference in the distribution was only 10% (4 missing). Most patients (58%) presented with one reason for encounter and the most common reason was back pain.

The interview themes
Three overall themes emerged from the interview data: *1) Advantages and disadvantages of using a clinical coding system in chiropractic practice, 2) ICPC-2 PLUS terminology issues for chiropractic practice, and 3) Implementation of a coding system into chiropractic practice.* The themes are described in the following section along with illustrative quotes from the participating chiropractors. For additional quotes see Additional file 2.

Table 2 Patient demographics and encounter reasons

Patient characteristics (N = 135)	No.	%
Age [missing]	[7]	5
18-30	24	18
31-45	38	28
46-70	61	45
70+	5	4
Gender [missing]	[5]	4
Male	58	43
Female	72	53
Number of reasons for encounter per patient: [missing]	[3]	2
1	77	57
2	40	30
3	15	11
Reasons for encounter: [missing]	[7]	5
Neck pain	46	22
Back pain	76	38
Check up/maintenance	27	13
Other*	53	26
Total number of reasons for encounter	202	
Total number of diagnoses provided by the chiropractors	167	

*Examples of other: Headache, shoulder pain, arm pain, leg pain.
Note: The number of patients, the number of reasons for encounter and the number of diagnoses varied. Patients could report up to three reasons for encounter, which meant that some patients could have multiple diagnoses. In other cases the chiropractor combined some of a patient's reasons for encounter into one diagnosis thus for these patients there could be more reasons for encounter than diagnoses.

Theme 1) Advantages and disadvantages of using a clinical coding system in chiropractic practice

Most of the chiropractors were positive towards to the idea of using diagnostic coding in chiropractic practice and they suggested many possible advantages. Some talked about how this could streamline their own clinical practice. Many suggested the possibility of creating a database of coded clinical practice information. They suggested that this database could be used to produce research more efficiently and to ensure the clinical relevance of the research produced.

However, some of the chiropractors did not see the relevance or purpose of ICPC-2 PLUS in chiropractic practice. An issue mentioned by many was that the terminology would not fit into what they called the "wellness-based approach" of some chiropractors. Some chiropractors suggested that the use of ICPC-2 PLUS in chiropractic practice could "medicalise" the profession. On the other hand many chiropractors discussed how diagnostic coding could create a common language that could facilitate better communication between the different musculoskeletal health professions. Some chiropractors also mentioned how this could lead to integration

into the mainstream healthcare system. Some illustrative quotes demonstrating these issues follows:

"The advantages are quite evident, what it can create is a very good database for epidemiological studies and for further research and getting a better appreciation of the type of presentations and you got a lot of data that then could be stored, collected and accessed and drawn upon for future research" [ID1, 48 years old, 16 years in practice, Metro].

"The minute I start doing this [coding exercise] *with trying to match their reported reason for encounter that then assumes that what you are doing on that day is a treatment for that reason for encounter right? And I can understand why you would have this if you are in medicine because that is what they do right? But that's not what we do. So someone might have a presenting complaint: "okay let's check you, let's see if you are subluxated, if you are then I'll adjust you, whether or not you've got that presenting complaint, it's irrelevant okay.. So I don't know how you could fit this* [ICPC-2 PLUS] *into the way I have just explained it, if there was a way that would be great."* [ID8, 43 years old, 19 years in practice, Metro].

"If it's going to create a language that helps through - not just the chiropractic profession communicating well with each other, but chiropractic profession communicating with the rest of the medical industry - medical - well, rather, the health world. Then that's good for everybody. So, that's a great role and if we're talking about chiropractic - getting a larger level of research towards it and integrating itself into a mainstream system more. I think that would be actually essential. So, yeah there's certainly a role for it." [ID13, 30 years old, 5 years in practice, Metro].

Theme 2) ICPC-2 PLUS terminology issues for chiropractic practice

The terminology in ICPC-2 PLUS was a topic mentioned frequently by the chiropractors. Many of the chiropractors mentioned that there were too many *terms* to choose from, but also that the *terms* were not specific enough to reflect chiropractic clinical practice. They believed that there were not enough relevant *terms* for the stage of the problem/diagnosis, for example the limited possibilities to describe if a problem/diagnoses was acute or chronic or somewhere between the two. Some illustrative quotes demonstrating these issues follows:

"Obviously they are not specific enough, it doesn't tell you the state of whether it's acute, chronic or what have you. Again it might tell you the region you are

looking at but not the anything specific of what you are looking at" [ID2, 50 years old, 28 years in practice, Metro]

"It wasn't easy cause 27000 things for the same thing (laughs) almost, yes too many choices and not specific enough or they are trying to be too specific which then makes it a bit harder to find exactly what is going on." [ID6, 46 years old, 11 years in practice, Rural]

Theme 3) Implementation of a coding system into chiropractic practice

Many chiropractors thought that implementation of ICPC-2 PLUS into chiropractic clinical practice would be feasible after some practice. Some of the issues mentioned were getting ICPC-2 PLUS into the existing electronic clinical record systems and that not all chiropractors use electronic clinical practice records. Some chiropractors mentioned that implementing a system like ICPC-2 PLUS would have to start at the undergraduate level. One chiropractor stated that the idea was good but the motivation for clinicians was not great enough to make implementation of ICPC-2 PLUS possible. Some illustrative quotes demonstrating these issues follows:

It got easier. I guess part of it is just being familiar with what your options are. " [ID12, 38 years old, 16 years in practice, Rural]

"When you familiarize yourself with it, it would be great." [ID1, 48 years old, 16 years in practice, Metro]
"I really think it's gotta start at the undergraduate level. To start teaching people this is the way of the future. And through training sessions and seminars disseminating it to the field practitioners." [ID7, 49 years old, 25 years in practice, Metro]

Coding exercise and agreement analysis

The 135 included patients provided 202 reasons for encounter. The chiropractors spent between 30 seconds to 20 minutes choosing a code for a particular diagnosis/problem.

Each of the 14 participating chiropractors recorded 10 patient encounters. For each of these patient encounters, the chiropractor could list up to 3 diagnoses. The total number of diagnostic codes provided by the chiropractors, and used in the agreement analysis, was 167 (Table 3). See Figure 1 for flow of participant and data in the study.

As presented in Table 3 the overall percentage agreement between the coder and the chiropractors on the ICPC-2 *Rubric level* (three-character code) was just over 50% agreement. On ICPC-2 PLUS *term level* (six-character code) the agreement was just over 30%. The level of

Table 3 Level of agreement

Chiropractor ID	Number of diagnoses coded	Agreement on *rubric level* (%)	Agreement on **term level* (%)
1	9	89	67
2	20	15	10
3	12	92	50
4	15	60	0
5	14	29	29
6	9	67	56
7	14	29	7
8	10	100	100
9	16	44	31
10	11	82	73
11	10	100	10
12	11	27	18
13	12	0	0
14	4	75	0
Overall agreement %		52	35
Agreement expected by chance		17	6
Overall agreement (Cohen's Kappa)	Total number of codes: 167	0.4 (95% CI 0.3-0.7)***	0.3 (95% CI 0.2-0.5)***

Rubric level: ICPC-2 classifies symptoms/complaints, problems/diagnoses and process of care using three character codes called a rubric. The first character, a letter, represents a chapter or a body system and the two additional characters, a number, represent a concept within this body system.
***Term level*: To allow for greater specificity, the ICPC-2 PLUS terminology was developed. Each PLUS *term* is classified to ICPC-2. ICPC-2 PLUS uses a six-character identifier by adding another three digits (a code) to the ICPC-2 rubric, to which the *term* has been classified.
***CI = 95% confidence interval.

agreement beyond chance was moderate with a Kappa score 0.4 (95% CI 0.3-0.7) on the ICPC-2 *Rubric level*, and fair with a Kappa score 0.3 (95% CI 0.2-0.5) on the ICPC-2 PLUS *term level*.

Discussion

This paper provides a first insight into views and perspectives of chiropractors about diagnostic coding in chiropractic practice. ICPC-2 PLUS was chosen as the example of a diagnostic coding system in this study because it has been proven to have a good reliability and validity for musculoskeletal diagnosis, which is the most common conditions treated in chiropractic practice. Also, it is already used in hospital settings/ secondary sector, the COAST data was coded with this particular classification and alongside the process a set of *terms* for chiropractic practice is under development ICPC-2 PLUS (Chiro) [7].

Most chiropractors were positive toward using a diagnostic coding system in their daily practice but some of

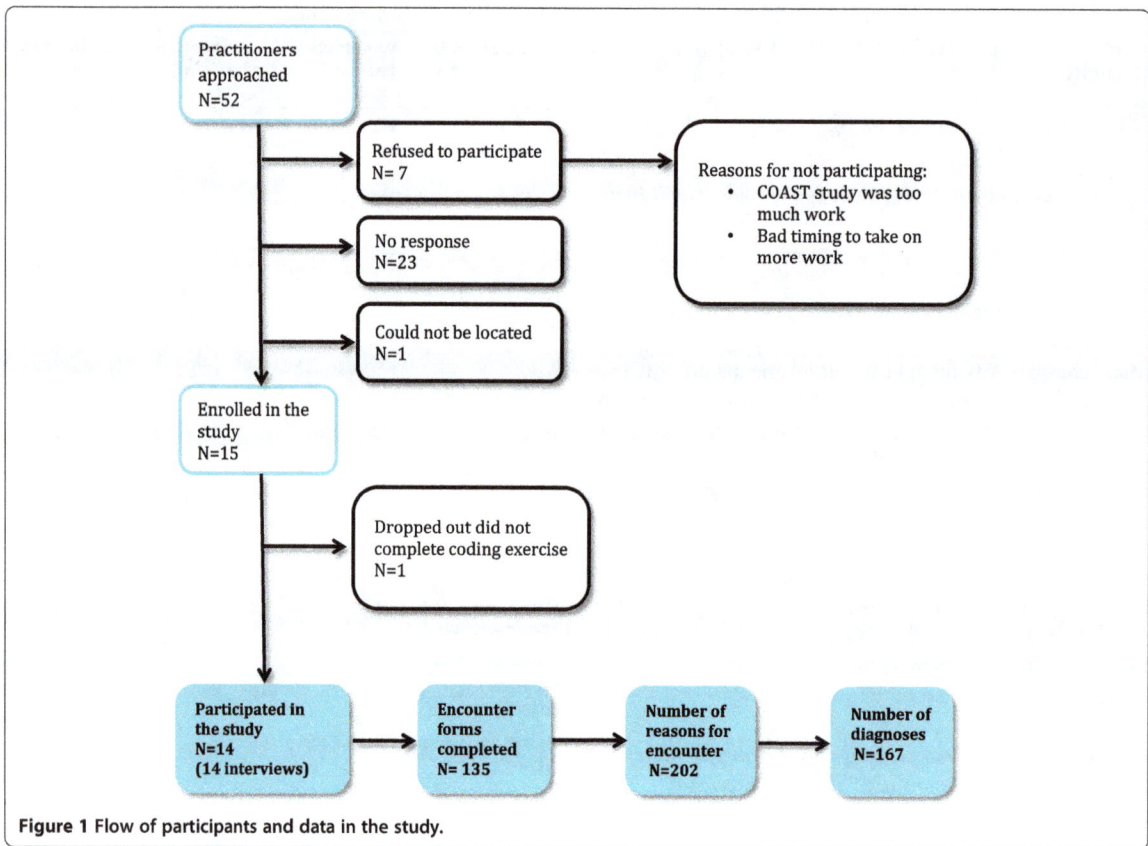

Figure 1 Flow of participants and data in the study.

those chiropractors did not see the relevance of the ICPC-2 PLUS for their practice. The chiropractors who described themselves as *wellness chiropractors* typically expressed the view that the terms available were not adequate to describe their clinical practice. The main issue here was the fact that they did not have a particular focus on specific symptoms. They said that it was obvious that ICPC-2 PLUS terms were made for medical practice, and that it would be better to make a new system for chiropractic practice with more relevant terms. Coding with the current terms in ICPC-2 PLUS may therefore not be relevant for all practice types. The terminology issue was also addressed alongside the conduct of COAST and resulted in a chiropractic-specific coding system being developed, ICPC-2 PLUS (Chiro) [7]. Many however agreed that with some training, ICPC-2 PLUS might be a useful system to have in chiropractic practice, especially to facilitate producing more clinically relevant research.

For the coding exercise if agreement between the chiropractor and coder was high, this would provide some support that ICPC-2 PLUS was potentially a good choice for diagnostic coding in chiropractic practice. If the agreement was low it would tell us that something

needed improvement. Either ICPC-2 PLUS was not a good fit for chiropractic practice, or the encounter forms the chiropractors completed did not provide enough information for the coder to agree with the chiropractors' choice of code.

The agreement between the coder and the chiropractors was higher than agreement expected by chance at both the ICPC-2 *Rubric level* and the ICPC-2 PLUS *term level*. However, the agreement was only fair to moderate and this could be due to a number of reasons. First, none of the chiropractors were familiar with the *terms* available for coding when they completed the encounter forms. The amount of time spent to get familiar with the *terms* available before the coding exercise differed considerably. The practitioners spent between 30 seconds to 20 minutes choosing a *term* for a particular diagnosis/ problem. Some of the participating chiropractors mentioned that they would have preferred some prior knowledge about the available *terms* before filling out the encounter forms. To avoid adding to the burden for the participating chiropractors, we decided not to include the list of *terms* in the study materials they received prior to the interviews. We do not know whether this would have improved the level of agreement or had an influence on their overall view on the idea of diagnostic coding in chiropractic practice.

For the agreement on ICPC-2 *rubric* level two chiropractors had 100% agreement with the coder, eight chiropractors had over 50% agreement with the coder. But the two chiropractors who achieved 100% agreement with the coder had only chosen one *term* for all the diagnoses. Despite a variation in their patients' reasons for encounter, the diagnoses, written by the chiropractor on the encounter form, were all the same. All other chiropractors had used at least three different *terms* when coding. In order to conduct the agreement analysis the participating chiropractors had to choose a *term* for every one of their diagnoses. They were asked to choose the *term* that came closest to describing the diagnosis, rather than being given an option of not choosing a *term*. This might have resulted in these two chiropractors choosing the same *term* for all the diagnoses.

Even the chiropractor who did not agree with the coder on any of the *terms* chosen was positive to using ICPC-2 PLUS in practice. Another chiropractor had an 82% agreement rate with the coder but was negative to the idea of using ICPC-2 PLUS in practice and emphasized a lack of relevance of the coding system to their clinical work and therefore lacked of motivation to implement the system. This chiropractor did not have a wellness practice.

Limitations and strengths

The sample size for both chiropractors and patient participants were smaller than planned. We did not reach our intended number of practitioners (14 instead of 15) and therefore also less patient participants. This meant one interview less than expected and less data for the agreement analysis. However, this study being the first of its kind and therefore exploratory we do not know what effects this would have had on the results. Qualitative research is not meant to be representative, it is meant to provide in-depth information and this study offers some insight to what possibilities and challenges diagnostic coding could bring to chiropractic practice.

The qualitative interviews, as well as the analysis, were completed with an awareness of the first author's (CT) personal background as a chiropractic student with minimal clinical experience, and a preconception that diagnostic coding could potentially improve patient care. Being aware of this a neutral approach was emphasized when interviewing and when conducting the analysis.

Suggestions for further studies

This study was the first to examine the role of diagnostic coding using an established primary care coding system in chiropractic practice. To determine the applicability of ICPC-2 PLUS or another diagnostic coding system in

chiropractic practice, more research is needed. A study with a bigger sample would provide further information on this topic.

In Denmark an introduction of the Danish version of ICPC-2, ICPC-2-DK to chiropractic practice is currently underway. ICPC-2-DK has been part of the electronic medical records in Danish general medical practice since 2009 [1]. A similar study to this with a sample of Danish chiropractors to evaluate the use of ICPC-2-DK in chiropractic practice would provide valuable information and potentially ease the implementation process.

Conclusion

Most of the chiropractors in this study found the use of diagnostic coding both feasible and applicable in their practices but recommended specific training for chiropractors in the use of the coding system. However, there was a strong agreement that the terminology in ICPC-2 PLUS would not be applicable or desirable for those members of the chiropractic profession who do not focus on symptoms in their approach to clinical care. Clinically relevant research opportunities and further integration in the mainstream health care system were mentioned as some of the future perspectives of diagnostic coding.

Thus, this first insight into the use of diagnostic coding in chiropractic practice is encouraging, but more research is needed to determine if these results are applicable to chiropractic practice in other countries and to investigate possibilities for improving the chiropractic relevance of the terminology.

Additional files

> **Additional file 1: The encounter form.**
>
> **Additional file 2: Additional quotes.**

Competing interests
LH is a member Editorial Board of Chiropractic & Manual Therapies, and SF is an Associate Editor, however neither had any involvement in the editorial process of this manuscript. Otherwise the authors declare no competing interests.

Authors' contributions
The study was conducted as part of a one-year pre-graduate research project undertaken by CT. SF was the main supervisor on location and overlooked every step of the process. SF and LH conceived the study. All authors were responsible for the study design. CT performed the data collection. CT and SF undertook the analyses. CT was responsible for drafting the manuscript. All authors read and approved the final manuscript.

Acknowledgements
We thank the participating chiropractors and patients, including Peter Werth and Tini Pham who participated in a pilot of the study. We would also like to thank the team in the Department of General Practice, at the University of Melbourne for their invaluable support, especially Melanie Charity and Patty Chondros for their help with the quantitative component as well as Victoria Palmer for her help with the qualitative component. Funding support for the first author (CT) to travel to Melbourne and conduct this study came from

the Nordic Institute for Chiropractic and Clinical Biomechanics (NIKKB). The University of Southern Denmark funded the vast majority of interview transcription and the Department of General Practice, the University of Melbourne, funded the transport to and from the clinics.

Author details
[1]Nordic Institute of Chiropractic and Clinical Biomechanics and Institute of Sports Science and Biomechanics, University of Southern Denmark, Odense, Denmark. [2]General Practice and Primary Health Care Academic Centre, University of Melbourne, Melbourne, VIC, Australia. [3]School of Rehabilitation Therapy, Faculty of Health Sciences, Queen's University, Kingston, Ontario, Canada.

References
1. Rosendal M, Falkoe E. Diagnostic classification in Denmark with emphasis on general practice. Ugeskr Laeger. 2009;171(12):997–1000. Danish.
2. ICPC-2 PLUS: The BEACH coding system Sydney, University of Sydney [updated 5 September 2012]. Available from: http://sydney.edu.au/medicine/fmrc/classifications/index.php.
3. Nielsen MN, Aaen-Larsen B, Vedsted P, Nielsen CV, Hjollund NH. Diagnosis coding of the musculoskeletal system in general practice. Ugeskr Laeger. 2008;170(37):2881–4.
4. French SD, Charity MJ, Forsdike K, Gunn JM, Polus BI, Walker BF, et al. Chiropractic Observation and Analysis Study (COAST): providing an understanding of current chiropractic practice. Med J Aust. 2013;199 (10):687–91.
5. Classification Committee of the World Organization of Family Doctors (WONCA) ICPC-2. International classification of primary care. Oxford: Oxford University Press; 1998.
6. Britt H, Miller GC, Henderson J, Charles J, Valenti L, Harrison C et al. General practice activity in Australia 2011–12. 2012;General practice series no. 31.
7. Charity MJ, French SD, Forsdike K, Britt H, Polus B, Gunn J. Extending ICPC-2 PLUS terminology to develop a classification system specific for the study of chiropractic encounters. Chiropr Man Therap. 2013;21(1):4.
8. ICPC-2 PLUS - Demonstrator Sydney, Australia: University of Sydney; 2002–2013 [updated 20 January 2013]. Available from: http://sydney.edu.au/medicine/fmrc/icpc-2-plus/demonstrator/index.php.
9. Kings N, Horrocks C. Interviews in Qualitative Research: SAGE Publications. 2010.
10. Patton M. Qualitative research and evaluation methods. 3rd ed. California, USA: Sage Publications, Inc.; 2002.
11. Hansen E. Successful qualitative health research. NSW, Australia: Allen and Unwin; 2006.
12. Landis JR, Koch GG. The measurement of observer agreement for categorical data. Biometrics. 1977;33(1):159–74.
13. National Statement on Ethical Conduct in Human Research Australia: National Health and Medical Research Council, NHMRC; 2013 [cited 2013 20 December 2013]. Available from: http://www.nhmrc.gov.au/guidelines/publications/e72.

16

Patients' experiences and expectations of chiropractic care: a national cross-sectional survey

Hugh MacPherson[1*], Elizabeth Newbronner[2], Ruth Chamberlain[3] and Ann Hopton[1]

Abstract

Background: Not enough is understood about patients' views of chiropractic care. The aims of this research were to explore patients' experiences and expectations, their perceptions of benefits and risks, and the implications for chiropractors' continuing fitness to practise.

Methods: Survey questions were formulated from existing literature, published guidance on good practice from the General Chiropractic Council, and from 28 telephone interviews and a small focus group with chiropractic patients using a semi-structured topic guide. In its final form, the survey elicited patients' ratings on expectations regarding 33 aspects of care. In a national cross-sectional survey, a number of sampling methods were required as a consequence of the low practitioner response rate.

Results: In total, 544 completed questionnaires were received from chiropractic patients, a lower response rate than expected (8%). The two main benefits that patients reported regarding their chiropractic care were reduced pain (92%) and increased mobility (80%). Of respondents, 20% reported unexpected or unpleasant reactions to their treatment, most commonly tiredness or fatigue (32%), and extra pain (36%). In most cases they expressed low levels of concern about these reactions. Patients' expectations were met for most aspects of care. The four aspects of practice where expectations were least well met comprised: having more information on the cost of the treatment plan at the first consultation (80%); the chiropractor contacting the patient's general practitioner if necessary (62%); having a discussion about a referral to another healthcare practitioner (62%); and providing a method for confidential feedback (66%).

Conclusions: Overall, patients reported a high level of satisfaction with the benefits of their chiropractic care, although there is a likelihood of bias towards patients with a positive experience of chiropractic. There were no serious adverse reactions; however, patients reported concern about pain, tingling and numbness in the limbs after chiropractic. In general, patients' expectations were being well met.

Keywords: Chiropractic, Patients' expectations, Patients' experiences, Risk, Benefit, Fitness to practice

Background

There is a growing body of research into patients' expectations and experiences (including adverse reactions) of complementary therapies. The OPEn Study [1] funded by the UK's General Osteopathic Council explored patients' expectations and experiences in relation to the benefits, risks and side effects of osteopathic treatment. It prioritised five areas of practice for the profession and the regulator to consider: the clinic environment; professionalism; treatment; relationship; and outcomes. It found a high level of satisfaction amongst patients consulting osteopaths working in private practice and most of the more widely held expectations were being met. Many of these related to the overall 'customer experience' but others were concerned with the therapeutic process and included the importance of "informing patients about what to expect in relation to treatment and outcomes including side effects" [1]. The study identified some gaps between expectations and delivery of care which could have a negative effect on the outcomes of care, and suggested that these gaps could be reduced by improving care and/or managing expectations better.

* Correspondence: hugh.macpherson@york.ac.uk
[1]Department of Health Sciences, University of York, York, UK
Full list of author information is available at the end of the article

There has been relatively little work on the expectations of patients of chiropractic. One study conducted in Sweden [2] found that whilst patients and chiropractors had similar expectations in relation to key areas such as the chiropractor diagnosing and explaining the nature of the problems to the patients, there were other important areas where expectations differed. In particular, patients were more likely than their chiropractor to expect a rapid (i.e. within one to two treatments) improvement in their condition. They were also more likely to expect to be given advice about how to manage their problem and exercises to do between treatments. Interestingly, the OPEn Study highlighted this as an area where the level of unmet positive expectation was relatively high.

In a Dutch study [3] on the benefits and risks of chiropractic care for neck pain, 529 patients provided data that showed that adverse reactions are rarely severe in nature and for most patients the benefits outweighed the risks. Two studies [4] commissioned by the UK's General Chiropractic Council (GCC) in 2009/10 brought together information from clinical research about the risks of chiropractic, and examined the possible costs of adverse reactions and sub-optimal outcomes. They concluded that 'suboptimal outcomes', such as delayed or missed diagnosis, missed recognition of contra-indications, inadequate care-management and poor record keeping, were of more concern (and had greater cost implications) than significant adverse reactions.

Whilst much can be learned from these and other studies, both from their direct work with patients and the wider literature reviews, the GCC identified an evidence gap in relation to UK chiropractic patients' views and expectations. Moreover the GCC was also reviewing its approach to the revalidation of registrants, and as part of this process wanted to gain a fuller understanding of patients' views of chiropractic care, in particular people's assessment of the risks and benefits of chiropractic treatment, their expectations of chiropractors, and their experience of them. In this context, the GCC commissioned independent researchers from Firefly Research & Evaluation, in partnership with the Department of Health Sciences at the University of York, to carry-out research with a focus on the experiences and expectations of patients and the extent to which these expectations were met. The results of the research outlined in this report were designed to inform the GCC's work on revalidation. This paper presents an overview of the survey results.

Methods
Design and setting of the qualitative interviews and focus group
We used qualitative methods as a preparation for designing and conducting a national survey. Three areas (Cardiff, the Scottish Borders, and Mansfield/Chesterfield) were chosen for the interviews and focus group to reflect city, town and rural communities. The chiropractors in each area were asked to assist with the study by inviting up to 10 of their current and former patients (including as far as possible a mix of age, gender, ethnicity and condition or disability) to take part in either a focus group, a telephone interview or face-to-face interview. In total, 12 chiropractors agreed to be involved and through them 30 patients gave written consent to take part in the study: 56% of these patients were female and 73% were aged under 65. Twenty-eight patients chose to take part in individual telephone interviews and two attended a focus group (in Mansfield/Chesterfield). The interviews and focus group were conducted by two experienced female health services researchers (LN, RC), using a semi-structured topic guide covering four main topics: 'choosing your chiropractor'; 'expectations'; 'risks and benefits'; and 'fitness to practice'. The topic guide used in the interviews provided an initial framework which was then expanded. The interviews were digitally recorded and typically lasted around 40 minutes. The interviews and focus group recordings were transcribed in full and the data were then analysed thematically [5] by two researchers (LN, RC). Ethical approval was obtained from the Research Governance Committee of the University of York's Department of Health Sciences (Ref no. HSRGC/2012/06)

Development of the questionnaire
The questionnaire used in the national cross-sectional survey was developed from reviewing the existing literature about patients' experiences and expectations of manual therapies, the General Chiropractic Code of Practice and Standard of Proficiency [6] and the telephone interviews and the focus group, as described above. The sections of the questionnaire were informed by five questions that were set out by the GCC to inform the research:

- What do patients of chiropractors see as the benefits of receiving chiropractic care?
- What do patients see as the potential risks of receiving chiropractic care?
- Has their perception of benefits and risks changed over time? If so, how?
- What has influenced their perceptions of the benefits and risks?
- Once a chiropractor is on the GCC register, what do patients expect will happen to assure an Individual chiropractor's continuing fitness to practise?

The core of the questionnaire focused on patients' experiences and expectations of chiropractic care and treatment at different stages in their contact with the chiropractor. We also asked patients directly about benefits, adverse reactions and what systems would reassure them that their chiropractor was keeping their knowledge and skills up to date. We tested the first draft of the questionnaire with a small number of patients who had taken part in the interviews and volunteered to assist us at this stage. Building on their comments and following discussions with colleagues at the GCC and within the research team, we developed a second draft of the questionnaire with was then tested with a sample of patients from a single chiropractic practice. Following this second pilot, the final version of the questionnaire was developed and agreed with colleagues at the GCC. A copy of the final questionnaire is attached in Additional file 1.

Survey participants

During November 2012 a random sample of 600 chiropractors (drawn from the GCC's database of registrants; n =960) were invited to participate in a national cross-sectional survey by distributing a questionnaire (available in paper-based form or electronically) to at least 10 of their current and former patients: four to current patients who were receiving regular chiropractic care over the past three months or more; two to new patients (i.e. at their first consultation); two to former patients who ceased treatment within the past 6 months by mutual agreement with the chiropractor and/or because the presenting problem was resolved; two to former patients who ceased treatment within the past 6 months but who ended their treatment unilaterally (i.e. before, in the chiropractor's view, the presenting problem was resolved). Practitioners were also asked to try to include a mix of age, gender, ethnicity and disability. In the first approach involving 600 practitioners, 47 chiropractors agreed to take part (8%). We subsequently contacted an additional sample of 360 chiropractors and of these 21 agreed to take part (6%). A further two chiropractors volunteered to be involved when the British Chiropractic Association (BCA) sent an email to its members. This resulted in a total of 70 chiropractors who agreed to help recruit patients for the survey. Information about the survey was also circulated by email to chiropractic patients registered with Care Response, an organisation that supports the collection of routine patient-related data (http://www.careresponse.co.uk/)

Data analysis

Data was entered onto an Excel spreadsheet and two researchers (Martin Baxter, Liz Newbronner) conducted a random audit of 10% of questionnaires to check for accuracy. Analysis of the survey data was conducted to characterise the survey respondents to assess the distribution of age within the sample, and the analysis included calculation of the mean, median and interquartile range values and the calculation of Z scores to assess the distribution of ages. Demographic data, comprising sex, ethnicity,

educational attainment, living environment and nationality, were analysed using frequencies and proportions. Other survey data regarding the experiences and expectations of chiropractic treatment were also analysed using frequencies and proportions. Associations between adverse reactions were analysed using Chi-squared statistics. Questions that were not answered (i.e. missing data) were also reported as frequencies and proportions.

Results

Patient participation rates and patient profile

We sent 1075 information sheets and questionnaires to the 70 recruited chiropractors and asked them to distribute these to their patients. This generated 401 usable questionnaires, a 37% response rate. A total of 5167 patients registered with 36 Care Response member chiropractors were emailed and 112 (2%) patients completed the survey through this route. In addition, the Chiropractic Patients Association also informed its members of the survey (N = 350) and 27 (9%) members and four of their friends and family responded as a result of this. Together all these recruitment methods generated a total of 544 respondents. Excluding the four family and friends, for whom we have no denominator, this represents an overall response rate of 8% (540/6592). The majority of questions (82%) had been answered; however, five questions (questions 40–44) contained between 16% and 20% of missing data. These questions with the greater proportion of missing data corresponded with the less well met expectations.

Of the 544 respondents, 360 (66%) were women; 4 (0.7%) did not give their gender (Table 1). The age distribution showed a significant negative skew ($z = -2.12$). The median age of respondents was 54.5 years (interquartile range = 43–71); yet when examined more closely, the age profile for women followed a normal distribution whilst the age profile for men showed a significant negative skew ($z = -2.810$) whereby 70% of the male participants were aged 50 and over. The majority of respondents lived in England (89%), classified their ethnic origin as white (96%), and lived within a city or town environment (58%). With regard to their highest level of educational qualification, 50% of the respondents had either first degrees or second degrees. This compares with 30% of the UK working age population having a first degree or higher [7].

Experiences of chiropractic care

Before receiving chiropractic treatment, 58% of patients had limited knowledge of what the treatment involved, 41% were unsure of the likely benefits and 71% had little knowledge of the possible reactions to treatment (Table 2). Over half (53%) attended every other month, 25% were no longer receiving treatment and 59% no

Table 1 Demographic of chiropractic patients surveyed (Total n = 544)

Questions asked		
What is your age? (n = 544)	**Years**	
Range =	16-87	
Median=	54.50	
Interquartile range 1; Interquartile range 3 =	43 ; 71	
Missing	0	
Are you? (n = 540)	**n =**	**(%)**
Male	180	33%
Female	360	66%
Missing	4	0.7%
What is your ethnicity? (n = 543)		
White	519	96%
Black or Black British	6	1%
Asian or Asian British	6	1%
Chinese or Chinese British	2	0.4%
Mixed heritage	0	0
Other ethnic group	8	1.4%
Missing	1	0.2%
Do you consider yourself to have a disability? (n =536)		
Yes	44	8%
No	492	91%
Missing	8	1.4%
What is your highest level of academic education/attainment? (n = 527)		
No academic qualifications	38	7%
GCSE or equivalent (e.g. O level, CSE, NVQ1)	96	18%
A levels or equivalent (e.g. NVQ2-3, BTec certificate, City and Guilds crafts)	117	22%
BA or BSC degree or equivalent (e.g. NVQ4, BTEC diploma, City and Guilds level 3+, nursing or teaching qualifications)	193	36%
Master's Degree, PhD, Post graduate certificate or NVQ level 5	79	15%
Other	4	0.7%
Missing	18	3%
How would you describe the area that you live in? (n = 534)		
City/Urban area	50	9%
Town or suburb	267	49%
Village or rural area	217	41%
Missing	10	1.8%
Which of the four UK nations do you live in? (n = 535)		
England	484	90%
Scotland	13	2%
Wales	28	5%
Northern Ireland	8	1.4%
Missing	9	1.6%

Table 2 Experiences of chiropractic treatment (n = 544)

Statements		
Before you first had chiropractic treatment, how much did you know about:		
a. What the treatment involved	**n =**	**%**
I knew very little	318	58%
Some knowledge	148	27%
I knew a lot	75	14%
Missing	2	0.4%
b. The likely benefits of the treatment		
I knew very little	224	41%
Some knowledge	182	33%
I knew a lot	134	25%
Missing	2	0.4%
c. Possible reactions to the treatment		
I knew very little	387	71%
Some knowledge	112	21%
I knew a lot	41	7%
Missing	2	0.4%
Approximately how many chiropractic treatments have you had in the last 12 months?	**n = treatments**	
Range =	0-55	
Median =	6	
Interquartile range 1; Interquartile range 3 =	4 ; 10	
Are you currently receiving treatment?	**n =**	**%**
YES	409	75%
NO	135	25%
Reasons given in answer to the question, "If 'NO', why did you stop chiropractic treatment?" (n = 135)		
	n =	**%**
The problem being treated improved/got better, I no longer needed treatment	79	59%
The problem being treated has improved and I am currently able to manage it myself	47	35%
I did not feel the treatment was benefitting me	6	4%
I was unhappy with the chiropractor's approach/manner	2	1.5%
I had an unpleasant reaction to treatment	0	0%
I was unhappy with the cost of treatment	3	2%
I am currently unable to afford treatment	7	5%
Other health problems have prevented me from having chiropractic treatment	1	0.7%
NB. 10 people (7%) gave more than one reason for stopping chiropractic treatment	145	107%

longer needed treatment. One third of the patients had changed their chiropractor at some point in the past with the main reasons being: linked to the patient moving to a new area; finding a chiropractor at a more convenient location; or the chiropractor moving away. Eight people (5%) said that the approach or manner of the chiropractor did not suit them or the treatment was not benefiting them.

Experiences of benefits and adverse reactions

The majority of patients surveyed reported benefits associated with chiropractic. These benefits included a reduction in the pain (92%) and an improvement in mobility (80%) (Table 3). More than half reported that chiropractic treatment had an ongoing effect of reducing future problems (55%) and provided a better understanding of their health problem (53%).

Approximately 20% (n = 110) of respondents reported one or more reactions to treatment that they found unexpected or unpleasant. Of a total of 153 reactions, among respondents 45% (n = 49) had one reaction, 34% (n = 37) had two reactions and the remainder had 3 or more (n = 15) (Table 4). Where patients reported on more than one type of reaction, they reported a single level of concern associated with their reactions. Extra pain and/or radiating pain was the symptom associated with the greatest level of concern (n = 19). Where patients had more than one reaction, extra pain was more commonly combined with tingling and stiffness.

Expectations of chiropractic care

Patients reported their expectations prior to the first consultation and what they experienced in practice (Table 5). Where patients responded 'Yes' to the question 'Did it happen' their expectation was met, but a response of 'No' signified their expectation was not met. For these questions, more than 80% of patients expected these aspects of care to happen and they did happen, which suggests there was a high level of satisfaction with this stage of the 'patient journey'.

Similar results were obtained for the patients' first consultation (Table 6). An area where there was a noticeable gap between expectations (86%) and experience (80%) was in regard to an explanation of the cost of the

Table 3 Experiences of chiropractic treatment: main benefits of treatment (n = 544)

	n =	%
It has reduced or removed the pain I was experiencing.	503	92%
It has increased my mobility/flexibility.	434	80%
It has helped me maintain my general health and wellbeing.	344	63%
It is helping to prevent or reduce future problems.	297	55%
It has given me a better understanding of my health problem.	286	53%
It has increased my ability/confidence to manage my health problem.	239	44%
It has enabled me to return to work, sport or other activities.	204	38%

treatment plan at the first consultation. Though there was a small difference of 3% between the expectation the chiropractor would talk about the possibility of adverse reactions and what happened, 13% of patients reported that this did not happen.

Questions were asked of respondents about on-going treatment processes (Table 7). In most cases, more than 90% of patients' expectations and experiences corresponded well. In some areas, chiropractors exceeded their patients' expectations, for example by displaying information about their length of time in practice and about their special interests or additional skills. In the survey, 99% of the respondents expected that their chiropractor would allow sufficient time for their consultation and this expectation was largely met, with 97% saying that it had happened. People responding to the survey had slightly lower expectations (85%) relating to when treatment should be reviewed.

When considering referral to other agencies, 86% of survey respondents expected that the chiropractor would refer them to other healthcare practitioners if appropriate and 87% expected them to contact their general practitioner, should this be needed (Table 8). In both cases, nearly two-thirds (62%) said this happened although 20% and 18% respectively did not answer the questions (q40, q41). It is not clear whether this relates to the expectation not being delivered or whether a referral was not required. Another area where there appeared to be a gap between expectations (76%) and experiences (66%) was with regard to a system for patients to provide confidential feedback; between 16% and 20% of patients did not answer these questions. A high percentage (97%) of survey respondents expected the chiropractor to provide advice on how to manage symptoms between treatments and this expectation was largely met, with 96% of respondents saying they had been given this type of support.

Expectations with regard to fitness to practice

With regards to the chiropractors' fitness to practice, almost half of the patients responding to the survey (49%) would feel reassured if patients were provided with information about the chiropractors' on-going training and development, whereas 19% disagreed and 30% were undecided. Between half and two-thirds of patients (61%) agreed that chiropractors should review their practice regularly (61%), be assessed by an independent assessor (66%) and have a practice-level system for gathering and showing patient feedback (59%). Half (50%) agreed that there should be a national system for gathering patient feedback and that patients could access.

Discussion

In a survey comprising 544 patients, the positive experiences reported were the benefits of reduced pain and increased mobility and an understanding of how to

Table 4 Experiences of chiropractic treatment: frequency of adverse reactions and reported level of concern (n = 110 of 544 patients)

Reaction	Level of concern (n =)		
	Of lower concern (1,2)	Of greater concern (3,4,5)	Total number of reactions
Tiredness or fatigue	33	2	35
Headache	19	4	23
Extra Pain and/or Radiating Pain	21	19	40
Tingling/numbness in legs or arms	3	9	12
Stiffness	13	7	20
Dizziness or light headedness	13	6	19
Nausea	1	3	4
Total	103	50	153

NB. Where patients reported on more than one type of reaction, they reported a single level of concern associated with their reactions.

maintain the improvements gained. There were no serious adverse reactions. Regarding minor reactions to treatment, some people reported greater concern about extra pain, tingling and numbness, whereas tiredness, fatigue and headache were of low concern. The survey showed that the patients' expectations of advice on how to manage symptoms between treatments were largely met. There were four areas where patients had relatively high expectations (i.e. >75% expected an aspect of care to happen) but these were not met for a significant proportion of patients (between 10 to 25%). These were: if necessary and with consent, the chiropractor would contact the patient's general practitioner; if the problem is not improving or the patient has other health needs the chiropractor will discuss referral to another healthcare practitioner; having the cost of the treatment plan explained at the first consultation; and the chiropractic practice having a system for patients to provide confidential feedback.

Strengths and limitations of the study

In terms of strengths, the study was conducted by a research group that was independent of associations or regulatory bodies associated with chiropractic. This independence meant that the study was not biased by prior agendas or partiality towards particular styles of chiropractic. The use of interviews with patients receiving chiropractic care prior to the national survey helped shape a more appropriate and targeted questionnaire. The piloting of the survey questions helped clarify the focus of the survey and reduced ambiguity. Nevertheless, the survey did require patients to recall their first consultation and so there is a risk of recall bias.

For many questions the level of expectation is high and the estimation of expectations being met may be reflected accurately. However, where the level of expectation is below 80% there may be a possibility of a substantial over-estimation of expectations being met. Furthermore, the missing data on questions relating to

Table 5 Expectations of chiropractic care: responses to questions related to 'before seeing the chiropractor' (n = 544); n/a = not answered

Statements	Expected			Did it happen?		
	Yes	No	n/a	Yes	No	n/a
Q11. Before seeing the Chiropractor I expect to be given general information about chiropractic treatment and what it involves.	91%	8%	1%	92%	7%	1%
Q12. Before seeing the Chiropractor I expect to be given general information about possible reactions (both positive and negative) to chiropractic treatment.	82%	15%	3%	82%	15%	3%
Q13. Before seeing the Chiropractor I expect to be given information about what will happen at my first consultation.	91%	7%	2%	91%	7%	2%
Q14. Before seeing the Chiropractor I expect to be told about the cost of treatments.	97%	2%	1%	95%	4%	1%
Q15. Before seeing the Chiropractor I expect to be told how long the first consultation is likely to last.	90%	8%	1%	91%	7%	2%
Q16. Before seeing the Chiropractor I expect to fill-in and sign a consent form for the first consultation.	83%	13%	3%	90%	6%	4%
Q17. Before seeing the Chiropractor I expect to provide my General Practitioner's name and contact details.	83%	15%	2%	91%	6%	3%

Table 6 Expectations of chiropractic care: responses to questions about the first consultation (n = 544); n/a = not answered

Statements	Expected			Did it happen?		
	Yes	No	n/a	Yes	No	n/a
Q18. At the First Consultation I expect to be given time to tell the chiropractor about my problem and how it was affecting me.	99%	0%	1%	99%	0%	1%
Q19. At the First Consultation I expect the chiropractor to take a detailed account of my personal case history.	96%	3%	1%	96%	1%	2%
Q20. At the First Consultation I expect to be given a gown and/or towels to cover up if I had to undress.	83%	12%	4%	84%	9%	7%
Q21. At the First Consultation I expect to be able to undress and dress in privacy.	90%	6%	5%	88%	5%	7%
Q22. At the First Consultation I expect the chiropractor to explain why any further investigations (e.g. X-Rays) were necessary and any risks associated with them.	72%	18%	10%	67%	20%	14%
Q23. At the First Consultation I expect the chiropractor to give me a diagnosis or rationale for my care.	93%	5%	2%	95%	3%	3%
Q24. At the First Consultation I expect the chiropractor to explain what treatment I will need (e.g. the type, frequency and duration of treatment).	97%	2%	1%	94%	4%	2%
Q25. At the First Consultation I expect the chiropractor to talk to me about any possible adverse reactions to the treatment.	87%	9%	3%	83%	13%	3%
Q26. At the First Consultation I expect the chiropractor to talk to me about the likely success of the treatment.	93%	6%	2%	91%	7%	2%
Q27. At the First Consultation I expect the chiropractor to explain what the cost of the agreed treatment plan would be.	86%	12%	3%	80%	17%	3%
Q28. At the First Consultation I expect the chiropractor to give me time to ask questions about the proposed treatment plan.	96%	3%	1%	94%	4%	2%

referral and the patients' complaint procedure may also reflect that the question was not applicable to them, because they had not previously considered the questions and therefore found it difficult to answer whether or not they expected to be told of either referral or complaints procedures.

A limitation of the survey was related to the difficulty we had in engaging chiropractors in the study, though we did eventually recruit 70, two of whom were not contacted directly. We only achieved a response rate of 7% (n = 68) from the 960 chiropractors that we contacted directly.

Moreover the response rate from their patients was also poor, with 37% of the questionnaires sent to chiropractors returned in paper form or on-line by their patients. It is possible that, despite the guidance provided by the research team, the chiropractors could have selected patients who they felt would provide a positive response, thereby biasing the sample. Therefore it could be argued that among respondents, largely consisting of patients selected by their own chiropractor or those who have joined a Chiropractic Patient's Association, attitudes towards chiropractic were biased towards being more favourable.

Table 7 Expectations of chiropractic care: responses to questions related to on-going treatment (n = 544); n/a = not answered

Statements	Expected			Did it happen?		
	Yes	No	n/a	Yes	No	n/a
Q29. I expect to be given time to tell the chiropractor about how I felt after my last treatment, and discuss any problems or concerns.	98%	1%	0%	97%	1%	1%
Q30. I expect the chiropractor to ask me if there has been any change in my condition, general health or medication.	97%	2%	1%	97%	2%	1%
Q31. I expect the chiropractor to allow sufficient time for the consultation.	99%	0%	1%	97%	2%	1%
Q32. I expect the chiropractor to talk to me about further treatment options.	91%	6%	2%	87%	9%	4%
Q33. I expect the chiropractor to allow me time to decide what I wish to do about future treatment.	92%	5%	3%	91%	5%	4%
Q34. I expect the chiropractor to agree with me when my treatment should be reviewed.	85%	11%	4%	84%	10%	6%
Q35. I expect the chiropractor to give me advice about how I manage my problems/symptoms between treatments.	97%	2%	1%	96	3%	1%

Table 8 Expectations of chiropractic care: assuring chiropractors are 'Fit to practice' responses to questions related to the chiropractor's knowledge and experience; (n=544); n/a = not answered

Statements	Expected			Did it happen?		
	Yes	No	n/a	Yes	No	n/a
Q36. I expect that information about the chiropractor's qualifications and registration will be displayed in the clinic/available in leaflets/included on the practice website.	90%	8%	2%	95%	4%	2%
Q37. I expect that information about the chiropractor's experience (e.g. length of time in practice) will be displayed in the clinic/available in leaflets/included on the practice website.	76%	22%	3%	82%	13%	6%
Q38. I expect that information about the chiropractor's special interests or additional skills (e.g. soft tissue massage) will be displayed in the clinic/available in leaflets/included on the practice website.	69%	26%	5%	75%	17%	9%
Q39. I expect that information about how the chiropractor is maintaining/improving their professional knowledge (e.g. further training) will be displayed in the clinic/included on the practice website.	56%	38%	6%	59%	28%	13%
Q40. I expect that if my problem is not improving with chiropractic treatment and/or I have other health needs, the chiropractor will discuss referral to another healthcare practitioner.	86%	8%	6%	62%	18%	20%
Q41. I expect that, if necessary, and with my consent, the chiropractor will contact my GP.	87%	10%	4%	62%	20%	18%
Responses to statements related to patient feedback and complaints						
Q42. I expect the chiropractic practice to have a clear system to enable me to provide confidential feedback (whether positive or negative).	76%	20%	4%	66%	18%	16%
Q43. I expect to be given information about the practice's complaints procedure.	54%	39%	7%	44%	38%	18%
Q44. I expect to be told about my right to refer a complaint to the General Chiropractic Council and be given the GCC's contact details.	51%	41%	9%	40%	40%	20%

There is some research evidence [8] that the overall population of chiropractic patients is fairly evenly split between women and men. We also noted the relatively high proportion of participants with either first degrees or second degrees compared to the UK working age population and speculate that this may reflect an affordability issue, in that chiropractic is more likely to be used by professional classes. In terms of how representative the patients involved in this study are of all patients who seek chiropractic care, it is important to sound a note of caution. The nature of this study means that most of the patients who contributed were either currently receiving treatment or had had on-going chiropractic care in the recent past. Those patients who ceased chiropractic care after a small number of treatments, perhaps because they were unhappy with their care may well be underrepresented. Nevertheless, our study data also suggests that where patients are unhappy with their treatment, this does not necessarily deter them from seeking further treatment from another chiropractor.

Comparison to previous literature

The positive experiences related to expectations of chiropractic care reported in this study are consistent with a previous quantitative study of expectations related to osteopathic treatment,[9] in which the majority of people were satisfied with the treatment they received

and their expectations of care were largely met. Also consistent with qualitative evidence within the osteopathic literature is that the most important expectations relate to the themes of individual agency, professional expertise, customer experience, therapeutic process and interpersonal relationships [10]. In a survey of chiropractic patients in Sweden, patients were found to have lower expectations of the chiropractic treatment than the chiropractors had, but higher expectations of being given advice and exercises than the chiropractors had [2]. Moreover, patients expected to get better faster than the chiropractors expected them to. We found that patients' expectations about being given advice about managing symptoms were largely met. In another study involving chiropractic patients, the researcher found that patients had an inaccurate or rudimentary understanding of the mechanisms that underpin chiropractic treatment, were not particularly interested in how it worked and despite the explanations of the chiropractor, patients showed only a limited understanding of the mechanisms [11]. In our study more than 90% expected to be given information about chiropractic and what it involved and to be given a diagnosis and rationale for their treatment. However, our survey did not ask whether the patients understood any of the information provided. There remains a gap in the literature, as previously identified [2], on whether unmet expectations contribute to lower levels of effectiveness.

Implications for practice

With regard to clinical practice, the less well met expectations can provide guidance on how chiropractic care could be improved from the perspective of patients. These areas where there could be some improvement include: allowing sufficient time for the consultation; being told about the cost of treatments; having the treatment needed explained; being given time to ask questions about the treatment plan; being told about the likely success of the treatment and adverse reactions; being told about further treatment options; and being able to undress and dress in privacy. A more substantial expectation/experience gap that could be addressed by changes in practice include: if necessary and with consent, the chiropractor would contact the patient's general practitioner; if the problem is not improving or the patient has other health needs the chiropractor will discuss referral to another healthcare practitioner; having the cost of the treatment plan explained at the first consultation; and the chiropractic practice having a system for patients to provide confidential feedback. These gaps between expectations and delivery of care are mostly a consequence of poor communication and may lead to negative effects on outcomes of care and/or patient dissatisfaction. By closing the gaps, chiropractors individually and as a profession can improve their clinical practice. In terms of future research, this paper provides a platform from which a more comprehensive survey can be conducted, with better methods of recruiting chiropractic patients to improve the response rate and to limit selection bias.

Conclusion

In general, patients reported a high level of satisfaction with the benefits of their chiropractic care, most commonly related to reduced pain and increased mobility. There were no serious adverse reactions. Among the minor reactions reported, there was greater concern about extra pain, tingling and numbness attributed to chiropractic and a lower level of concern about reactions of tiredness or fatigue. As reported by patients, expectations were largely met for most of the 33 aspects of practice. The areas where expectations were less well met were mostly due to inadequate or limited communication. By addressing these areas, chiropractors can improve the quality of their clinical practice and delivery of patient care.

Additional files

Additional file 1: Questionnaire for national survey -final.pdf, 339 K
http://www.chiromt.com/imedia/1336971084126552/supp1.pdf.

Competing interests
The authors declare that they have no competing interests.

Authors' contributions
HM is a senior research fellow specialising in the effectiveness, cost-effectiveness, mechanisms and safety in the evaluation of complementary medicine. He provided academic supervision for the study, drafted the article and gave final approval for publication. LN is an independent health and social care researcher whose research focuses on long term conditions, disability and self-management. She conducted the interviews and analysis, managed the survey, interpreted the data and helped revise the article. RC is an independent health and social care researcher who specialises in qualitative research. She conducted the interviews and analysis. AH is a research fellow from a nursing background whose research focuses on the non-pharmacological management of chronic pain and depression. She contributed to the design of the survey and revised the article. All authors read and approved the final manuscript.

Acknowledgements
We would like to thank all the patients who kindly agreed to be interviewed for this study and those who took the time to complete the survey. We are also very grateful to the chiropractors who agreed to assist us with the research as without their help in recruiting patients for the interviews and distributing the survey the study would not have been possible. We would also like to thank those professional associations who assisted us by publicising the study. Lastly we are indebted to Carol Latto from Chiropractic Plus for all her help and advice throughout the study, to Jonathan Field who distributed information about the survey to the Care Response patients from consenting practices, to Martin Baxter who provided technical support in managing the data from the survey and to Janet Eldred for her copy-editing.

Funding statement
The General Chiropractic Council, 44 Wicklow Street, London WC1X 9HL, UK commissioned and funded the independent research organisation, Firefly Research & Evaluation, North Yorkshire, to conduct this study. The GCC provided practical assistance in sampling from their database of registered chiropractors but had no involvement in the sampling decisions. The data collection, analysis and interpretation of the data of the project and the preparation, review and final approval of the manuscript were undertaken independently of the GCC by Firefly Research and by the Complementary Medicine Evaluation Group at the University of York.

Author details
[1]Department of Health Sciences, University of York, York, UK. [2]Firefly Research & Evaluation and Visiting Fellow, Department of Health Sciences, University of York, York, UK. [3]Firefly Research & Evaluation, North Yorkshire, UK.

References
1. Leach J, Cross V, Fawkes C, Mandy A, Hankins M, Fiske A, et al. Investigating osteopathic patients' expectations of osteopathic care: the OPEn project. Brighton: University of Brighton; 2011 [http://www.osteopathy.org.uk/resources/Research-and-surveys/GOsC-research/Osteopathic-patient-expectations-study/]
2. Sigrell H. Expectations of chiropractic treatment: what are the expectations of new patients consulting a chiropractor, and do chiropractors and patients have similar expectations? J Manip Physiol Ther. 2002;25(5):300–5.
3. Rubinstein SM, Leboeuf-Yde C, Knol DL, De Koekkoek TE, Pfeifle CE, Van Tulder MW. The benefits outweigh the risks for patients undergoing chiropractic care for neck pain: a prospective, multicenter, cohort study. J Manip Physiol Ther. 2007;30(6):408–18.
4. European Economics for the GCC: Report to the General Chiropractic Council and Counterfactual for Revalidation – Report to the General Chiropractic Council. General Chiropractic Council; 2010.
5. Braun V, Clarke V. Using thematic analysis in psychology. Qual Res Psychol. 2006;3:77–101.
6. General Chiropractic Code of Practice and Standard of Proficiency. General Chiropractic Council; 2010 [cited 2014 Apr 7]. [http://www.gccuk.org/UserFiles/Docs/COPSOP_2010.pdf]
7. Office for National Statistics. Census Population of working age by level of highest qualification, second quarter 2009. 2012, [http://www.ons.gov.uk/ons/publications/re-reference-tables.html?edition=tcm%3A77-363799]

8.   Pedersen P, Breen AC. An overview of European chiropractic practice. J Manip Physiol Ther. 1994;17(4):228–37.

9.   Leach C, Mandy A, Hankins M, Bottomley LM, Cross V, Fawkes CA, et al. Patients' expectations of private osteopathic care in the UK: a national survey of patients. BMC Comp Altern Med. 2013;13(1):122.

10. Cross V, Leach CMJ, Fawkes CA, Moore AP. Patients' expectations of osteopathic care: a qualitative study. Health Expect; 2013 May. doi:10.1111/hex.12084

11. Hennius BJ. Contemporary chiropractic practice in the UK: a field study of a chiropractor and his patients in a suburban chiropractic clinic. Chiropr Man Ther. 2013;21(1):25.

17

Chiropractic care and the risk of vertebrobasilar stroke: results of a case–control study in U.S. commercial and Medicare Advantage populations

Thomas M Kosloff[1*†], David Elton[1†], Jiang Tao[2†] and Wade M Bannister[2†]

Abstract

Background: There is controversy surrounding the risk of manipulation, which is often used by chiropractors, with respect to its association with vertebrobasilar artery system (VBA) stroke. The objective of this study was to compare the associations between chiropractic care and VBA stroke with recent primary care physician (PCP) care and VBA stroke.

Methods: The study design was a case–control study of commercially insured and Medicare Advantage (MA) health plan members in the U.S. population between January 1, 2011 and December 31, 2013. Administrative data were used to identify exposures to chiropractic and PCP care. Separate analyses using conditional logistic regression were conducted for the commercially insured and the MA populations. The analysis of the commercial population was further stratified by age (<45 years; ≥45 years). Odds ratios were calculated to measure associations for different hazard periods. A secondary descriptive analysis was conducted to determine the relevance of using chiropractic visits as a proxy for exposure to manipulative treatment.

Results: There were a total of 1,829 VBA stroke cases (1,159 – commercial; 670 – MA). The findings showed no significant association between chiropractic visits and VBA stroke for either population or for samples stratified by age. In both commercial and MA populations, there was a significant association between PCP visits and VBA stroke incidence regardless of length of hazard period. The results were similar for age-stratified samples. The findings of the secondary analysis showed that chiropractic visits did not report the inclusion of manipulation in almost one third of stroke cases in the commercial population and in only 1 of 2 cases of the MA cohort.

Conclusions: We found no significant association between exposure to chiropractic care and the risk of VBA stroke. We conclude that manipulation is an unlikely cause of VBA stroke. The positive association between PCP visits and VBA stroke is most likely due to patient decisions to seek care for the symptoms (headache and neck pain) of arterial dissection. We further conclude that using chiropractic visits as a measure of exposure to manipulation may result in unreliable estimates of the strength of association with the occurrence of VBA stroke.

Keywords: Chiropractic, Primary care, Cervical manipulation, Vertebrobasilar stroke, Adverse events

* Correspondence: thomas.kosloff@optum.com
†Equal contributors
[1]Optum Health – Clinical Programs at United Health Group, 11000 Optum Circle, Eden Prairie MN 55344, USA
Full list of author information is available at the end of the article

Background

The burden of neck pain and headache or migraine among adults in the United States is significant. Survey data indicate 13% of adults reported neck pain in the past 3 months [1]. In any given year, neck pain affects 30% to 50% of adults in the general population [2]. Prevalence rates were reportedly greater in more economically advantaged countries, such as the USA, with a higher incidence of neck pain noted in office and computer workers [3]. Similar to neck pain, the prevalence of headache is substantial. During any 3-month timeframe, severe headaches or migraines reportedly affect one in eight adults [1].

Neck pain is a very common reason for seeking health care services. "In 2004, 16.4 million patient visits or 1.5% of all health care visits to hospitals and physician offices, were for neck pain" [4]. Eighty percent (80%) of visits occurred as outpatient care in a physician's office [4]. The utilization of health care resources for the treatment of headache is also significant. "In 2006, adults made nearly 11 million physician visits with a headache diagnosis, over 1 million outpatient hospital visits, 3.3 million emergency department visits, and 445 thousand inpatient hospitalizations" [1].

In the United States, chiropractic care is frequently utilized by individuals with neck and/or headache complaints. A national survey of chiropractors in 2003 reported that neck conditions and headache/facial pain accounted respectively for 18.7% and 12% of the patient chief complaints [5]. Chiropractors routinely employ spinal manipulative treatment (SMT) in the management of patients presenting with neck and/or headache [6], either alone or combined with other treatment approaches [7-10].

While evidence syntheses suggest the benefits of SMT for neck pain [7-9,11-13] and various types of headaches [10,12,14-16], the potential for rare but serious adverse events (AE) following cervical SMT is a concern for researchers [17,18], practitioners [19,20], professional organizations [21-23], policymakers [24,25] and the public [26,27]. In particular, the occurrence of stroke affecting the vertebrobasilar artery system (VBA stroke) has been associated with cervical manipulation. A recent publication [28] assessing the safety of chiropractic care reported, "...the frequency of serious adverse events varied between 5 strokes/ 100,000 manipulations to 1.46 serious adverse events/ 10,000,000 manipulations and 2.68 deaths/10,000,000 manipulations". These estimates were, however, derived from retrospective anecdotal reports and liability claims data, and do not permit confident conclusions about the actual frequency of neurological complications following spinal manipulation.

Several systematic reviews investigating the association between stroke and chiropractic cervical manipulation have reported the data are insufficient to produce definitive conclusions about its safety [28-31]. Two case–control studies [32,33] used visits to a chiropractor as a proxy for SMT in their analyses of standardized health system databases for the population of Ontario (Canada). The more recent of these studies [32] also included a case-crossover methodology, which reduced the risk of bias from confounding variables. Both case–control studies reported an increased risk of VBA stroke in association with chiropractic visits for the population under age 45 years old. Cassidy, et al. [32] found, however, the association was similar to visits to a primary care physician (PCP). Consequently, the results of this study suggested the association between chiropractic care and stroke was noncausal. In contrast to these studies, which found a significant association between chiropractic visits and VBA stroke in younger patients (<45 yrs.), the analysis of a population-based case-series suggested that VBA stroke patients who consulted a chiropractor the year before their stroke were older (mean age 57.6 yrs.) than previously documented [34].

The work by Cassidy, et al. [32] has been qualitatively appraised as one of the most robustly designed investigations of the association between chiropractic manipulative treatment and VBA stroke [31]. To the best of our knowledge, this work has not been reproduced in the U.S. population. Thus, the main purpose of this study is to replicate the case–control epidemiological design published by Cassidy, et al. [32] to investigate the association between chiropractic care and VBA stroke; and compare it to the association between recent PCP care and VBA stroke in samples of the U.S. commercial and Medicare Advantage (MA) populations. A secondary aim of this study is to assess the utility of employing chiropractic visits as a proxy measure for exposure to spinal manipulation.

Methods

Study design and population

We developed a case–control study based on the experience of commercially insured and MA health plan members between January 1, 2011 and December 31, 2013. General criteria for membership in a commercial or MA health plan included either residing or working in a region where health care coverage was offered by the insurer. Individuals must have Medicare Part A and Part B to join a MA plan. The data set included health plan members located in 49 of 50 states. North Dakota was the only State not represented.

Both case and control data were extracted from the same source population, which encompassed national health plan data for 35,726,224 unique commercial and 3,188,825 unique MA members. Since members might be enrolled for more than one year, the average

Chiropractic care and the risk of vertebrobasilar stroke: results of a case–control study...

163

annual commercial membership was 14.7 million members and the average annual MA membership was 1.4 million members over the three year study period, which is comparable to ~5% of the total US population based on the data available from US Census Bureau [35]. Administrative claims data were used to identify cases, as well as patient characteristics and health service utilization.

The stroke cases included all patients admitted to an acute care hospital with vertebrobasilar (VBA) occlusion and stenosis strokes as defined by ICD-9 codes of 433.0, 433.01, 433.20, and 433.21 during the study period. Patients with more than one admission for a VBA stroke were excluded from the study. For each stroke case, four age and gender matched controls were randomly selected from sampled qualified members. Both cases and controls were randomly sorted prior to the matching using a greedy matching algorithm [36].

Exposures
The index date was defined as the date of admission for the VBA stroke. Any encounters with a chiropractor or a primary care physician (PCP) prior to the index date were considered as exposures. To evaluate the impact of chiropractic and PCP treatment, the designated hazard period in this study was zero to 30 days prior to the index date. For the PCP analysis, the index date was excluded from the hazard period since patients might consult PCPs after having a stroke. The standard health plan coverage included a limit of 20 chiropractic visits. In rare circumstances a small employer may have selected a 12-visit limit. An internal analysis (data not shown) revealed that 5% of the combined (commercial and MA) populations reached their chiropractic visit limits. Instances of an employer not covering chiropractic care were estimated to be so rare that it would have had no measureable impact on the analysis. There were no limits on the number of reimbursed PCP visits per year.

Analyses
Two sets of similar analyses were performed, one for the commercially insured population and one for the MA population. In each set of analyses, conditional logistic regression models were used to examine the association between the exposures and VBA strokes. To measure the association, we estimated the odds ratio of having the VBA stroke and the effect of total number of chiropractic visits and PCP visits within the hazard period. The analyses were applied to different hazard periods, including one day, three days, seven days, 14 days and 30 days for both chiropractic and PCP visits. The results of the chiropractic and PCP visit analyses were then compared to find evidence of excess risk of having stroke for patients with chiropractic visits during the

hazard period. Previous research has indicated that most patients who experience a vertebral artery dissection are under the age of 45. Therefore, in order to investigate the impact of exposure on the population at different ages, separate analyses were performed on patients stratified by age (under 45 years and 45 years and up) for the study of the commercial population. The number of visits within the hazard period was entered as a continuous variable in the logistic model. The chi square test was used to analyze the proportion of co-morbidities in cases as compared to controls.

A secondary analysis was performed to evaluate the relevance of using chiropractic visits as a proxy for spinal manipulation. The commercial and MA databases were queried to identify the proportions of cases of VBA stroke and matched controls for which at least one chiropractic spinal manipulative treatment procedural code (CPT 98940 – 98942) was or was not recorded. The analysis also calculated the use of another manual therapy code (CPT 97140), which may be employed by chiropractors as an alternative means of reporting spinal manipulation.

Ethics
The New England Institutional Review Board (NEIRB) determined that this study was exempt from ethics review.

Results
The commercial study sample included 1,159 VBA stroke cases over the three year period and 4,633 age and gender matched controls. The average age of the patients was 65.1 years and 64.8% of the patients were male (Table 1). The prevalence rate of VBA stroke in the commercial population was 0.0032%.

There were a total of 670 stroke cases and 2,680 matched controls included in the MA study. The average patient age was 76.1 years and 58.6% of the patients were male (Table 2). For the MA population, the prevalence rate of VBA stroke was 0.021%.

Claims during a one year period prior to the index date were extracted to identify comorbid disorders. Both the commercial and MA cases had a high percentage of comorbidities, with 71.5% of cases in the commercial study and 88.5% of the cases in the MA study reporting at least one of the comorbid conditions (Table 3). Six comorbid conditions of particular interest were identified, including hypertensive disease (ICD-9 401–404), ischemic

Table 1 Age and gender of cases and controls (Commercial)

Variable	Cases (n = 1159)	Controls (n = 4633)
Age: mean (median)	65.1 (64.7)	65.1 (64.7)
Males: n (%)	751 (64.8)	3001 (64.8)

Table 2 Age and gender of cases and controls (Medicare)

Variable	Cases (n = 670)	Controls (n = 2680)
Age: mean (median)	76.1 (76.2)	76.1 (76.2)
Males: n (%)	393 (58.6)	1572 (58.6)

heart disease (ICD-9 410–414), disease of pulmonary circulation (ICD-9 415–417), other forms of heart disease (ICD-9 420–429), pure hypercholesterolemia (ICD-9 272.0) and diseases of other endocrine glands (ICD-9 249–250). There were statistically significant differences (p = <0.05) between groups for most comorbidities. Greater proportions of comorbid disorders (p = <0.0001) were reported in the commercial and MA cases for hypertensive disease, heart disease and endocrine disorders (Table 3). The commercial cases also showed a larger proportion of diseases of pulmonary circulation, which was statistically significant (p = 0.0008). There were no significance differences in pure hypercholesterolemia for either the commercial or MA populations. Overall, cases in both the commercial and MA populations were more likely (p = <0.0001) to have at least one comorbid condition.

Among the commercially insured, 1.6% of stroke cases had visited chiropractors within 30 days of being admitted to the hospital, as compared to 1.3% of controls visiting chiropractors within 30 days prior to their index date. Of the stroke cases, 18.9% had visited a PCP within 30 days prior to their index date, while only 6.8% of controls had visited a PCP (Table 4). The proportion of exposures for chiropractic visits was lower in the MA sample within the 30-day hazard period (cases = 0.3%; controls = 0.9%). However, the proportion of exposures for PCP visits was higher, with 21.3% of cases having PCP visits as compared to12.9% for controls (Table 5).

The results from the analyses of both the commercial population and the MA population were similar (Tables 6, 7 and 8). There was no association between chiropractic visits and VBA stroke found for the overall sample, or for samples stratified by age. No estimated odds ratio was significant at the 95% confidence level. MA data were insufficient to calculate statistical measures of association for hazard periods less than 0–14 days for chiropractic visits. When stratified by age, the data were too sparse to calculate measures of association for hazard periods less than 0–30 days in the commercial population. The data were too few to analyze associative risk by headache and/or neck pain diagnoses (data not shown).

These results showed there is an association existing between PCP visits and VBA stroke incidence regardless of age or length of hazard period. A strong association was found for those visits close to the index date (OR 11.56; 95% CI 6.32-21.21) for all patients with a PCP visit within 0–1 day hazard period in the commercial sample. There was an increased risk of VBA stroke associated with each PCP visit within 30-days prior to the index date for MA patients (OR 1.51; 95% CI 1.32-1.73) and commercial patients (OR 2.01; 95% CI 1.77-2.29).

The findings of the secondary analysis showed – that of 1159 stroke cases from commercial population – there were a total of 19 stroke cases associated with chiropractic visits for which 13 (68%) had claims documentation indicating chiropractic SMT was performed. For the control group of the commercial cohort, 62 of 4633 controls had claims of any kind of chiropractic visits and 47 of 4633 controls had claims of SMT. In the commercial control group, 47 of 62 DC visits (76%) included SMT in the claims data. Only 1 of 2 stroke cases in the MA population included SMT in the claims data. For the MA cohort, 21 of 24 control chiropractic visits (88%) included SMT in the claims data (Table 9).

None of the stroke cases in either population included CPT 97140 as a substitute for the more conventionally reported chiropractic manipulative treatment procedural codes (98940 – 98942). For the control groups, there were three instances where CPT 97140 was reported without CPT 98940 – 98942 in the commercial population. The CPT code 97140 was not reported in MA control cohort.

Table 3 Comorbid conditions

Conditions n (%)	Commercial			Medicare		
	Cases (n = 1159)	Controls (n = 4633)	p-value	Cases (n = 670)	Controls (n = 2680)	p-value
Hypertensive disease	767 (66.2)	2078 (44.9)	<0.0001	554 (82.7)	1721 (64.2)	<0.0001
Ischemic heart disease	300 (25.9)	638 (13.8)	<0.0001	258 (38.5)	563 (21.0)	<0.0001
Diseases of pulmonary circulation	29 (2.5)	55 (1.2)	0.0008	18 (2.7)	70 (2.6)	0.9140
Other forms of heart disease	357 (30.8)	800 (17.3)	<0.0001	306 (45.7)	713 (26.6)	<0.0001
Pure Hypercholesterolemia	9 (0.8)	24 (0.5)	0.2957	6 (0.9)	26 (1.0)	0.8590
Diseases of other endocrine glands	319 (27.5)	754 (16.3)	<0.0001	285 (42.5)	740 (27.6)	<0.0001
At least one of the conditions	829 (71.5)	2317 (50.0)	<0.0001	593 (88.5)	1885 (70.3)	<0.0001

Table 4 Chiropractic and PCP visits prior to the index date (Commercial)

Exposures	All		Age <45 yr		Age ≥45 yr	
	Cases (n = 1159)	Controls (n = 4633)	Cases (n = 98)	Controls (n = 392)	Cases (n = 1061)	Controls (n = 4241)
Most recent DC Visit						
0-1 day: n (%)	3 (0.3)	11 (0.2)	*	*	3 (0.3)	11 (0.3)
0-3 days: n (%)	6 (0.5)	21 (0.5)	*	1 (0.3)	6 (0.6)	20 (0.5)
0-7 days: n (%)	8 (0.7)	31 (0.7)	*	1 (0.3)	8 (0.8)	30 (0.7)
0-14 days: n (%)	9 (0.8)	44 (0.9)	*	3 (0.8)	9 (0.8)	41 (1.0)
0-30 days: n (%)	19 (1.6)	62 (1.3)	2 (2.0)	7 (1.8)	17 (1.6)	55 (1.3)
Most recent PCP Visit						
1-1 day: n (%)	41 (3.5)	15 (0.3)	4 (4.1)	1 (0.3)	37 (3.5)	14 (0.3)
1-3 days: n (%)	78 (6.7)	41 (0.9)	8 (8.2)	2 (0.5)	70 (6.6)	39 (0.9)
1-7 days: n (%)	115 (9.9)	93 (2.0)	10 (10.2)	4 (1.0)	105 (9.9)	89 (2.1)
1-14 days: n (%)	157 (13.5)	165 (3.6)	12 (12.2)	15 (3.8)	145 (13.7)	150 (3.5)
1-30 days: n (%)	219 (18.9)	316 (6.8)	23 (23.5)	29 (7.4)	196 (18.5)	287 (6.8)

*Insufficient data to compute an estimate.

Discussion

The primary aim of the present study was to investigate the association between chiropractic manipulative treatment and VBA stroke in a sample of the U.S. population. This study was modelled after a case–control design previously conducted for a Canadian population [32]. Administrative data for enrollees in a large national health care insurer were analyzed to explore the occurrence of VBA stroke across different time periods of exposure to chiropractic care in comparison with PCP care.

Unlike Cassidy et al. [32] and most other case–control studies [33,37,38], our results showed there was no significant association between VBA stroke and chiropractic visits. This was the case for both the commercial and MA populations. In contrast to two earlier case–control studies [32,33], this lack of association was found to be

Table 5 Chiropractic and PCP visits prior the index date (Medicare)

Exposures	Cases (n = 670)	Controls (n = 2680)
Most recent DC Visit		
0-1 day: n (%)	*	4 (0.1)
0-3 days: n (%)	*	8 (0.3)
0-7 days: n (%)	*	9 (0.3)
0-14 days: n (%)	1 (0.1)	15 (0.6)
0-30 days: n (%)	2 (0.3)	24 (0.9)
Most recent PCP Visit		
1-1 day: n (%)	16 (2.4)	18 (0.7)
1-3 days: n (%)	30 (4.5)	36 (1.3)
1-7 days: n (%)	55 (8.2)	97 (3.6)
1-14 days: n (%)	90 (13.4)	183 (6.8)
1-30 days: n (%)	143 (21.3)	346 (12.9)

*Insufficient data to compute an estimate.

irrespective of age. Although, our results (Table 8) did lend credence to previous reports that VBA stroke occurs more frequently in patients under the age of 45 years. Additionally, the results from the present study did not identify a relevant temporal impact. There was no significant association, when the data were sufficient to calculate estimates, between chiropractic visits and stroke regardless of the hazard period (timing of most recent visit to a chiropractor and the occurrence of stroke).

There are several possible reasons for the variation in results with previous similar case–control studies. The younger (<45 yrs.) commercial cohort that received chiropractic care in our study had noticeably fewer cases. The 0–30 days hazard period included only 2 VBA stroke cases. There were no stroke cases for other hazard periods in this population. In contrast, earlier studies reported sufficient cases to calculate risk estimates for most hazard periods [32,33].

Another factor that potentially influenced the difference in results concerns the accuracy of hospital claims data in the U.S. vs. Ontario, Canada. The source population in the Province of Ontario was identified, in part, from the Discharge Abstract Database (DAD). The DAD includes hospital discharge and emergency visit diagnoses that have undergone a standardized assessment by a medical records coder [39]. To the best of our knowledge, similar quality management practices were not routinely applied to hospital claims data used in sourcing the population for our study.

An additional reason for the disparity in results may be due to differences in the proportions of chiropractic visits where SMT was reportedly performed. Our study showed that SMT was not reported by chiropractors in more than 30% of commercial cases. It is plausible that a number of the cases in earlier studies also did not

Table 6 Estimated odds ratios and 95% confidence interval (Commercial)

Exposures	All		Age < 45 yr		Age > =45 yr	
	Odds ratio	95% CI	Odds ratio	95% CI	Odds ratio	95% CI
Any DC Visit						
0-1 day	1.09	0.30-3.91	*	*	1.09	0.30-3.91
0-3 days	1.14	0.46-2.83	*	*	1.20	0.48-2.30
0-7 days	1.03	0.48-2.25	*	*	1.07	0.49-2.33
0-14 days	0.82	0.40-1.68	*	*	0.88	0.43-1.81
0-30 days	1.23	0.73-2.06	1.14	0.24-5.50	1.24	0.72-2.14
Any PCP Visit						
1-1 day	11.56	6.30-21.21	16.00	1.79-143.2	11.22	5.96-21.11
1-3 days	7.75	5.29-11.35	16.00	3.40-75.35	7.31	4.93-10.86
1-7 days	5.23	3.95-6.93	10.00	3.14-31.88	5.00	3.73-6.68
1-14 days	4.24	3.36-5.35	3.72	1.62-8.53	4.29	3.37-5.46
1-30 days	3.22	2.66-3.89	4.08	2.17-7.68	3.14	2.58-3.83

*Insufficient data to compute an estimate.

include SMT as an intervention. Differences between studies in the proportion of cases reporting SMT may have affected the calculation of risk estimates.

Also, there were an insufficient number of cases having cervical and/or headache diagnoses in our study. Therefore, our sample population may have included proportionally less cases where cervical manipulation was performed.

Our results were consistent with previous findings [32,33] in showing a significant association between PCP visits and VBA stroke. The odds ratios for any PCP visit increase dramatically from 1–30 days to 1–1 day (Tables 6 and 7). This finding is consistent with the hypothesis that patients are more likely to see a PCP for symptoms related to vertebral artery dissection closer to the index date of their actual stroke. Since it is unlikely that the services provided by PCPs cause VBA strokes, the association

between recent PCP visits and VBA stroke is more likely attributable to the background risk related to the natural history of the condition [32].

A secondary goal of our study was to assess the utility of employing chiropractic visits as a surrogate for SMT. Our findings indicate there is a high risk of bias associated with using this approach, which likely overestimated the strength of association. Less than 70% of stroke cases (commercial and MA) associated with chiropractic care included SMT. A somewhat higher proportion of chiropractic visits included SMT for the control groups (commercial = 76%; MA = 88%).

There are plausible reasons that support these findings. Internal analyses of claims data (not shown) consistently demonstrate that one visit is the most common number associated with a chiropractic episode of care. The single visit may consist of an evaluation without treatment such as SMT. Further; SMT may have been viewed as contraindicated due to signs and symptoms of vertebral artery dissection (VAD) and/or stroke. This might explain the greater proportion of SMT provided to control groups in both the commercial and MA populations.

Overall, our results increase confidence in the findings of a previous study [32], which concluded there was no excess risk of VBA stroke associated chiropractic care compared to primary care. Further, our results indicate there is no significant risk of VBA stroke associated with chiropractic care. Additionally, our findings highlight the potential flaws in using a surrogate variable (chiropractic visits) to estimate the risk of VBA stroke in association with a specific intervention (manipulation).

Our study had a number of strengths and limitations. Both case and control data were extracted from the same source population, which encompassed national health plan data for approximately 36 million

Table 7 Estimated odds ratios and 95% CI (Medicare)

Exposures	Odds ratio	95% CI
Any DC Visit		
0-1 day	*	*
0-3 days	*	*
0-7 days	*	*
0-14 days	0.26	0.03-2.00
0-30 days	0.32	0.08-1.39
Any PCP Visit		
1-1 day	3.66	1.85-7.26
1-3 days	3.38	2.07-5.51
1-7 days	2.37	1.68-3.34
1-14 days	2.09	1.60-2.73
1-30 days	1.81	1.46-2.25

*Insufficient data to compute an estimate.

Table 8 Odds ratio and 95% CI for association between # of exposures during 30-day hazard period

Exposures	All cases		Age <45 yr		Age >45 yr	
	Odds ratio	95% CI	Odds ratio	95% CI	Odds ratio	95% CI
Commercial						
Any DC* visit	1.03	0.86-1.26	1.32	0.64-2.71	1.01	0.81-1.25
Any PCP visit	2.01	1.77-2.29	2.38	1.55-3.66	1.97	1.72-2.26
Medicare						
Any DC* visit	0.54	0.23-1.28				
Any PCP visit	1.51	1.32-1.73				

*DC = Chiropractic.

commercial and 3 million MA members. A total of 1,829 cases were identified, making this the largest case–control study to investigate the association between chiropractic manipulation and VBA stroke. Due to the nationwide setting and large sample size, our study likely reduced the risk of bias related to geographic factors. However, there was a risk of selection bias – owing to the data set being from a single health insurer – including income status, workforce participation, and links to health care providers and hospitals.

Our study closely followed a methodological approach that had previously been described [32], thus allowing for more confident comparisons.

The current investigation analyzed data for a number of comorbid conditions that have been identified as potentially modifiable risk factors for a first ischemic stroke [40]. The differences between groups were statistically significant for most comorbidities. Information was not obtainable about behavioural comorbid factors e.g., smoking and body mass. With the exception of hypertensive disease, there are reasons to question the clinical significance of these conditions in the occurrence of ischemic stroke due to vertebral artery dissection. A large multinational case-referent study investigated the association between vascular risk factors (history of vascular disease, hypertension, smoking, hypercholesterolemia, diabetes mellitus, and obesity/overweight) for ischemic stroke and the occurrence of cervical artery dissection [41]. Only hypertension had a positive association (odds ratio 1.67; 95% confidence interval, 1.32 to 2.1; P <0.0001) with cervical artery dissection.

While the effect of other unmeasured confounders cannot be discounted, there is reason to suspect the absence of these data was not deleterious to the results. Cassidy, et al. found no significant differences in the results their case-crossover design, which affords better control of unknown confounding variables, and the findings of their case–control study [32].

Our results highlight just how unusual VBA stroke is in the MA cohort (prevalence = 0.021%) and – even more so – for the commercial population (prevalence = 0.0032%). As a result, some limitations of this study related to the rarity of reporting VBA stroke events. Despite the larger number of cases, data were insufficient to calculate estimates and confidence intervals for seven measures of exposure (4 commercial and 3 MA) for chiropractic visits. Additionally, we were not able to compute estimates specifically for headache and neck pain diagnoses due to small numbers. Confidence intervals associated with estimates tended to be wide making the results imprecise [42].

There were limitations related to the use of administrative claims data. "Disadvantages of using secondary data for research purposes include: variations in coding from hospital to hospital or from department to department, errors in coding and incomplete coding, for example in the presence of comorbidities. Random errors in coding and registration of discharge diagnoses may dilute and attenuate estimates of statistical association" [43]. The recordings of unvalidated hospital discharge diagnostic codes for stroke have been shown to be less precise when compared to chart review [44,45] and validated patient registries

Table 9 Chiropractic (DC) visits with spinal manipulative treatment (SMT)

	Commercial			Medicare		
	DC visit with SMT	Any DC visit	Total # in sample	DC visit with SMT	Any DC visit	Total # in sample
Stroke cases	13	19	1159	1	2	670
Controls	47	62	4633	21	24	2680
All	60	81	5792	22	26	3350

[43,46]. Cassidy, et al. [32] conducted a sensitivity analysis to determine the effect of diagnostic misclassification bias. Their conclusions did not change when the effects of misclassification were assumed to be similarly distributed between chiropractic and PCP cases.

A particular limitation in using administrative claims data is the paucity of contextual information surrounding the clinical encounters between chiropractors/PCPs and their patients. Historical elements describing the occurrence/absence of recent trauma or activities reported in case studies [47-51] as potential risk factors for VBA stroke were not available in claims data. Confidence was low concerning the ability of claims data to provide accurate and complete reporting of other health disorders, which have been described in case–control designs as being associated with the occurrence of VBA stroke e.g., migraine [52] or recent infection [53]. Symptoms and physical examination findings that would have permitted further stratification of cases were not reported in the claims data.

The reporting of clinical procedures using current procedural terminology (CPT) codes presented additional shortcomings concerning the accuracy and interpretation of administrative data. One inherent constraint was the lack of anatomic specificity associated with the use of standardized procedural codes in claims data. Chiropractic manipulative treatment codes (CPT 98940 – 98942) have been formatted to describe the number of spinal regions receiving manipulation. They do not identify the particular spinal regions manipulated.

Also, treatment information describing the type(s) of manipulation was not available. When SMT was reported, claims data could not discriminate among the range of techniques including thrust or rotational manipulation, various non-thrust interventions e.g., mechanical instruments, soft tissue mobilizations, muscle energy techniques, manual cervical traction, etc. Many of these techniques do not incorporate the same biomechanical stressors associated with the type of manipulation (high velocity low amplitude) that has been investigated as a putative risk factor for VBA stroke [54-56]. It seems plausible that the utility of future VBA stroke research would benefit from explicit descriptions of the particular type of manipulation performed.

Moreover, patient responses to care – including any adverse events suggestive of vertebral artery dissection or stroke-like symptoms – were not obtainable in the data set used for the current study.

In the absence of performing comprehensive clinical chart audits, it is not possible to know from claims data what actually transpired in the clinical encounter. Further, chart notes may themselves be incomplete or otherwise fail to precisely describe the nature of interventions [57]. Therefore, manipulation codes represent surrogate measures, albeit more direct surrogate measures, than simply using the exposure to chiropractic visits.

Our study was also limited to replication of the case-control design described by Cassidy, et al. [32]. For pragmatic reasons, we did not attempt to conduct a case-crossover design. While the addition of a case-crossover design would have provided better control of confounding variables, Cassidy, et al. [32] showed the results were similar for both the case control and case crossover studies.

The findings of this case–control study and previous retrospective research underscore the need to rethink how to better conduct future investigations. Researchers should seek to avoid the use of surrogate measures or use the least indirect measures available. Instead, the focus should be on capturing data about the types of services and not the type of health care provider.

In alignment with this approach, it is also important for investigators to access contextual data (e.g., from electronic health records), which can be enabled by qualitative data analysis computer programs [58]. The acquisition of the elements of clinical encounters – including history, diagnosis, intervention, and adverse events – can provide the infrastructure for more actionable research. Because of the rarity of VBA stroke, large data sets (e.g., registries) containing these elements will be necessary to achieve adequate statistical power for making confident conclusions.

Until research efforts produce more definitive results, health care policy and clinical practice judgments are best informed by the evidence about the effectiveness of manipulation, plausible treatment options (including non-thrust manual techniques) and individual patient values [20].

Conclusions

Our findings should be viewed in the context of the body of knowledge concerning the risk of VBA stroke. In contrast to several other case–control studies, we found no significant association between exposure to chiropractic care and the risk of VBA stroke. Our secondary analysis clearly showed that manipulation may or may not have been reported at every chiropractic visit. Therefore, the use of chiropractic visits as a proxy for manipulation may not be reliable. Our results add weight to the view that chiropractic care is an unlikely cause of VBA strokes. However, the current study does not exclude cervical manipulation as a possible cause or contributory factor in the occurrence of VBA stroke.

Competing interests

All authors are employees of UnitedHealth Group – a U.S based commercial health care company. The authors declare that they have no other competing interests.

Authors' contributions

DE conceived of the study, and participated in its design and coordination. JT participated in the design of the study, performed the statistical analysis and helped to draft the manuscript. TMK participated in the design and coordination of the study, and wrote the initial draft and revisions of the manuscript. WMB participated in the coordination of the study and the statistical analysis, and helped to draft the manuscript. All authors contributed to the interpretation of the data. All authors read and approved the final manuscript.

Author details

[1]Optum Health – Clinical Programs at United Health Group, 11000 Optum Circle, Eden Prairie MN 55344, USA. [2]Optum Health – Clinical Analytics at United Health Group, 11000 Optum Circle, Eden Prairie MN 55344, USA.

References

1. Paulose R, Hertz R. The burden of pain among adults in the United States. In Pfizer Facts. Edited by Pfizer Inc. 2008. [http://www.pfizer.com/files/products/PF_Pain.pdf] Accessed May 14, 2014.
2. Carroll L, Hogg-Johnson S, van der Velde G, Haldeman S, Holm L, Carragee E, et al. Bone and Joint Decade 2000–2010 Task Force on Neck Pain and Its Associated Disorders: Course and prognostic factors for neck pain in the general population: results of the Bone and Joint Decade 2000–2010 Task Force on Neck Pain and Its Associated Disorders. Spine (Phila Pa 1976). 2008;33(4 Suppl):S75–82.
3. Hoy D, Protani M, De R, Buchbinder R. The epidemiology of neck pain. Best Pract Res Clin Rheumatol. 2010;24(6):783–92.
4. Jacobs J, Andersson G, Bell J, Weinstein S, Dormans J, Gnatz S, et al. Spine: low back and neck pain. In The Burden of Musculoskeletal Diseases in the United States. Chapter 2. Edited by Bone and Joint Decade USA 2002–2011. Rosemont, IL: The American Academy of Orthopaedic Surgeons; 2008:21–56.
5. Christensen M, Kollasch M, Hyland J, Rosner A. Chapter 8 – Patient Conditions. In Practice Analysis of Chiropractic: A Project Report, Survey Analysis, and Summary of the Practice of Chiropractic Within the United States. Greeley, CO: The National Board of Chiropractic Examiners. 2010:95–120.
6. Christensen M, Kollasch M, Hyland J, Rosner A. Chapter 9 – Professional functions and treatment procedures. In Practice Analysis of Chiropractic: A Project Report, Survey Analysis, and Summary of the Practice of Chiropractic Within the United States. Greeley, CO: The National Board of Chiropractic Examiners. 2010:121–136.
7. D'Sylva J, Miller J, Gross A, Burnie S, Goldsmith G, Graham N, et al. Manual therapy with or without physical medicine modalities for neck pain: a systematic review. Man Ther. 2010;15(4):415–33.
8. Gross A, Miller J, D'Sylva J, Burnie S, Goldsmith G, Graham N, et al. Manipulation or mobilisation for neck pain: A Cochrane review. Man Ther. 2010;15(4):315–33.
9. Bryans R, Decina P, Descarreaux M, Duranleau M, Marcoux H, Potter B, et al. Evidence-based guidelines for the chiropractic treatment of adults with neck pain. J Manipulative Physiol Ther. 2014;37(1):42–63.
10. Bryans R, Descarreaux M, Duranleau M, Marcoux H, Potter B, Ruegg R, et al. Evidence-based guidelines for the chiropractic treatment of adults with headache. J Manipulative Physiol Ther. 2011;34(5):274–89.
11. Childs J, Cleland J, Elliott J, Teyhen D, Wainner R, Whitman J, et al. Neck pain: clinical practice guidelines linked to the International Classification of Functioning, Disability, and Health from the Orthopaedic Section of the American Physical Therapy Association. J Orthop Sports Phys Ther. 2008;38(9):A1–A34.
12. Clar C, Tsertsvadze A, Court R, Hundt G, Clarke A, Sutcliffe P. Clinical effectiveness of manual therapy for the management of musculoskeletal and non-musculoskeletal conditions: systematic review and update of UK evidence report. Chiropr Man Therap. 2014;22(1):12.
13. Vincent K, Maigne J, Fischhoff C, Lanlo O, Dagenais S. Systematic review of manual therapies for nonspecific neck pain. Joint Bone Spine. 2013;80(5):508–15.
14. Bronfort G, Assendelft W, Evans R, Haas M, Bouter L. Efficacy of spinal manipulation for chronic headache: a systematic review. J Manipulative Physiol Ther. 2001;24(7):457–66.
15. Chaibi A, Tuchin P, Russell M. Manual therapies for migraine: a systematic review. J Headache Pain. 2011;12(2):127–33.
16. Racicki S, Gerwin S, Diclaudio S, Reinmann S, Donaldson M. Conservative physical therapy management for the treatment of cervicogenic headache: a systematic review. J Man Manip Ther. 2013;21(2):113–24.
17. Cassidy J, Bronfort G, Hartvigsen J. Should we abandon cervical spine manipulation for mechanical neck pain? No BMJ. 2012;344, e3680.
18. Wand B, Heine P, O'Connell N. Should we abandon cervical spine manipulation for mechanical neck pain? Yes BMJ. 2012;344, e3679.
19. Moloo J. What's the Best Approach for Managing Neck Pain? NEJM Journal Watch 2012. [http://www.jwatch.org/jw201202090000004/2012/02/09/whats-best-approach-managing-neck-pain] Accessed May 14, 2014.
20. Schneider M, Weinstein S, Chimes G. Cervical manipulation for neck pain. PM&R. 2012;4(8):606–12.
21. Biller J, Sacco R, Albuquerque F, Demaerschalk B, Fayad P, Long P, et al. Cervical arterial dissections and association with cervical manipulative therapy: a statement for healthcare professionals from the American Heart Association/American Stroke Association. Stroke 2014, Epub ahead of print.
22. American Chiropractic Association: ACA Response to AHA Statement on Neck Manipulation. 2014 (Aug 7). [http://www.acatoday.org/press_css.cfm?CID=5534] Accessed August 15, 2014.
23. American Physical Therapy Association: APTA responds to American Heart Association cervical manipulation paper. 2014 (Aug 7). [http://www.apta.org/Media/Releases/Consumer/2014/8/7/] Accessed August 15, 2014.
24. Kardys JA. Declaratory ruling regarding informed consent. Connecticut State Board of Chiropractic Examiners – State of Connecticut Department of Public Health. 2010. [http://www.ctchiro.com/upload/news/44_0.pdf] Accessed May 14, 2014.
25. Wangler M, Fujikawa R, Hestbæk L, Michielsen T, Raven T, Thiel H, et al. Creating European guidelines for Chiropractic Incident Reporting and Learning Systems (CIRLS): relevance and structure. Chiropr Man Therap. 2011;19:9.
26. Berger S: How safe are the vigorous neck manipulations done by chiropractors? Washington Post 2014 (Jan. 6). [http://www.washingtonpost.com/national/health-science/how-safe-are-the-vigorous-neck-manipulations-done-by-chiropractors/2014/01/06/26870726-5cf7-11e3-bc56-c6ca94801fac_story.html] Accessed January 10, 2014.
27. Group wants provincial ban on some neck manipulation by chiropractors. Winnipeg Free Press 2012 (Oct 4). [http://www.winnipegfreepress.com/local/Group-wants-provincial-ban-on-some-neck-manipulation-by-chiropractors-172692471.htm] Accessed May 14, 2014.
28. Gouveia L, Castanho P, Ferreira J. Safety of chiropractic interventions: a systematic review. Spine (Phila Pa 1976). 2009;34(11):E405–13.
29. Carlesso L, Gross A, Santaguida P, Burnie S, Voth S, Sadi J. Adverse events associated with the use of cervical manipulation and mobilization for the treatment of neck pain in adults: a systematic review. Man Ther. 2010;15(5):434–44.
30. Chung C, Côté P, Stern P, L'Espérance G. The association between cervical spine manipulation and carotid artery dissection: a systematic review of the literature. J Manipulative Physiol Ther 2014, [Epub ahead of print].
31. Haynes M, Vincent K, Fischhoff C, Bremner A, Lanlo O, Hankey G. Assessing the risk of stroke from neck manipulation: a systematic review. Int J Clin Pract. 2012;66(10):940–7.
32. Cassidy J, Boyle E, Cote P, He Y, Hogg-Johnson S, Silver F, et al. Risk of vertebrobasilar stroke and chiropractic care: results of a population-based case–control and case-crossover study. Spine (Phila Pa 1976). 2008;33 Suppl 4:S176–83.
33. Rothwell D, Bondy S, Williams J. Chiropractic manipulation and stroke: a population-based case–control study. Stroke. 2001;32(5):1054–60.
34. Choi S, Boyle E, Côté P, Cassidy JD. A population-based case-series of Ontario patients who develop a vertebrobasilar artery stroke after seeing a chiropractor. J Manipulative Physiol Ther. 2011;34(1):15–22.
35. U.S. Census Bureau: State and County QuickFacts. Data derived from Population Estimates, American Community Survey, Census of Population and Housing, State and County Housing Unit Estimates, County Business Patterns, Nonemployer Statistics, Economic Census, Survey of Business Owners, Building Permits. 2014 (rev July 8). [http://quickfacts.census.gov/qfd/states/00000.html] Accessed August 19, 2014.
36. Kosanke J, Bergstralh E. GMatch Macro (SAS program): Mayo Clinic College of Medicine. 2004. [http://www.mayo.edu/research/departments-divisions/department-health-sciences-research/division-biomedical-statistics-informatics/software/locally-written-sas-macros] Accessed June 6, 2014.

37. Smith W, Johnston S, Skalabrin E, Weaver M, Azari P, Albers G, et al. Spinal manipulative therapy is an independent risk factor for vertebral artery dissection. Neurology. 2003;60(9):1424–8.

38. Engelter S, Grond-Ginsbach C, Metso T, Metso A, Kloss M, Debette S, et al. Cervical Artery Dissection and Ischemic Stroke Patients Study Group: Cervical artery dissection: trauma and other potential mechanical trigger events. Neurology. 2013;80(21):1950–7.

39. Ardal S, Baigent L, Bains N, Hay C, Lee P, Loomer S: The health analyst's toolkit. Ministry of Health and Long-Term Care Health Results Team - Information Management. Ontario (CA) 2006 (January) [http://www.health.gov.on.ca/transformation/providers/information/resources/analyst_toolkit.pdf] Accessed January 12, 2015.

40. Sacco RL, Benjamin EJ, Broderick JP, Dyken M, Easton JD, Feinberg WM, et al. American Heart Association Prevention Conference. IV. Prevention and rehabilitation of stroke. Risk factors. Stroke. 1997;28(7):1507–17.

41. Debette S, Metso T, Pezzini A, Abboud S, Metso A, Leys D, et al. Cervical Artery Dissection and Ischemic Stroke Patients (CADISP) Group: Association of vascular risk factors with cervical artery dissection and ischemic stroke in young adults. Circulation. 2011;123(14):1537–44.

42. Guyatt G, Oxman A, Kunz R, Brozek J, Alonso-Coello P, Rind D, et al. GRADE guidelines 6. Rating the quality of evidence – imprecision. J Clin Epidemiol. 2011;64(12):1283–93.

43. Krarup L, Boysen G, Janjua H, Prescott E, Truelsen T. Validity of stroke diagnoses in a National Register of Patients. Neuroepidemiology. 2007;28(3):150–4.

44. Goldstein L. Accuracy of ICD-9-CM coding for the identification of patients with acute ischemic stroke: effect of modifier codes. Stroke. 1998;29(8):1602–4.

45. Liu L, Reeder B, Shuaib A, Mazagri R. Validity of stroke diagnosis on hospital discharge records in Saskatchewan, Canada: implications for stroke surveillance. Cerebrovasc Dis. 1999;9(4):224–30.

46. Ellekjaer H, Holmen J, Krüger O, Terent A. Identification of incident stroke in Norway: hospital discharge data compared with a population-based stroke register. Stroke. 1999;30(1):56–60.

47. Braksiak R, Roberts D. Amusement park injuries and deaths. An Emerg Med. 2002;39(1):65–72.

48. Dittrich R, Rohsbach D, Heidbreder A, Heuschmann P, Nassenstein I, Bachmann R, et al. Mild mechanical traumas are possible risk factors for cervical artery dissection. Cerebrovasc Dis. 2007;23(4):275–81.

49. Mas J, Bousser M, Hasboun D, Laplane D. Extracranial vertebral artery dissection: a review of 13 cases. Stroke. 1987;18(6):1037–47.

50. Slankamenac P, Jesic A, Avramov P, Zivanovic Z, Covic S, Till V. Multiple cervical artery dissection in a volleyball player. Arch Neuro. 2010;67(8):1024–5.

51. Weintraub M. Beauty parlor stroke syndrome: report of five cases. JAMA. 1993;269(16):2085–6.

52. Tzourio C, Benslamia L, Guilllon B, Aïdi S, Bertrand M, Berthet K, et al. Migraine and the risk of cervical artery dissection: a case control study. Neurology. 2002;59(3):435–7.

53. Guillon B, Berthet K, Benslamia L, Bertrand M, Bousser M, Tzourio C. Infection and the risk of cervical artery dissection: a case–control study. Stroke. 2003;34(7):e79–81.

54. Symons B, Leonard TR, Herzog W. Internal forces sustained by the vertebral artery during spinal manipulative therapy. J Manip Physiol Ther. 2002;25(8):504–10.

55. Wuest S, Symons B, Leonard T, Herzog W. Preliminary report: biomechanics of vertebral artery segments C1-C6 during cervical spinal manipulation. J Manip Physiol Ther. 2010;33(4):273–8.

56. Herzog W, Leonard TR, Symons B, Tang C, Wuest S. Vertebral artery strains during high-speed, low amplitude cervical spinal manipulation. J Electromyogr Kinesiol. 2012;22(5):747–51.

57. Centers for Medicare & Medicaid: Comprehensive error rate testing (CERT). 2015 (Jan. 15). [http://www.cms.gov/Research-Statistics-Data-and-Systems/Monitoring-Programs/Medicare-FFS-Compliance-Programs/CERT/index.html?redirect=/cert] Accessed February 4, 2015.

58. Welsh E: Dealing with data: using NVivo in the qualitative data analysis process. Forum: Qualitative Social Research 2002, 3(2): Art. 26 [http://nbn-resolving.de/urn:nbn:de:0114-fqs0202260] Accessed February 4, 2015.

Absence of low back pain to demarcate an episode: a prospective multicentre study in primary care

Andreas Eklund[1*], Irene Jensen[1], Malin Lohela-Karlsson[1], Charlotte Leboeuf-Yde[2] and Iben Axén[1,2]

Abstract

Background: It has been proposed that an episode of low back pain (LBP) be defined as: "a period of pain in the lower back lasting for more than 24 h preceded and followed by a period of at least 1 month without LBP". Previous studies have tested the definition in the general population and in secondary care populations with distinctly different results. The objectives of this study (in a primary care population) were to investigate the prevalence of 1) the number of consecutive weeks free from bothersome LBP, 2) the prevalence of at least four consecutive weeks free from bothersome LBP at any time during the study period, and 3) the prevalence of at least four consecutive weeks free from bothersome LBP at any time during the study period among subgroups that reported >30 days or ≤30 days of LBP the preceding year.

Method: In this prospective multicentre study subjects with LBP ($n = 262$) were consecutively recruited from chiropractic primary care clinics in Sweden. The number of days with bothersome LBP was collected through weekly automated text messages. The maximum number of weeks in a row without bothersome LBP and the number of periods of at least four consecutive weeks free from bothersome LBP was counted for each individual and analysed as proportions.

Results: Data from 222 recruited subjects were analysed, of which 59 % reported at least one period of four consecutive weeks free from bothersome LBP. The number of consecutive pain free weeks ranged from 82 (at least one) to 31 % (9 or more). In subjects with a total duration of LBP of ≤ 30 days the previous year, 75 % reported a period of 4 consecutive weeks free from bothersome LBP during the study period whereas this was reported by only 48 % of subjects with a total duration of LBP of >30 days the previous year.

Conclusion: Prevalence of four consecutive pain free weeks is found in the majority of subjects in this population logically reflects duration of LBP within the sample and may be applied on patients in primary care to demarcate a LBP episode.

Keywords: Low back pain, LBP, Definition, Recovery, Episode, Demarcation, Primary care, Chiropractic, Absence, Non-episode

* Correspondence: andreas.eklund@ki.se
[1]Unit of Intervention and Implementation Research, Karolinska Institutet, Institute of Environmental Medicine, Nobels v 13, S-171 77 Stockholm, Sweden
Full list of author information is available at the end of the article

Background

Low back pain (LBP) is a prevalent condition [1, 2] often with an intermittent course [3, 4] with episodic flare-ups [5, 6] and periods without pain [7, 8]. A definition of what constitutes an episode of LBP is fundamental for the study of new episodes, risk factors, resolution, persistence and recurrence [9]. To specify when one episode ends and a new one begins, a period free from pain (in previous research described as a "non-episode" [7, 8]) is required. Recovery is a term that may be used to demarcate such a period with absence of pain following or preceding an episode of LBP. However, there is no evidence-based definition of recovery [10] to date. Such a definition would aid in the exploration of pain trajectories to subgroup individuals and possibly tailor interventions accordingly.

De Vet et al. [9] proposed a definition of an episode of LBP based on an extensive literature search and group discussions with researchers and clinicians. They proposed that an episode of LBP be defined as: "a period of pain in the lower back lasting for more than 24 h preceded and followed by a period of at least 1 month without LBP". In a recent [11] modified Delphi approach, it was agreed to incorporate de Vet's definition into the consensus definition of recovery.

Leboeuf-Yde et al. [7] investigated if part of de Vet's proposed definition, namely "at least 1 month without LBP" was applicable in two populations of LBP patients from secondary care. Using weekly data, the prevalence of periods of at least four consecutive weeks free from bothersome LBP was determined. It was found that only 18 and 20 % of the patients reported at least one period of a minimum of four consecutive weeks free from bothersome LBP during the 1-year study period.

Leboeuf-Yde et al. proposed that a relationship could exist between duration of pain and the absence of pain. Thus, one would expect patients with LBP of shorter duration to have longer consecutive pain free periods compared to patients with LBP of longer duration. The above described method was thus repeated in a sample from the general population and the prevalence of at least 4 consecutive weeks free from bothersome LBP was, as expected, found to be much higher, 83 %, during the 1-year study period [8]. The authors concluded that it would be possible to use 1 month of absence of bothersome LBP as a measure in order to study the occurrence of episodes in the general population. Whether the definition is applicable in a primary care population has not been tested, and doing so could reveal if it can be used as a demarcation of an episode. A logical relationship between the prevalence of four consecutive pain free weeks and duration of LBP would be expected.

The use of text messages is a novel and promising data collection method [12] for clinical research, as most people have a mobile phone and carry it with them at all times. This enables repeated and frequent measures without recall bias. Text messages have been used in many different settings in the investigation of diseases [7, 8, 12] and behaviours [13, 14]. Further, this type of data allow for an in depth analysis of the fluctuation of pain.

This study utilizes weekly text message data [12, 15] and replicates the method from the previous studies [7, 8]. The aim is to investigate the applicability of de Vet et al.'s [9] definition (as a demarcation of an episode of LBP) in a primary care population by estimating prevalence of 4 consecutive weeks free from bothersome pain during the study period.

Methods

Design

The data for this prospective multicentre study with a 6 month follow up period were collected in Sweden between May 2008 and June 2009 [12] with the primary aim of describing the clinical course of LBP. This report is based on a secondary analysis of those data. To effectively recruit patients, chiropractic clinics were chosen as LBP is the most common condition treated by chiropractors in Sweden [16]. Thirty-five chiropractors recruited up to 10 consecutive LBP patients each. To ensure sufficient academic and clinical standards, only members from the Swedish Chiropractic Association (SCA) were invited. The involved clinicians were representative of SCA's members in terms of age, sex, years in practice and have a geographical spread across Sweden with the highest densities around the major cities (Stockholm, Göteborg and Malmö) [12] .

Objectives

The objectives were to study the six months prevalence of:

1) The number of consecutive weeks free from bothersome LBP.
2) At least 4 consecutive weeks free from bothersome LBP at any time during the study period.
3) At least 4 consecutive weeks free from bothersome LBP at any time during the study period among subgroups that reported having had altogether >30 days or ≤30 days of LBP the preceding year.

We hypothesised our population to reflect that subjects with a previous history of longer LBP duration (>30 days of LBP the preceding year) would report fewer consecutive pain-free weeks as compared to those with a previous history of shorter duration of their LBP (≤30 days of LBP the preceding year).

Subjects and data

Subjects were recruited when they sought chiropractic care for non-specific LBP with or without leg pain. Participants were of working age and were excluded if pregnant, unable to understand Swedish, did not have a mobile phone, or were unable to send text messages from their mobile phones. Patients that had been under chiropractic care during the previous 3 months were also excluded as were those with specific LBP (i.e., where pathology was suspected or present). After receiving information about the study and signing informed consent forms, the study subjects filled in a baseline questionnaire with information on sex, age and occupation, as well as area, intensity, duration and frequency of the LBP. Treatment content was decided by the individual chiropractor and not regulated by the research protocol. To minimize the burden on the participating clinicians, data on screened but ineligible subjects were not collected. The data from this study is a secondary analysis of a convenience sample collected during 2008 (reported 2012). The recruitment and data collection process have been described in detail in a previous publication [12].

Text messages

SMS-Track® is a web-based system designed specifically for research to enable frequent data collection using text messages [15]. Previous studies have shown this to be an inexpensive method [17] that yields high response rates [12, 18], and good compliance. Compliance is not affected by age, sex or season [12]. The system uses a web-based interface, which can be accessed in real time to monitor compliance.

Measurements

The term "bothersomeness" has been used in previous studies as a measurement for the impact of pain [19–21]. The term has been shown to correlate well with self-rated health [22], pain intensity [18], disability, psychological health (anxiety, depression), prediction of future work absence and healthcare consultations [23], and has been suggested as a standard outcome measure in LBP research [21]. Choosing this term further aligns with the bio-psychosocial model of care [24, 25].

During the 6-month study period the subjects were monitored with a weekly text message asking: "How many days this previous week has your low back pain been bothersome?" (requiring an answer between 0 and 7, sent in a reply text message). The weekly data were used in this study to examine the definition of episode with regard to absence of bothersome LBP. To elicit information regarding previous duration, the study subjects were asked as part of the baseline questionnaire to state if they had experienced more or less than 30 days of pain during the past year. Previous research [26] has found this classification of duration to have prognostic value, as it predicts treatment outcome for chiropractic patients with LBP [26]. This classification has been used in number of studies [12, 18, 27–29] to subgroup LBP patients. Three possible answer categories were available in this study; ≤30 days; >30 days intermittently; >30 days with more or less daily pain. For the purpose of this study, the two latter choices were collapsed into one category.

Ethical considerations

Participation was voluntary and all participants received information regarding the study and signed informed consent forms. Ethics approval was granted by the ethics committee at Karolinska Institutet, 2007/ 1458-31/4.

Data analysis

The number of consecutive weeks free from LBP was counted using a programmed bespoke syntax in SPSS v20 (available from the authors upon request). To conform to one of the previous studies [7] only subjects who replied to the weekly text messages at least 50 % of the time were included to ensure reliable estimates. Missing cells were considered to be weeks with LBP in the main analysis (as in one of the previous studies [8]) in order to avoid over-estimation of the presence of consecutive weeks free from LBP. To assess the possible bias due to the imputation method, a sensitivity analysis to illustrate best case scenario was performed where the missing data were considered to be weeks free from LBP.

To investigate the applicability of de Vet et al.'s definition of LBP episodes, three main data analyses were performed with regard to the absence of LBP over 6 months: 1) The maximum number of consecutive weeks free from LBP, 2) the prevalence of at least four consecutive weeks free from LBP at any time during the study period, and 3) the same analyses among the subpopulations that reported either >30 or ≤30 days of LBP the previous year.

The data are reported as percentages with 95 % confidence intervals.

Results

A total of 262 subjects agreed to participate in the study but 18 (7 %) dropped out. Twenty-two subjects (8 %) replied to less than 50 % of the weekly text messages were excluded from the analyses. Overall the response rate was high and in the final dataset, 222 subjects were included (85 % of the source population providing 5772 data points) with a total of 654 (11 %) missing weekly data points. During week 1 and 26 there were 7 % (16 data points) and 15 % (33 data points) missing data respectively. Descriptive data of the study population are summarized in Table 1.

Table 1 Descriptive data of the study population

Variable	Dropouts	Excluded	Study sample
Number of subjects	18	22	222
Age in years, mean (SD[a])	43 (11)	41 (14)	44 (11)
Sex distribution, %			
Men	56	64	50
Women	44	36	49
Main type of occupation, %:			
Sitting	38	29	43
Standing	13	19	22
Varying	37	28	28
Heavy	12	24	7
Pain intensity 0–10, mean (SD[a])	3.9 (3.1)	5.4 (2.3)	4.3 (2.2)
Presence of leg pain, %	59	47	49
Pain duration >30 days, %	33	57	59

[a]SD standard deviation

The distribution of the maximum number of consecutive LBP-free weeks in a row per individual is reported in Table 2. The vast majority, 82 % (CI: 71–93), experienced at least 1 week without LBP at some point during the study period. During the study, 59 % (CI: 51–67) of the subjects experienced at least one period of at least four consecutive weeks free from LBP.

Among the 92 subjects with shorter duration LBP (≤30 days) the previous year, 75 % (CI: 60–90) reported a period of at least 4 consecutive weeks free from LBP during the study period. Within the group of 130 subjects who reported longer duration of LBP (>30 days) the previous year, 48 % (CI: 40–56) reported a period of at least 4 consecutive weeks free from LBP during the study period.

The sensitivity analysis comparing the main analysis (worst case scenario) to a secondary analysis where missing data was imputed as weeks without LBP (best case

Table 2 Distribution of weeks free from bothersome pain

Maximum number of consecutive weeks free from bothersome pain	% (95 % CI[a]) N = 222
0	18 (16–20)
1	9 (8–10)
2	5 (4–6)
3	9 (8–10)
4	8 (7–9)
5	6 (5–7)
6	5 (4–6)
7	4 (3–5)
8	5 (4–6)
9 or more	31 (27–35)

[a]CI confidence interval

scenario), showed a maximum difference of 10–15 % of consecutive weeks free from LBP across all measurements. See Fig. 1.

Discussion

In line with de Vet et al's definition, this is the first study to investigate the applicability of 4 weeks with absence of pain as a demarcation of an episode of LBP [9] in a primary care population. The results of this study support this definition as a demarcation of an episode in this population. Consecutive weeks free from pain occur at some point in a vast majority of our sample and inversely mirrors the duration of pain the previous year. The data support the use of de Vet's definition as they reflect the expected variability of episodes in a primary care sample.

In this study, a third of the subjects reported 9 consecutive weeks free from LBP or more, while a fifth never reported a single week free from LBP. The presence of at least 4 consecutive weeks free from LBP at any time during the study period was found in a majority (82 %) of the subjects, i.e., it was more prevalent than in the secondary care populations [7], but less prevalent than the general population [8] (see Table 3). This relationship between a history of longer duration of pain and fewer consecutive weeks free from bothersome pain is confirmed when our sample is dichotomized according to previous duration. Thus prevalence of consecutive weeks free from pain seems to reflect previous duration of LBP in a logical manner.

The high response rate and low recall bias of the repeated measures are the main strengths of the study and are a result of using weekly text messages [17]. Furthermore, the same data collection method and measurement were used in Leboeuf-Yde et al's two previous studies [7, 8], which allows the results to be compared.

However, chiropractic subjects may differ somewhat from other primary care patients, perhaps limiting generalizability of the results. Recent research (2013) from Australia compared chiropractic patients to other patient groups in the primary care sector [30] and found that they are less disadvantaged but more likely to suffer from depression and other chronic health problems. This sample of patients has not received financial reimbursement of their chiropractic visits in contrast to other primary care consultations within the traditional Swedish healthcare system (where fees are normally subsidized). It is therefore possible that these patients differ in socioeconomic class compared to other primary care populations, which in turn may have resulted in a different psychological profile (possibly higher self-efficacy and better general health) compared to patients seen by physiotherapists or in general medical practice. Given the aim of the study, this does not pose a major problem

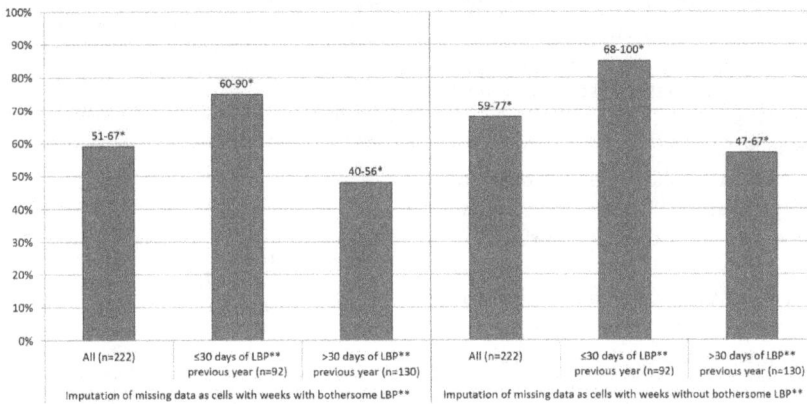

Fig. 1 Sensitivity analysis comparing imputation of missing data as cells with or without weeks with bothersome pain in a best case and a worst case scenario. The Y-axis is displaying the percentage of the population with at least four consecutive weeks free from bothersome pain. *CI, Confidence Interval

as this particular population was selected specifically because it is likely to be different to those investigated in the previous two studies [7, 8].

The use of mobile-phones may pose a risk of selection bias across age groups. However the penetration of such technology is widespread in Sweden and during 2008 it was used by 94 % of the population [31]. Further, this study involved only people of working ages. Therefore this is not considered a source for bias in this study.

In Sweden, there are two different professional chiropractic organisations. All members of the SCA have been educated at an accredited institution (outside of Sweden) and hold an academic degree. The SCA members are probably not representative of all chiropractors in Sweden. However, the SCA members were chosen for reasons of comparability with other clinicians with similar academic standard within and outside of Sweden (such as Denmark where the two previous studies were conducted [7, 8]).

Missing data were treated as days with pain to avoid overestimating the LBP free periods. Similar to the study from the secondary care sector [7], only subjects who responded to more than 50 % of text messages were included which resulted in a limited number of missing values. Because of the high response rate, and good compliance, the sensitivity analysis showed only minor changes in the results and did not change the interpretation of the results.

The fact that "bothersomeness" was used as a measure of LBP may also affect the generalizability of our data when comparing to other studies where the presence of even minor LBP has been used [32]. One may argue that in reporting bothersome LBP, the result may overestimate weeks without LBP. De Vet et al. [9] explicitly refer to the "presence of pain" and reject "disabling pain" in the operational definition. However, although bothersomeness incorporates function it also closely correlates with pain intensity [18, 23]. Therefore, "bothersome pain" is distinctly different to "disabling pain" by also capturing pain that is not disabling but still relevant for the individual. Therefore, the deviation from de Vet et al's operational definition is deemed reasonable, should not raise any methodological issues and should result in the reporting of mainly relevant levels of LBP. This study, along with the other two in this field [7, 8], is in fact using a more

Table 3 Comparison with other study samples from general population and secondary care

Variable	General population [8]	Chiropractic primary care population [This study]	Secondary care [7] (Two study samples)
Proportion of at least 4 consecutive weeks free from bothersome pain during the study period, % (95 % CI[a])	83 (78–88)	59 (51–67)	20 (11–29), 18 (13–23)
Proportion women, %	54	49	68, 54
Age mean	50	44	46, 38
Pain intensity 0–10, mean	-	4.3	5.3, 4.9
Study period	12 months	6 months	12 months
Text message interval	Fortnightly	Weekly	Weekly

[a]CI confidence interval

comprehensive term for LBP [9]. However, future research may investigate the correlation of consecutive weeks free from pain with other outcomes such as pain intensity, activity limitation, self-rated health and psychological factors.

Comparing the results from the chiropractic primary care patients to the previous studies from secondary care [7] and the general population [8] posed one potential major limitation. The data were collected during different follow-up periods, 6 months in our study compared to 12 months in the others, which limits the direct comparability between the cohorts and may have resulted in an underestimation of four consecutive weeks free from LBP in the present study population.

Research has shown that individuals with LBP may be clustered in specific trajectories [27]. Future research may investigate the usefulness of the duration of absence of pain as another variable that could be added to identify trajectories.

Four consecutive weeks free from LBP may also be useful as an outcome measure in clinical studies. A positive outcome may thus be defined in terms of frequency and duration of episodes of being free from LBP. Future research should test 4 consecutive weeks free from LBP for further clinical relevance and value as an outcome measure.

Conclusions

A logical relationship exists between the prevalence of four consecutive pain free weeks and the study population, it being most common in the general population, followed by the primary care population and least common in the secondary care sector Further, absence of LBP is less common in patients from the primary care sector with a previous long duration of pain than in those with previous shorter pain duration. Therefore, a period of four consecutive pain free weeks may be applied both for research purposes and in clinical practice to demarcate a LBP episode.

Competing interests
The authors declare that they have no competing interests.

Authors' contributions
AE, IJ, MLK, CLY and IA have been involved in the planning and design of the study. AE has been the main author, and all of the authors have been involved in critical revision and intellectual improvement of the manuscript. All authors read and approved the final manuscript.

Acknowledgements
The study was partly funded by the Institute for Chiropractic and Neuro-Musculoskeletal Research (IKoN) as well as the European Chiropractors Union (ECU). Grateful acknowledgement to Jan Hagberg, PhD, and Professor Lennart Bodin for statistical support and guidance. The authors also wish to express their gratitude to the chiropractors who collected data and the subjects who participated in the study.

Author details
[1]Unit of Intervention and Implementation Research, Karolinska Institutet, Institute of Environmental Medicine, Nobels v 13, S-171 77 Stockholm, Sweden. [2]Research Department, Spine Center of Southern Denmark, Institute for Regional Health Research, Hospital Lillebælt, University of Southern Denmark, Østre Hougvej 55, DK-5500 Middelfart, Denmark.

References
1. Vassilaki M, Hurwitz EL. Insights in public health: perspectives on pain in the low back and neck: global burden, epidemiology, and management. Hawaii J Med Public Health. 2014;73(4):122–6.
2. Hoy D, Brooks P, Blyth F, Buchbinder R. The epidemiology of low back pain. Best Pract Res Clin Rheumatol. 2010;24(6):769–81. doi:10.1016/j.berh.2010.10.002.
3. Dunn KM, Jordan K, Croft PR. Characterizing the course of low back pain: a latent class analysis. Am J Epidemiol. 2006;163(8):754–61. doi:10.1093/aje/kwj100.
4. Chen C, Hogg-Johnson S, Smith P. The recovery patterns of back pain among workers with compensated occupational back injuries. Occup Environ Med. 2007;64(8):534–40. doi:10.1136/oem.2006.029215.
5. Von Korff M. Studying the natural history of back pain. Spine. 1994;19(18 Suppl):2041S–6.
6. Von Korff M, Saunders K. The course of back pain in primary care. Spine. 1996;21(24):2833–7. discussion 8–9.
7. Leboeuf-Yde C, Jensen RK, Axen I. Absence of low back pain in patients followed weekly over one year with automated text messages. Chiropr Man Therap. 2012;20(1):9. doi:10.1186/2045-709X-20-9.
8. Leboeuf-Yde C, Lemeunier N, Wedderkopp N, Kjaer P. Absence of low back pain in the general population followed fortnightly over one year with automated text messages. Chiropr Man Therap. 2014;22(1):1. doi:10.1186/2045-709X-22-12045-709X-22-1.
9. de Vet HC, Heymans MW, Dunn KM, Pope DP, van der Beek AJ, Macfarlane GJ, et al. Episodes of low back pain: a proposal for uniform definitions to be used in research. Spine. 2002;27(21):2409–16. doi:10.1097/01.BRS. 0000030307.34002.BE.
10. Kamper SJ, Stanton TR, Williams CM, Maher CG, Hush JM. How is recovery from low back pain measured? A systematic review of the literature. Eur Spine J. 2011;20(1):9–18. doi:10.1007/s00586-010-1477-8.
11. Stanton TR, Latimer J, Maher CG, Hancock MJ. A modified Delphi approach to standardize low back pain recurrence terminology. Eur Spine J. 2011;20(5):744–52. doi:10.1007/s00586-010-1671-8.
12. Axen I, Bodin L, Bergstrom G, Halasz L, Lange F, Lovgren PW, et al. The use of weekly text messaging over 6 months was a feasible method for monitoring the clinical course of low back pain in patients seeking chiropractic care. J Clin Epidemiol. 2012;65(4):454–61. doi:10.1016/j.jclinepi. 2011.07.012.
13. Smith KL, Kerr DA, Fenner AA, Straker LM. Adolescents just do not know what they want: a qualitative study to describe obese adolescents' experiences of text messaging to support behavior change maintenance post intervention. J Med Internet Res. 2014;16(4), e103. doi:10.2196/jmir. 3113v16i4e103.
14. Park LG, Howie-Esquivel J, Chung ML, Dracup K. A text messaging intervention to promote medication adherence for patients with coronary heart disease: a randomized controlled trial. Patient Educ Couns. 2014;94(2):261–8. doi:10.1016/j.pec.2013.10.027S0738-3991(13)00468-0.
15. SMS-Track. https://www.sms-track.com/.
16. Leboeuf-Yde C, Hennius B, Rudberg E, Leufvenmark P, Thunman M. Chiropractic in Sweden: a short description of patients and treatment. J Manipulative Physiol Ther. 1997;20(8):507–10.
17. Johansen B, Wedderkopp N. Comparison between data obtained through real-time data capture by SMS and a retrospective telephone interview. Chiropractic & Osteopathy. 2010;18(1):10. doi:10.1186/1746-1340-18-10.
18. Kongsted A, Leboeuf-Yde C. The Nordic back pain subpopulation program: course patterns established through weekly follow-ups in patients treated for low back pain. Chiropr Osteopat. 2010;18:2. doi:10.1186/1746-1340-18-2.
19. Cherkin DC, Deyo RA, Battie M, Street J, Barlow W. A comparison of physical therapy, chiropractic manipulation, and provision of an educational booklet for the treatment of patients with low back pain. N Engl J Med. 1998; 339(15):1021–9. doi:10.1056/NEJM199810083391502.

20. Daltroy LH, Cats-Baril WL, Katz JN, Fossel AH, Liang MH. The North American spine society lumbar spine outcome assessment Instrument: reliability and validity tests. Spine. 1996;21(6):741–9.

21. Deyo RA, Battie M, Beurskens AJ, Bombardier C, Croft P, Koes B, et al. Outcome measures for low back pain research. A proposal for standardized use. Spine. 1998;23(18):2003–13.

22. Patrick DL, Deyo RA, Atlas SJ, Singer DE, Chapin A, Keller RB. Assessing health-related quality of life in patients with sciatica. Spine. 1995;20(17):1899–908. discussion 909.

23. Dunn KM, Croft PR. Classification of low back pain in primary care: using "bothersomeness" to identify the most severe cases. Spine. 2005;30(16):1887–92.

24. Gatchel RJTD. Psychosocial factors in pain: critical perspectives. New York: Guilford Press; 1999.

25. Weiner BK. Spine update: the biopsychosocial model and spine care. Spine. 2008;33(2):219–23. doi:10.1097/BRS.0b013e318160457200007632-200801150-00017.

26. Leboeuf-Yde C, Axen I, Jones JJ, Rosenbaum A, Lovgren PW, Halasz L, et al. The Nordic back pain subpopulation program: the long-term outcome pattern in patients with low back pain treated by chiropractors in Sweden. J Manipulative Physiol Ther. 2005;28(7):472–8. doi:10.1016/j.jmpt.2005.07.003.

27. Axen I, Bodin L, Bergstrom G, Halasz L, Lange F, Lovgren PW, et al. Clustering patients on the basis of their individual course of low back pain over a six month period. BMC Musculoskelet Disord. 2011;12:99. doi:10.1186/1471-2474-12-99.

28. Axen I, Bodin L. The Nordic maintenance care program: the clinical use of identified indications for preventive care. Chiropr Man Therap. 2013;21(1):10. doi:10.1186/2045-709X-21-102045-709X-21-10.

29. Leboeuf-Yde C, Rosenbaum A, Axen I, Lovgren PW, Jorgensen K, Halasz L, et al. The Nordic Subpopulation Research Programme: prediction of treatment outcome in patients with low back pain treated by chiropractors-does the psychological profile matter? Chiropr Osteopat. 2009;17:14. doi:10.1186/1746-1340-17-14.

30. French SD, Densley K, Charity MJ, Gunn J. Who uses Australian chiropractic services? Chiropr Man Therap. 2013;21(1):31. doi:10.1186/2045-709X-21-312045-709X-21-31.

31. Jönsson C. The Swedish population's use of the internet and telephones - an individual survey 2. Stockholm: Swedish National Post and Telecom Agency; 2008. p. 24.

32. McGorry RW, Webster BS, Snook SH, Hsiang SM. The relation between pain intensity, disability, and the episodic nature of chronic and recurrent low back pain. Spine. 2000;25(7):834–41.

19

The chiropractic profession in Denmark 2010–2014: a descriptive report

Orla Lund Nielsen[1]*, Alice Kongsted[1,2] and Henrik Wulff Christensen[1]

Abstract

Background: The chiropractic profession has been well established in Denmark for several decades with state authorization, partial reimbursement by the state and a formal academic education. Biennial systematic data collections among all chiropractors and clinics have been performed since 2010 in order to provide exact information on the profession to The Danish Chiropractic Association (DCA). It is the aim of this study to outline the major characteristics and developments of the chiropractic profession in Denmark to make this information accessible to other stakeholders, domestic as well as foreign.

Methods: Using contact information from the DCA, two questionnaires were distributed electronically to all individual members of the association actively working as chiropractors and all clinics respectively in 2010, 2012 and 2014. The questions asked were developed for this specific survey.

Results: Response rates varied between 59 and 78 % for the clinic questionnaires and 75 to 86 % for the individual questionnaires. Almost half the Danish chiropractors were educated in Denmark and a small majority was female. The average Danish chiropractor of 2014 was 44 years old, graduated 17 years earlier, and worked full time in a primary care clinic with at least one colleague. Half the chiropractors spent more than 20 h a year on continued professional development. Danish chiropractic clinics had a median of 3 treatment rooms, most had digital X-ray equipment, around 6 out of 10 had exercise facilities, and 1 out of 4 employed a physiotherapist. Three out of 4 clinics employed a secretary, too. The average duration of a consultation was 40 min for a new patient and 13 min for a follow-up consultation. Virtually all Danish chiropractors working in the primary sector made use of manipulation as one of their treatment modalities.

Conclusion: This is the first study to describe the state and latest development of the chiropractic profession in Denmark using repeated surveys. Displaying various characteristics of both clinics and individual chiropractors, the image emerging is one of a stable profession where rapid or drastic changes are not taking place over short intervals of time.

Keywords: Chiropractic, Clinical practice pattern, PrimaryHealth Care, Denmark

Background

Organisation of chiropractic in Denmark

The first chiropractor in Denmark started practising in 1920. Since then a profession has emerged and it has been an acknowledged and accepted part of the official Danish health care system for several decades by now. Although only to a limited degree, partial reimbursement of expenses for chiropractic care was acceded to in 1978 by the Danish government, and in 1992 a state authorization for practicing as a chiropractor was

introduced as the final step towards full recognition of the profession [1–3].

A 5-year academic chiropractic education was introduced in 1994 at what is now called The University of Southern Denmark (SDU) in Odense, and since 1999 when the first students completed their education approximately 300 Danish chiropractors (by 2014) have joined the profession after graduating at SDU largely supplanting United Kingdom and USA as the most common place of education [1].

The Danish Chiropractors' Association (DCA) was established in 1925. Since then, it has been the sole chiropractic professional organisation in Denmark except for a two-year period in the late 1940s. Affiliation

* Correspondence: o.nielsen@nikkb.dk
[1]The Nordic Institute of Chiropractic and Clinical Biomechanics, Campusvej 55, DK-5230 Odense M, Denmark
Full list of author information is available at the end of the article

to the association is a requirement for receiving reimbursement from the national health insurance because the DCA negotiates the agreement with the Danish health authorities (The Regions' Board for Wages and Tariffs) on behalf of the profession. Negotiations take place every three years and includes agreements on payment to chiropractors, regulations related to the profession, and which developmental initiatives the profession should take on. State reimbursement amounts to approximately 20 % of the treatment fee.

The association organizes clinic owners, chiropractic employees in both the primary and the secondary sector, researchers and university lecturers with a chiropractic background, and retired chiropractors as non-active members.

Patients either self-refer to chiropractors or are advised about chiropractic care by a general practitioner. There is no formal referral from general practice and patient costs are the same whether self-referring or being advised to seek chiropractic care by a general practitioner.

In 1987, the DCA established The Foundation for Chiropractic Research and Post Graduate Education in collaboration with The Regions' Board for Wages and Tariffs (RBWT). Among the objectives of the foundation is to provide financially support for research projects, international stipends, and quality development projects within the field of clinical biomechanics as well as supporting continued professional development. One third of the foundation's yearly income is provided by RBWT while two thirds is drawn directly from the state reimbursements to the clinics.

Study background

In 2010 a desire to investigate the major characteristics of the now fairly well established profession and to initiate an on-going monitoring of its further development caused the launching of the first systematic data collection on the chiropractic profession in Denmark. The main purpose of the initiative was to provide comprehensive information to The Danish Chiropractors' Association to help the organisation in its effort to refine and develop the profession even further. However, we regard this information to be relevant to chiropractors, healthcare professionals, officials, and chiropractic associations in other countries too.

Over the past decade, similar descriptive reports on the chiropractic profession have been issued from a number of our neighbouring countries, mainly displaying characteristics of the individual country at a specific time. A majority of these deal with chiropractic communities somewhat smaller than the Danish profession and presents comparatively few responders (Germany $n = 49$ [4], Finland $n = 44$ [5], Belgium $n = 80$ [6], The Netherlands $n = 113$ [7]), and one of them deals with chiropractors'

beliefs and professional opinions rather than a quantitative description of the profession [8]. A Norwegian study very similar to the Danish survey and actually based on the Danish questionnaires obtained 320 responses from individual chiropractors in 2011 [9], and a study from Switzerland based on 183 participants explicitly aimed at comparing data with data from other countries [10]. Finally a comprehensive American analysis included data from a number of surveys performed in USA over a period of nearly 20 years, the latest of which is from 2009 and had close to 2.300 responders [11].

The primary objective of this report is to describe the chiropractic profession in Denmark in 2014, tentatively outlining developments since 2009 when possible. However, due to the short intervals between the surveys, some data will only be reported for 2014.

Though it is not a main objective of this study to present an exhaustive comparison between countries, in cases where conspicuous similarities or differences call for attention details from previously published reports will be taken into account in the discussion.

Method

Between 2010 and 2014, three cross-sectional data collections were carried out among Danish chiropractors using contact information obtained from the DCA. Two separate questionnaires were distributed electronically in each survey: one directed at all individual chiropractors who were registered members of the DCA and actively working as chiropractors at the time of initiating the data collection, and one addressed to each separate physical clinic. Hence one owner from each clinic was required to answer both questionnaires.

Designing the project, data collection and analysis were anchored at the Nordic Institute of Chiropractic and Clinical Biomechanics (NIKKB). Mails with a short introduction to the survey signed by a senior researcher at NIKKB and a link to the questionnaire itself were distributed via the licensed online survey database SurveyXact [12]. Analysis was performed in STATA14 [13]. Non-responders and responders who had only filled out part of the questionnaires automatically received reminders one and two weeks later. One or two further reminders were sent manually to non-responders and after approximately five weeks the data collection was closed.

The questions asked were developed for this specific survey and were not previously validated. *Years since education, Physical size of the clinic, Number of treatment rooms, No. of chiropractors* and all questions concerning the duration of consultations were collected as continuous variables. Answer categories to the other questions appear from the tables. Average age was calculated on the basis of 10-year age groups.

According to Danish legislation stipulated in Act on Research Ethics Review of Health Research Projects, section 14, subsection 1–2, approval from The Health Research Ethics Committee System in Denmark was not required as the questionnaires do not ask for personal information and all data were collected anonymously [14].

Results

Response rates and geographical representativeness

The response rates for the surveys are shown in Table 1. Some of the questionnaires were only partially completed, which accounts for the "missing" category in the majority of the tables.

Assessment of representativeness could be based on the actual regional distribution of the clinics in 2014 known from the DCA mailing list. A comparison with responses to the clinic questionnaires that same year (Fig. 1) showed the Capital Region of Denmark (Region Hovedstaden) and the Central Denmark Region (Region Midtjylland) to be slightly underrepresented in the survey. A similar pattern was seen in 2012.

Demographic data

In the 2014 survey, 252 of the 454 (56 %) respondents were female representing a slight increase compared to the earlier surveys (Table 2). Almost half the respondents were 40 years old or younger in 2010 while only 40 % of the responders belonged to this age group in 2014. In the same period of time the percentage of chiropractors aged more than 50 years increased from 23 to 30 %. The calculated average age increased from 41.7 years in 2010 over 42.6 in 2012 to 44.2 years in 2014.

Denmark was the most common place of education with a little less than half the responders having graduated here, some 20 % in the United Kingdom and 30 % in the USA. Only small differences could be seen from 2010 to 2014.

In line with a smaller proportion of chiropractors belonging to the youngest age groups, the proportion of responders having graduated less than a decade ago steadily decreased over the study period (Table 2). However, the last survey suffered from some missing values on this particular topic.

Clinic characteristics

The proportion of clinics covered by the agreement with The Danish health authorities ensuring partial reimbursement was 86 % (173/201) in the 2014 survey.

Table 1 Response rates

Questionnaire type	2010	2012	2014
Clinic questionnaire	59 % (143/244)	77 % (193/250)	78 % (201/258)
Individual questionnaire	75 % (393/524)	86 % (469/547)	82 % (454/551)

The average Danish chiropractic clinic had 4 treatment rooms in 2014 and a size of 223 m^2 which is roughly the same as in the previous years (Table 3). The proportion of medium sized clinics with 3–5 treatment rooms rose slightly to nearly half the clinics in 2014. Very large clinics with more than 10 treatment rooms made up 2 % equalling 5 clinics in 2014. The previous surveys listed 3 and 2 such clinics respectively.

Approximately half the clinics offered the use of movable exercise equipment to their patients. The proportion of clinics with a separate exercise room located on the same address remained relatively stable around 30 % (Table 3).

The proportion of clinics with digital X-ray equipment increased across the survey time points at the same time as the prevalence of analogue X-ray equipment went down. Proportions with diagnostic ultrasound varied little across surveys (Table 3).

Staffing

Clinics manned by one chiropractor only accounted for little more than one third of the total number (Table 4, no information available for 2010). One out of twenty clinics employed five chiropractors or more.

A majority of the clinics employed secretaries. Among other health practitioners masseurs were the group most frequently employed, while physiotherapists were engaged in about one fourth of the clinics.

More than half the clinics had some kind of health practitioner other than a chiropractor employed, e.g. masseurs, physiotherapists, acupuncturists, dieticians or medical doctors etc. (Table 4).

Employment, working hours and continuing professional development

When looking at the chiropractors' occupational status in general, i.e. both primary and secondary jobs as a whole, practising in the primary sector is by far the most frequent type of employment (Table 5). Almost two thirds of the practitioners are owners. The proportion of chiropractors employed by the health insurance companies decreased across the survey period.

In terms of each chiropractor's primary job only (not reported in the tables) as opposed to employment in general, 11 individuals (2 %) did clinical work at a hospital in the secondary sector, another 11 were engaged by a health insurance company, and 16 chiropractors (4 %) were employed in research and/or teaching in 2014 (*n* = 454). In 2014 the respondents were given the opportunity to state administrational tasks or management as their primary function too and 9 individuals (2 %) did so.

Nearly one out of five chiropractors had two or three employments related to the profession (83 in 2014, 89 in 2012 and 72 in 2010). Teaching formed the largest single

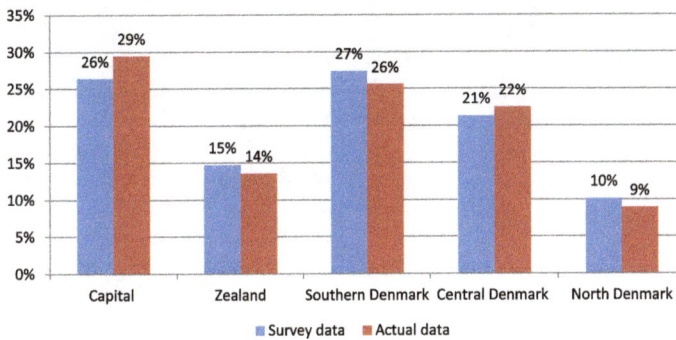

Fig. 1 Regional distribution of clinics in Denmark 2014. Survey data compared to the actual distribution of chiropractic clinics in Denmark on the five Regions

job function among this group and was done by 35 % in 2014 (34 % in 2012 and 38 % in 2010).

Most Danish chiropractors worked full time or more (Table 5). Lack of employment was rare with six chiropractors (2 %) declaring not being occupied as a chiropractor in 2010 decreasing to four in 2012 and only one chiropractor lacking employment in 2014.

Table 2 Demographic data

Gender	2010 (n = 393)	2012 (n = 469)	2014 (n = 454)
Male	46 %	44 %	43 %
Female	54 %	54 %	56 %
Missing	0 %	2 %	1 %
Age group	2010 (n = 393)	2012 (n = 469)	2014 (n = 454)
21–30 years	12 %	9 %	8 %
31–40 years	39 %	36 %	32 %
41–50 years	26 %	31 %	29 %
51–60 years	18 %	18 %	22 %
61–70 years	5 %	6 %	8 %
>70 years	<1 %	<1 %	<1 %
Place of graduation	2010 (n = 393)	2012 (n = 469)	2014 (n = 454)
Denmark	47 %	47 %	46 %
United Kingdom	19 %	20 %	19 %
USA	31 %	29 %	29 %
Canada	2 %	3 %	2 %
Other countries	0 %	1 %	1 %
Missing	1 %	1 %	2 %
Years since graduation	2010 (n = 393)	2012 (n = 469)	2014 (n = 454)
0–10 years	42 %	35 %	28 %
11–20 years	19 %	24 %	24 %
21–30 years	24 %	25 %	24 %
>30 years	15 %	14 %	13 %
Missing	0 %	2 %	10 %

Owners of a clinic tended to work more than their employees. Figures from 2014 showed that 40 % of the clinic owners reported to work more than 37 h a week in total versus 12 % of the chiropractors in the primary sector who were not self-employed. The proportion of owners working 25–29 h and less than 25 h weekly was 10 and 5 % respectively, whereas the corresponding percentages for employees were 15 and 12 %.

Data on the effort dedicated to continued professional development (CPD) by each respondent was only available from the two latest surveys (Table 5). Half the chiropractors reported more than 20 h a year dedicated to CPD in 2014.

Working in the primary sector
Chiropractors working in a clinic, whether that may be as their primary or secondary job, naturally spent the vast majority of their working capacity on patient consultations. An average of 29 h weekly was dedicated by these chiropractors to the treatment of patients in 2014, and a little less than 4 h and 2 h were spent on administration and communication with other parties of the Danish health care sector respectively.

The duration of the various kinds of consultations seems remarkably constant (Table 6).

Virtually all Danish chiropractors working in the primary sector make use of manipulation while trigger point treatment and other soft tissue techniques are offered by 85-90 % and exercise instructions by more than 80 %. The Danish surveys did not ask about the proportion of patients the various treatment modalities were given to.

Discussion
General findings
The average Danish chiropractor of 2014 is 44 years old, graduated 17 years ago and works full time in a primary care clinic with at least one colleague. Danish chiropractic clinics have a median of 3 treatment rooms, most have digital X-ray equipment, around 6 out of 10 have exercise

Table 3 Physical characteristics of the clinic

Physical size of the clinic	2010 (n = 143)	2012 (n = 193)	2014 (n = 201)
Average size (m²)	226 m²	216 m²	223 m²
<100 m²	10 %	10 %	12 %
100–199 m²	39 %	44 %	37 %
200–299 m²	22 %	25 %	23 %
300–399 m²	10 %	8 %	12 %
≥400 m²	10 %	9 %	10 %
Missing	9 %	4 %	5 %
Number of treatment rooms	2010 (n = 143)	2012 (n = 193)	2014 (n = 201)
1–2	32 %	37 %	35 %
3–5	43 %	44 %	48 %
6–10	15 %	15 %	11 %
>10	2 %	1 %	2 %
Missing	8 %	4 %	3 %
Exercise facilities[a]	2010 (n = 143)	2012 (n = 193)	2014 (n = 201)
Separate exercise room at the clinic	31 %	22 %	29 %
Gym machines	16 %	15 %	15 %
Movable exercise equipment	52 %	47 %	51 %
Shower	14 %	9 %	12 %
No facilities	39 %	48 %	41 %
Missing	8 %	4 %	4 %
Average size of exercise rooms (m²)	113 m²	122 m²	123 m²
Diagnostic imaging facilities[a]	2010 (n = 143)	2012 (n = 193)	2014 (n = 201)
Digital X-ray equipment	57 %	63 %	70 %
Analogue X-ray equiment	25 %	15 %	5 %
Ultrasound	18 %	19 %	17 %
MR imaging	7 %	1 %	1 %
None	9 %	13 %	17 %
Missing	10 %	5 %	4 %

[a]The possibility to give more than one answer was explicitly stated in the questionnaire

facilities, and 1 out of 4 employs a physiotherapist. The described profile of the Danish chiropractic profession did not undergo large changes from 2010 to 2014.

Quality of the data

A response rate above 75 % as seen in five out of the six questionnaires is considered satisfactory, and matches or exceeds comparable studies from our neighbouring countries [4–7, 9–11]. Two of the individual questionnaires even obtain response rates of 82 and 86 %. Only a single question in one of the surveys had more than 10 % missing values.

With contact information made available by the only chiropractic association in Denmark, we were able to contact practically all Danish chiropractors. However, we do not know if non-responders to the surveys may represent a group of clinicians with a certain profile.

Negatively affecting the response rate for the clinic questionnaire may be that owners were required to answer both questionnaires, perhaps mistakenly leading them to believe the questionnaire to be already answered when they got to the second one. A similar effect may have been caused by the fact that the data source was physical clinics which implied that a clinic working from several addresses received several questionnaires probably even using the same email address. However, the results, especially from the 2012- and 2014-surveys, can be viewed as confidently reflecting the actual state of the Danish chiropractic profession.

The Danish chiropractor

Distinguishing the Danish profession most clearly from the Norwegian, Swiss, Belgian, Dutch or Finnish profession is the very high proportion of female practitioners of 56 % compared to 20–36 % in the said countries. With 43 % female chiropractors, the United Kingdom is the only country relatively close to the Danish gender distribution [5–10].

The American survey displays a female proportion changing from 13 % in 1991 to 22 % in 2009 [11]. A certain increase has been taking place in Denmark too over the years covered by the Danish survey, but due to the short time span it shows somewhat less markedly. Future increase in the proportion of female chiropractors is expected with a majority of Danish chiropractor students being females (from 2010–2014 59–67 % of admitted students were females [15]).

In terms of average age the Danish chiropractor seems to be growing older too. From 2010 to 2014 the proportion of chiropractors still in their twenties has decreased from 12 to 8 % while the 61–70 years age group has increased from 5 to 8 %. At the same time the surveys display a decrease in the proportion of responders with a maximum of 10 years since the date of their graduation from 42 % in 2010 over 35 % in 2012 to just 28 % in 2014, but due to a comparatively high number of missing values in the latest survey on this specific issue we are unable to ascertain to what extent the apparent change may be caused by selection bias.

Chiropractic clinics, the owners and their employees

Significant changes in the size or characteristic of the average Danish chiropractic clinic cannot be detected over the past four years.

Table 4 Staffing

No. of chiropractors (incl. owners)	2010 (n = 143)	2012 (n = 193)	2014 (n = 201)
1	Not available	37 %	36 %
2	Not available	26 %	25 %
3	Not available	13 %	19 %
4	Not available	10 %	8 %
≥5	Not available	6 %	5 %
Missing	Not available	8 %	6 %
Percentage of clinics employing other staff groups than chiropractors	2010 (n = 143)	2012 (n = 193)	2014 (n = 201)
Secretaries	69 %	79 %	76 %
Physiotherapists	27 %	25 %	25 %
Masseurs	43 %	46 %	48 %
Medical doctors	1 %	1 %	1 %
Other practitioners	19 %	14 %	19 %
No other employees	9 %	7 %	11 %
Missing	9 %	6 %	5 %
Multidisciplinary setting[a]	52 %	55 %	56 %

[a]Understood as the percentage of clinics employing at least one health practitioner (not secretaries) of any kind

Table 5 Employment, working hours and continued professional development (CPD)

General employment[a]	2010 (n = 393)	2012 (n = 469)	2014 (n = 454)
Owner of a clinic	56 %	58 %	58 %
Employed by a private clinic	32 %	32 %	30 %
Employed in the public sector	11 %	10 %	12 %
Employed by health insurance comp.	13 %	7 %	6 %
Other	8 %	4 %	3 %
Missing	1 %	1 %	4 %
Total working hours pr. week	2010 (n = 393)	2012 (n = 469)	2014 (n = 454)
More than 37 h	30 %	32 %	31 %
30–37 h	48 %	46 %	46 %
25–29 h	13 %	12 %	12 %
20–24 h	4 %	5 %	4 %
Less than 20 h	2 %	3 %	4 %
Missing	4 %	2 %	3 %
Hours of CPD pr. year	2010 (n = 388)	2012 (n = 469)	2014 (n = 454)
0 h	Not available	1 %	5 %
1–10 h	Not available	13 %	21 %
11–20 h	Not available	16 %	22 %
21–30 h	Not available	20 %	18 %
31–40 h	Not available	12 %	11 %
41–50 h	Not available	6 %	6 %
More than 50 h	Not available	20 %	15 %
Missing	Not available	13 %	3 %

[a]The possibility to give more than one answer was explicitly stated in the questionnaire

Clinics with 3–5 treatment rooms comprise nearly half the total number of clinics in 2014 which may represent a certain tendency towards medium sized clinics.

The prevalence of diagnostic imaging facilities forms the most distinct development in relation to the physical appearance of the clinic. The proportion of clinics with digital X-ray facilities rose from 57 % in 2010 over 63 % in 2012 to 70 % in 2014. Even more significant is the decrease in the prevalence of analogue X-ray equipment in the same period of time from 25 % over 15 to 5 %. Considered together with the increase in the number of clinics reporting to have no such facilities at all from 9 % over 13 to 17 % we see that whereas a growing number of the clinics acquire digital imaging facilities of their own not all the discarded analogue equipment is substituted by digital facilities. Some clinics simply choose to refer their patients to somewhere else for imaging.

Though a tendency towards bigger clinics cannot be ascertained based on physical size, more clinics find themselves in need of secretaries or a receptionist. Co-habitation or sharing facilities with other kinds of health practitioners such as masseurs or physiotherapists is widespread and more than half the clinics have formally employed health practitioners other than chiropractors. This proportion has increased from 52 % in 2010 to 56 % in 2014.

Comparison with other countries in this respect must be looked upon with some reservation due to the considerable variation in the way related questions are posed. The Swiss survey from 2009 has 10 % of its respondents reporting to "practice in a multidisciplinary office" [10], and in The Netherlands the proportion of chiropractors who "shared facilities with providers from other health-care professions" was likewise 10 % in 2004. In Finland 14 % employed "a non-chiropractic assistant" according to the data from 2002 [5]. Only unpublished data from the Norwegian survey reveals a proportion of multidisciplinary setting close to the Danish level as 44 % of the clinics state to have at least one additional health practitioner at the clinic.

Despite the lack of homogeneity of the data, however, it seems safe to conclude that the co-habitation is far more developed in Denmark compared to most other countries, although further information on this subject as well as on the actual level of interdisciplinary collaboration is desirable.

The chiropractic consultation

Looking at the average duration of a patient consultation, a remarkably stable pattern is revealed. Neither

Table 6 Work in the primary sector

Minutes allotted to a new patient	2010 (n = 332)	2012 (n = 403)	2014 (n = 400)
Average	40 min.	40 min.	40 min.
≤15 min.	1 %	0 %	0 %
16–30 min.	33 %	33 %	33 %
31–45 min.	47 %	49 %	52 %
46–60 min.	16 %	15 %	12 %
>60 min	0 %	0 %	1 %
Missing	2 %	3 %	2 %
Minutes allotted to known patients presenting with a new problem	2010 (n = 332)	2012 (n = 403)	2014 (n = 400)
Average	25 min.	26 min.	26 min.
≤15 min.	17 %	11 %	12 %
16–30 min.	73 %	77 %	77 %
31–45 min.	7 %	7 %	8 %
46–60 min.	2 %	2 %	1 %
>60 min	0 %	0 %	0 %
Missing	2 %	3 %	2 %
Minutes allotted follow-up consultations	2010 (n = 332)	2012 (n = 403)	2014 (n = 400)
Average	13 min.	13 min.	13 min.
≤5 min.	3 %	1 %	2 %
6–10 min.	50 %	49 %	46 %
11–15 min.	37 %	40 %	40 %
16–30 min.	8 %	6 %	9 %
>60 min	0 %	0 %	0 %
Missing	2 %	3 %	3 %
Which treatment modalities do you make use of?[a]	2010 (n = 332)	2012 (n = 403)	2014 (n = 400)
Manipulation	97 %	97 %	98 %
Trigger point	93 %	93 %	90 %
Other soft tissue techniques	86 %	88 %	86 %
Activator	45 %	50 %	48 %
Shockwave	8 %	11 %	13 %
Acupuncture/dry-needling	38 %	40 %	48 %
Exercise instruction	85 %	83 %	81 %
Laser	Not available	Not available	25 %
Missing	2 %	2 %	1 %

[a]The possibility to give more than one answer was explicitly stated in the questionnaire

the first consultation with a new patient nor the follow-up consultations display any variation in length at all over the three surveys (40 min and 13 min respectively). In 2014 85 % of the chiropractors allotted 16–45 min to a new patient and approximately the same proportion allotted 6–15 min to follow-up consultations suggesting that Danish chiropractors have reached a rather firm concept of their individual treatment procedure.

The average duration of consultations does not differ very much across countries. In The Netherlands and Belgium an appointment with a new patient takes on average 41 and 36 min respectively, and follow-up consultations are done in 15 min in both countries [6, 7]. A comparison with Humphreys et al. suggests slightly longer consultations in Switzerland as new patients are seen 16–30 min by 23 % and 31–45 min by 60 % (Denmark: 33 and 52 %) and follow-up consultations are done in 6–10 min by 29 % and 11–15 min by 58 % (Denmark: 46 and 40 %). However very short first consultations with new patients of 15 min or less are not registered in Denmark but comprise 3 % of the Swiss consultations [10].

A similar pattern with comparatively long consultations is also seen in the other Nordic countries although different time categories make a one-on-one comparison impossible. In Norway 80 % dedicates 30–49 min to a new patient and 60 % see a follow-up patient for 15–20 min [9] while 80 % of the Finnish chiropractors allot 30–45 min to new patients and 15–30 min to follow-up patients respectively [5].

Conclusions

This is the first study to describe the state and latest development of the chiropractic profession in Denmark using several consecutive surveys. Displaying various characteristics of both clinics and individual chiropractors, the image emerging is one of a stable profession where rapid or drastic changes are not taking place over short intervals of time.

The typical Danish chiropractor works in primary care, she is in her mid-forties with some 17 years of working experience. About half the profession graduated from University of Southern Denmark. The average clinic has 3–5 treatment rooms, is equipped with digital X-ray facilities and offers exercise facilities too. It employs at least one secretary, more than one chiropractor and, unlike clinics in our neighbouring countries, very often other health practitioners too. The average duration of the consultations, however, resembles that of other countries in the North-Western Europe, and it has been quite stable across all three surveys on 40 min for a new patient and 13 min for a follow-up consultation. Virtually all Danish chiropractors use manipulation as one of their treatment modalities.

Competing interests
The authors declare that they have no competing interests.

Authors' contribution
HWC and AK designed the original survey, helped designing the study and drafting the manuscript. OLN collected and analysed the data, designed the study and drafted the manuscript. All authors assisted in interpreting the data, critically revising the manuscript and approving it.

Acknowledgment
The study was carried out as a part of NIKKB's on-going survey of the chiropractic profession in Denmark. NIKKB is funded by The Foundation for Chiropractic Research and Post Graduate Education, which neither participated in the study nor had any influence on analysis or reporting of the results.

Author details
[1]The Nordic Institute of Chiropractic and Clinical Biomechanics, Campusvej 55, DK-5230 Odense M, Denmark. [2]Department of Sports Science and Clinical Biomechanics, University of Southern Denmark, Campusvej 55, 5230 Odense M, Denmark.

References
1. Jørgensen P. Kiropraktikkens historie i Danmark. Odense: Syddansk Universitetsforlag; 2014. p. 195–248.
2. Lov om Kiropraktorer m.v. af 06/06/1991. Available from: https://www.retsinformation.dk/Forms/R0710.aspx?id=46942.
3. Myburgh C. A qualitative exploration of key informant perspectives regarding the nature and impact of contemporary legislation on professional development: a grounded theory study of chiropractic in Denmark. J Manip Physiol Ther. 2014;37(6):383–95.
4. Schwarz I, Hondras MA. A survey of chiropractors practicing in Germany: practice characteristics, professional reading habits, and attitudes and perceptions toward research. Chiropractic Osteopathy. 2007;15:6.
5. Malmqvist S, Leboeuf-Yde C. Chiropractors in Finland–a demographic survey. Chiropractic Osteopathy. 2008;16:9.
6. Ailliet L, Rubinstein SM, de Vet HC. Characteristics of chiropractors and their patients in Belgium. J Manip Physiol Ther. 2010;33(8):618–25.
7. Imbos N, Langworthy J, Wilson F, Regelink G. Practice characteristics of chiropractors in The Netherlands. Clin Chiropr. 2005;8:7–12.
8. Pollentier A, Langworthy J. The scope of chiropractic practice: A survey of chiropractors in the UK. Clin Chiropr. 2007;10:147–55.
9. Kvammen OC, Leboeuf-Yde C. The chiropractic profession in Norway 2011. Chiropractic Manual Therapies. 2014;22(1):44.
10. Humphreys BK, Peterson CK, Muehlemann D, Haueter P. Are Swiss chiropractors different than other chiropractors? Results of the job analysis survey 2009. J Manip Physiol Ther. 2010;33(7):519–35.
11. Christensen GM, Kollasch MW, Hyland JK. Practice analysis of chiropractic 2010 - A project report, survey analysis, and summary of the practice of chiropractic within the United States. Greeley, Colorado: National Board of Chiropractic Examiners 2010.
12. SurveyXact. Available from: www.surveyxact.dk.
13. STATA. Available from: www.stata.com.
14. Act on Research Ethics Review of Health Research Projects. Available from: http://www.cvk.sum.dk/English/actonabiomedicalresearch.aspx.
15. Danish Ministry of Higher Education and Science. Available from: http://ufm.dk/uddannelse-og-institutioner/statistik-og-analyser/sogning-og-optag-pa-videregaende-uddannelser/grundtal-om-sogning-og-optag/ansogere-og-optagne-fordelt-pa-kon-alder-og-adgangsgrundlag/ansogere-og-optagne-fordelt-pa-kon-alder-og-adgangsgrundlag

20

Does cervical lordosis change after spinal manipulation for non-specific neck pain? A prospective cohort study

Michael Shilton[1], Jonathan Branney[2,3*], Bas Penning de Vries[1] and Alan C. Breen[3]

Abstract

Background: The association between cervical lordosis (sagittal alignment) and neck pain is controversial. Further, it is unclear whether spinal manipulative therapy can change cervical lordosis. This study aimed to determine whether cervical lordosis changes after a course of spinal manipulation for non-specific neck pain.

Methods: Posterior tangents of C2 and C6 were drawn on the lateral cervical fluoroscopic images of 29 patients with subacute/chronic non-specific neck pain and 30 healthy volunteers matched for age and gender, recruited August 2011 to April 2013. The resultant angle was measured using 'Image J' digital geometric software. The intra-observer repeatability (measurement error and reliability) and intra-subject repeatability (minimum detectable change (MDC) over 4 weeks) were determined in healthy volunteers. A comparison of cervical lordosis was made between patients and healthy volunteers at baseline. Change in lordosis between baseline and 4-week follow-up was determined in patients receiving spinal manipulation.

Results: Intra-observer measurement error for cervical lordosis was acceptable (SEM 3.6°) and reliability was substantial ICC 0.98, 95 % CI 0.962–0991). The intra-subject MDC however, was large (13.5°). There was no significant difference between lordotic angles in patients and healthy volunteers ($p = 0.16$). The mean cervical lordotic increase over 4 weeks in patients was 2.1° (9.2) which was not significant ($p = 0.12$).

Conclusions: This study found no difference in cervical lordosis (sagittal alignment) between patients with mild non-specific neck pain and matched healthy volunteers. Furthermore, there was no significant change in cervical lordosis in patients after 4 weeks of cervical spinal manipulation.

Keywords: Neck pain, Spinal manipulation, Cervical lordosis, Sagittal alignment

Background

Neck pain is a common complaint that will affect three quarters of people at some point in their lives [1]. It is one of the most commonly reported reasons for ambulatory health care visits with 12 month prevalence rates ranging from 30 to 50 % [2]. At the societal level, neck pain significantly impacts economically in terms of work absenteeism and health care expenditure [3–5].

* Correspondence: jbranney@bournemouth.ac.uk
[2]Faculty of Health and Social Sciences, Bournemouth University, Bournemouth House, Bournemouth BH1 3LH, UK
[3]Institute of Musculoskeletal Research and Clinical Implementation, Anglo-European College of Chiropractic, 13-15 Parkwood Road, Bournemouth BH5 2DF, UK
Full list of author information is available at the end of the article

In general, despite technological advancements, an accurate diagnosis of neck pain remains elusive [6], but it has been proposed that the amount of lordosis (sagittal alignment) in the cervical spine is important for treatment and prognosis [7, 8]. However, the importance of cervical lordosis in relation to neck pain is controversial and has yet to be substantiated by high quality prospective research.

It has been suggested that lordosis can change following trauma or due to disc degeneration [9] and reduced cervical lordosis has been associated with neck pain in acute and chronic neck pain patients [7, 10–12]. However, one study used retrospective data from radiographs ranging from 1988 to 2003 [12], giving rise to concerns about measurement standardisation. Given the time frame, it seems reasonable to suggest that positioning may not have been standardised across time. In addition, others [13–18] found no association between lordosis and neck pain, and in a literature review Gay [16] concluded that the curve of the cervical spine had little prognostic significance. Further, a more recent systematic review concluded that an association between cervical lordosis and spinal pain was not supported by the epidemiological evidence, albeit much of the research reviewed was found to be of low methodological quality [19].

Harrison et al. [7, 11] reported increases in cervical lordosis after treatment (consisting of spinal manipulative therapy (SMT) and cervical traction) in 30 neck pain patients and found this to be consistent with a reduction in pain. However, the authors [7] conceded that their study design fell short of allowing them to suggest that one has caused the other. In addition, if a systematic change in lordosis after treatment is found, this change cannot be attributed to the treatment intervention if there is a lack of (i) a control group with which to compare differences in change or (ii) an estimate of measurement error.

Closer inspection reveals further design problems with these studies [7, 11]. Although they incorporated a standardised radiographic positioning protocol consisting of obtaining two flexion and extension positions reached with eyes closed, this may involve a considerable repositioning error due to patients not being re-positioned in exactly the same way as for the first measurement. Furthermore, one study [11] involved only patients with a reduced lordosis at baseline and in the other [7] subjects were excluded if they had a cervical kyphosis, either segmentally or throughout the neck. This calls into question the generalisability of the findings.

According to Cooperstein and Gleberzen [20], there is a paucity of evidence investigating the ability of SMT to alter the shape of spinal curves and to our knowledge, no one has established a mimimum detectable change (MDC) to allow one to distinguish real changes from natural variation. Although the Cobb angle analysis has been the method of choice for measurement of overall lordosis and kyphosis of the sagittal spinal curves on lateral radiographs, it has been claimed that the posterior tangent method is superior in terms of measurement error (standard error of measurement) and face validity by avoiding over or under-estimation of lordosis [7, 11, 21].

This present study aimed to explore the effects of cervical manipulation on lordosis as measured using the posterior tangent method.

The study objectives were:

1. To determine the intra-observer and intra-subject repeatability (measurement error and reliability) for cervical lordosis measurement in healthy volunteers

2. To determine whether cervical lordosis changes (change equal to or larger than the MDC calculated from untreated healthy volunteers) after a course of spinal manipulation for non-specific neck pain.

Methods

Study design

The data for this study were collected as part of a prospective cohort study [22] (the 'parent study') investigating the effect of spinal manipulation on inter-vertebral motion. In that study, fluoroscopic imaging sequences of cervical flexion/extension were recorded at baseline and 4-week follow-up in neck pain patients receiving SMT and healthy volunteers not receiving any treatment using a standardised positioning protocol (Fig. 1). From those sequences, initial static neutral images were extracted as Audio Video Interleaved (AVI) files from which to measure cervical lordosis in this present study.

The sample size of 30 in each group was a realistic recruitment target given time and resource constraints and would allow adequate opportunity for normal distributions of interval data if present [23]. The sample provided a 90 % power to detect a 6° (SD 10) change in cervical lordosis in patients at the 95 % level of significance, hence the possibility of detecting changes far smaller than those previously reported in response to manual treatment in the literature [7]. Figure 2 provides an overview of the study design.

An intra-observer repeatability study was undertaken to test the repeatability (measurement error and reliability) of the measurement instrument in healthy volunteers ($n = 30$) [24]. The cervical lordoses of non-specific neck pain patients were compared at baseline with healthy volunteers and a baseline to follow-up comparison in healthy volunteers was used to calculate the MDC. Changes in cervical lordosis at follow-up in patients were then identified with respect to the MDC. The acquisition set up of the parent study is shown in Fig. 3.

Measurements of the positioning apparatus at baseline were taken and recorded (Figs. 3 and 4) so that the configuration could be faithfully replicated at 4-week follow-up.

Participants

All participants were recruited from August 2011 to April 2013. Data were collected from 30 patients (21 female) attending the Anglo-European College of Chiropractic (AECC) out-patient clinic with a new episode of non-specific neck pain of at least 2 weeks' duration and 30 pain-free healthy volunteers age and gender-matched with the patients and recruited from staff and students of AECC and the Faculty of Health and Social Sciences (formerly the School of Health & Social Care), Bournemouth University. One patient's

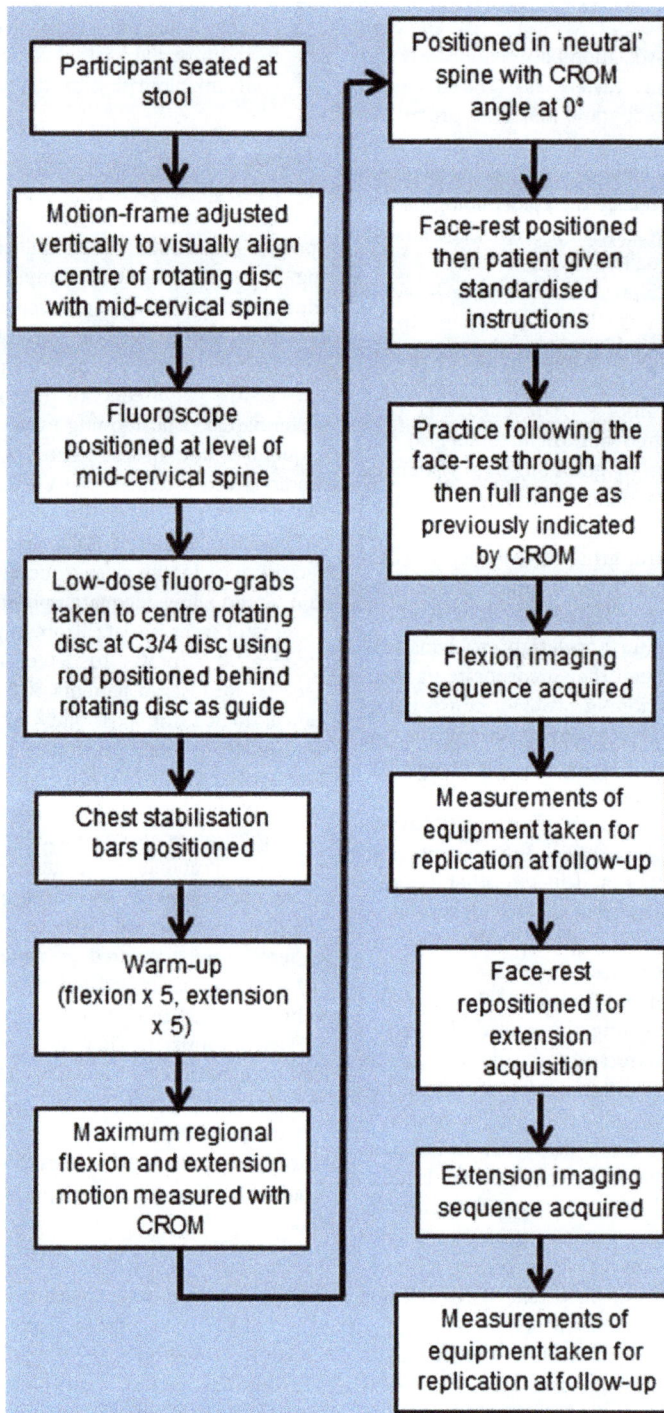

Fig. 1 Fluoroscopic image acquisition protocol

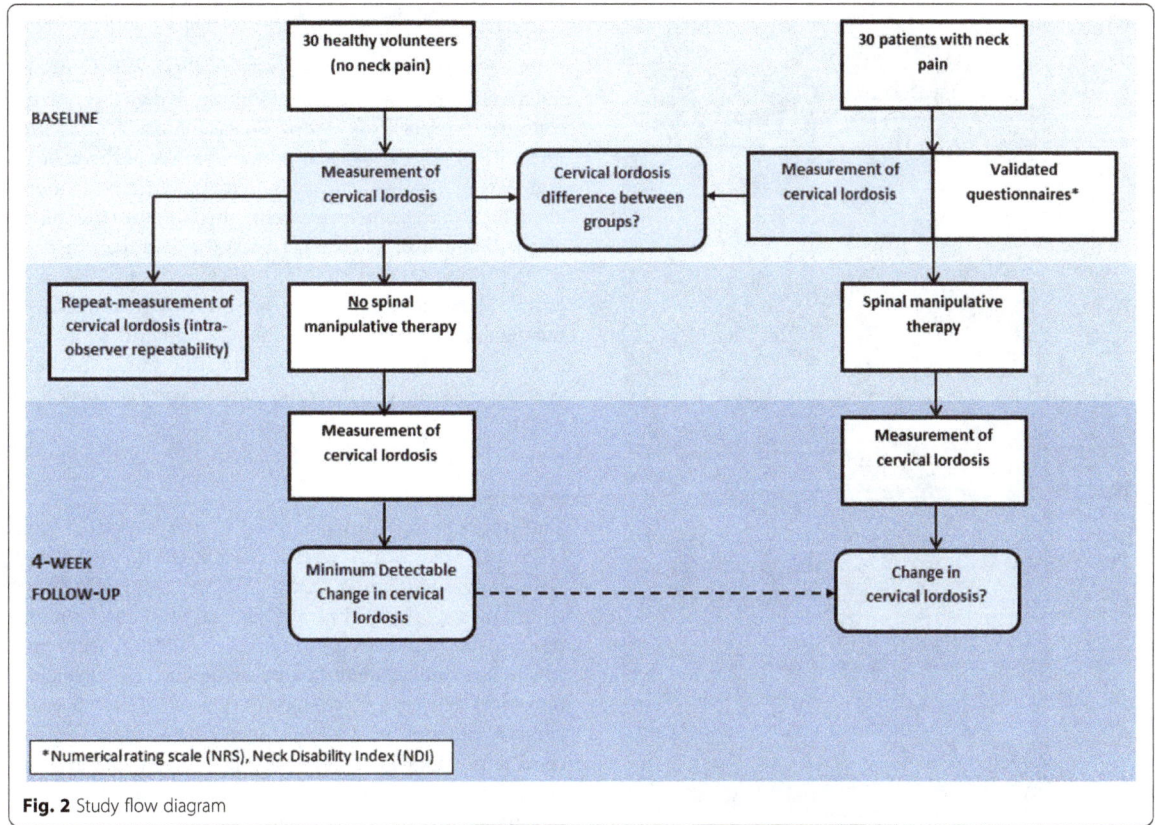

Fig. 2 Study flow diagram

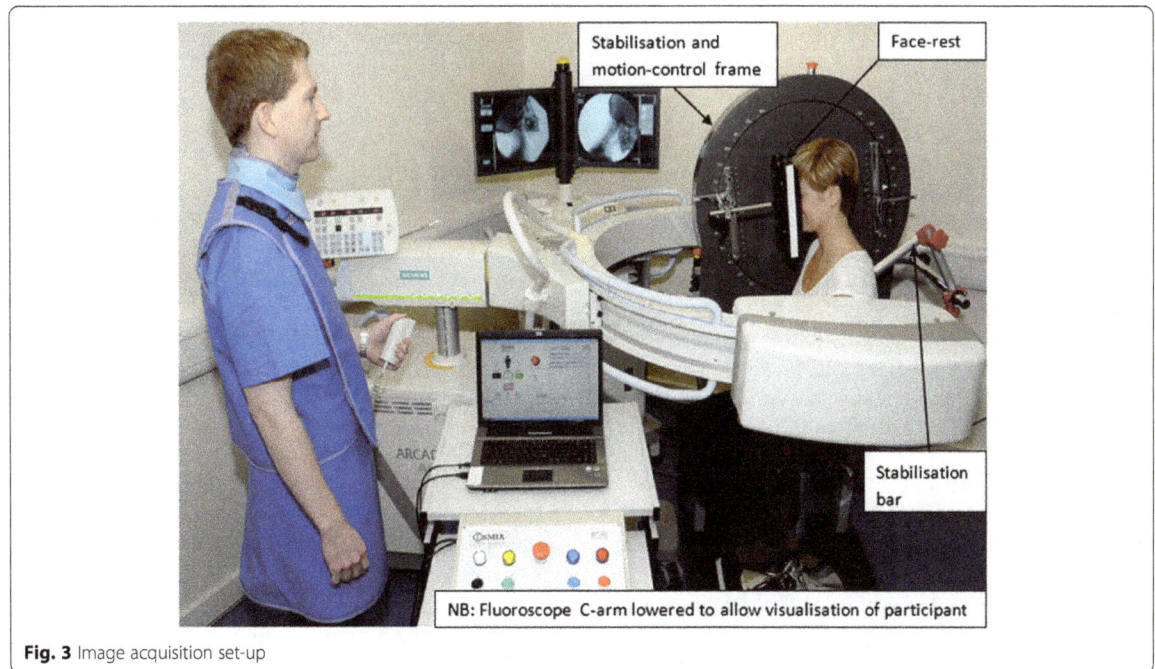

Fig. 3 Image acquisition set-up

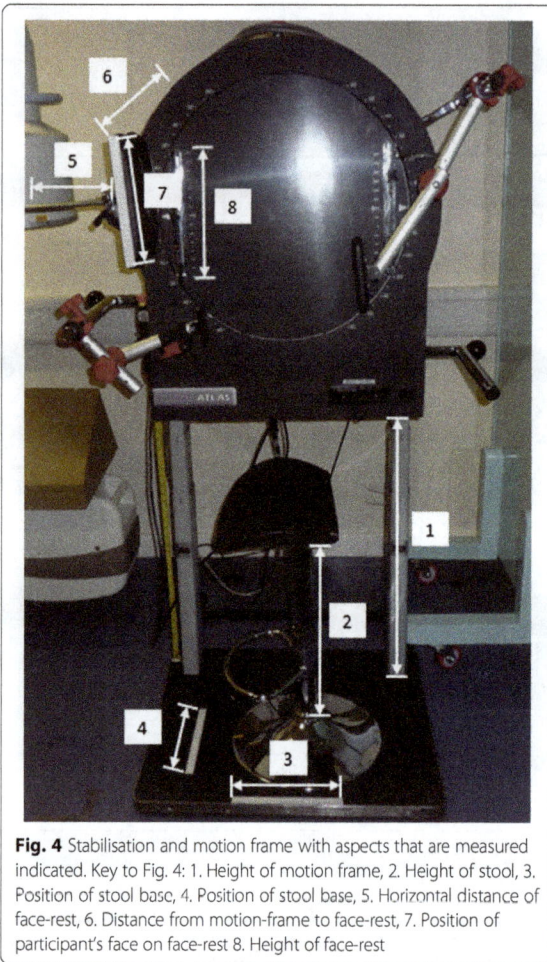

Fig. 4 Stabilisation and motion frame with aspects that are measured indicated. Key to Fig. 4: 1. Height of motion frame, 2. Height of stool, 3. Position of stool base, 4. Position of stool base, 5. Horizontal distance of face-rest, 6. Distance from motion-frame to face-rest, 7. Position of participant's face on face-rest 8. Height of face-rest

imaging sequence was not available due to a technical error which reduced the patient sample to 29.

The inclusion criteria for patients were: non-specific neck pain (reproducible by neck movement/provocation tests), of at least two weeks' duration, a self-reported pain rating of 3 or more on a 11 point numerical rating scale (NRS) and no suspected pathology.

The inclusion criteria for the healthy volunteers were that they should not have any current neck pain, dizziness or vertigo or any neck pain that limited activity for more than 24 h in the last 12 months.

Image measurement

For this study, the method of Gore was used for image measurement to be consistent with other studies [7, 8, 11, 14] for comparison and because Harrison et al. [21] found it to be superior to the Cobb method in terms of the measurement error (SEM). This method involves measuring the angle between lines drawn parallel

to the posterior surface of the vertebral bodies of C2 and C7 (Fig. 5).

The image measurement was facilitated by importing the fluoroscopic images into 'Image J' digital geometric software (available from: http://imagej.nih.gov/ij/ [Accessed June 2013]). As C7 was not visualised in six of the patients and two of the healthy volunteers the vertebral bodies chosen for this measurement throughout the study were C2 and C6. The image used was reduced to 75 % of the original size before marking. Using the program's drawing tool, a line was drawn posteriorly to the vertebral bodies of C2 and C6 and the protractor tool was then used to measure the angle between them. Kyphotic and lordotic angles were recorded as negative and positive values, respectively.

Interventions

The intervention involved SMT of the cervical region twice per week for 4 weeks. Manipulation was a high velocity low amplitude thrust (HVLA) using diversified techniques [25] as clinically indicated (based on patient history and exam findings including segmental pain/restriction as identified by static and motion palpation) and delivered by a chiropractor of at least 5 years' clinical experience. Patients received a mean of 1.3 cervical manipulations per visit (SD 0.4) and 10.7 over the course of the study (SD 3.5) [22]. Final year chiropractic interns also administered trigger point therapy and light massage (both received at least once by 27 patients) to the neck as clinically indicated. Seven patients reported using hot or cold packs during the study period, and 18 used over the counter pain-relieving medication [22]. The outcome measure for this present study was the angle of cervical lordosis.

Data analysis

Analysis was carried out using IBM SPSS Statistics (V210 and Stats Direct (V2.7.7). Baseline and follow-up lordoses for both patients and healthy volunteers were assessed for normality using the Shapiro-Wilk test. Provided the data were normally distributed, an unpaired two-tailed t-test was used to evaluate whether there was a statistically significant difference (significance level $\alpha = 0.05$) in mean cervical lordosis at baseline between patients and healthy volunteers. Baseline to follow-up comparisons in patients were performed using paired two-tailed t-tests (significance level $\alpha = 0.05$).

Repeatability encompasses measurement error (agreement) and reliability [24]. Measurement error was quantified by the SEM and repeatability coefficients were calculated to represent the MDC [26]. The SEM and MDC in healthy volunteers were calculated using the following formulae:

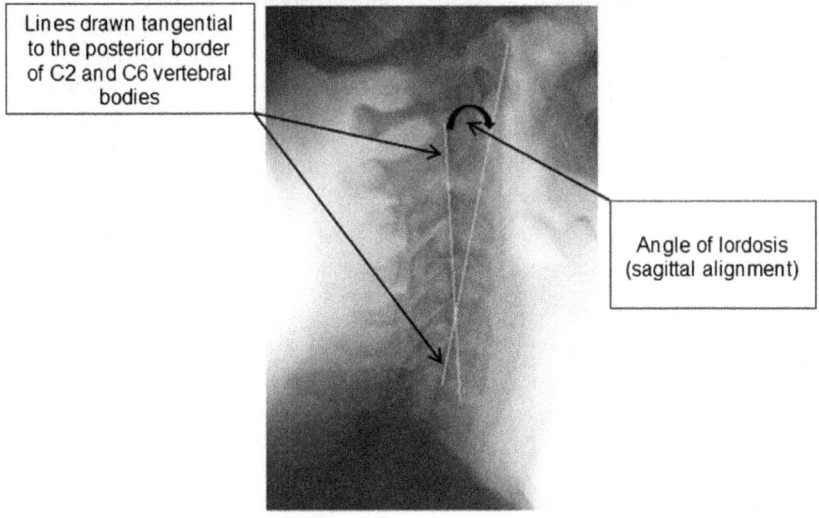

Fig. 5 Posterior tangent method of measuring cervical sagittal alignment

$$SEM_{agreement} = \sqrt{MSW} = S_w$$
$$MDC = S_w \cdot \sqrt{2} \cdot 1.96$$

Here, S_w and MSW denote the within-subject standard deviation and within-subjects mean square, respectively. For the intra-*observer* repeatability study, one observer repeated two measurements of cervical lordosis per healthy volunteer from one fluoroscopic image, at least 24 h apart. For the intra-*subject* repeatability study, calculations were based on baseline and follow-up lordosis measurements from each healthy volunteer as obtained by one observer.

Intraclass correlation coefficients (ICC) were used to quantify intra-observer reliability [24]. Generally $ICC_{agreement}$ (A) is the better option over $ICC_{consistency}$ (C) as the first is sensitive to proportional and fixed bias while the later only to proportional bias [27]. Since measurements per subject could potentially differ in a systematic manner, a 2-way analysis of variance (ANOVA) was used to estimate the various components of the ICC parameters. The type of ICC calculated was ICC (3A,1) single measures as each target or object of measurement is rated by each of the same k observers, where $k = 1$, and it was assumed that this was the only observer of interest [28, 29]. Using SPSS, ICCs (3A, 1) and 95 % confidence intervals (CI) were obtained.

Results

Baseline and follow-up measurements of lordoses for both patients and healthy volunteers were normally distributed.

Participant baseline characteristics

Table 1 shows the baseline characteristics of the healthy volunteers and patients. There were no statistically significant differences between the groups in terms of their gender, age or cervical lordosis, although patients tended to have greater lordotic curves.

Repeatability (measurement error and reliability) of cervical lordosis measurement

Table 2 shows the intra-observer and intra-subject repeatability in healthy volunteers.

An intra-observer MDC of 9.9° indicates that two measurements performed by one observer within 24 h and using one radiograph are expected to differ by no more than 9.9° in 95 % of subjects [24]. Similarly, an intra-subject MDC of 13.5° indicates that over a 4-week period subjects' lordosis measurements are expected to change no more than 13.5°. Only changes greater than

Table 1 Baseline characteristics of participants

	Patients	Healthy volunteers	Significance (p)
N	29	30	
Female	21	21	
Age, years	39.6 (12.8)	40.5 (12.7)	0.72[*]
NRS score/10	5.1 (1.4)		
NDI score/50	12.7 (6.6)		
Cervical lordosis, degrees	9.5 (13.5)	4.4 (14.0)	0.16[*]

Mean (SD) unless otherwise stated; *NRS* 11-point numerical rating scale; *NDI* neck disability index
[*]p-values for unpaired two-tailed t-tests

Table 2 Intra-observer and intra-subject repeatability in healthy volunteers

	Intra-observer repeatability	Intra-subject repeatability
SEM$_{agreement}$	3.6°	4.9°
MDC	9.9°	13.5°
ICC (3A,1), (95 % CI)	0.98 (0.962–0991)	0.87 (0.743–0.936)

SEM standard error of measurement; *MDC* minimum detectable change; *ICC (3A, 1)* intra-class correlation coefficient two-way single measures mixed effects model (agreement)

13.5° can, at least in part, be confidently associated with a factor (such as treatment) to which the healthy volunteers have not been exposed.

Changes to cervical lordosis in patients
Patients' lordoses increased, on average, from +9.5° (SD 13.5°, 95 % CI 4.6°–14.5°) to +11.6° (SD 11.8°, 95 % CI 7.3°–15.9°). These changes were not statistically significant ($p > 0.05$). The change in cervical lordosis was highly variable (range = 0.1–24.9°). In only 14 % (4/29) of patients was cervical lordosis increased by at least the MDC.

Discussion
Many researchers have suggested that a loss of cervical lordosis, as measured using plain-film radiographs, might be a cause of neck pain [7, 8, 10–12]. This has led some practitioners to place emphasis on the restoration of the lordotic curve as an important outcome measure for their treatment [8, 11, 30]. However, other researchers have suggested that a lack of lordosis is a normal variant and therefore not a cause of symptoms for neck pain [14–18].

In order to determine whether cervical lordosis changes because of treatment, a measurement tool of high repeatability is required to detect small differences. No studies were discovered in this review of the literature that found patients with neck pain to have a different cervical lordosis from asymptomatic subjects using a methodology that does not involve exclusion based on pre-existing cervical spine alignment or with highly standardised positioning.

The present investigation used images in which the cervical lordoses of clinically presenting neck pain patients matched with healthy volunteers were measured under highly standardised positioning at baseline and 4 week follow-up. In this way it was possible to more confidently investigate the association between cervical lordosis and pain and to test the repeatability of measuring cervical lordosis.

Intra-observer repeatability
The ICC (3A,1) of 0.981 (0.962–0991) indicates substantial reliability [31]. However, the intra-observer study demonstrated only modest levels of agreement with an SEM of 3.6°. This is higher than that reported by Gwinn et al. [32] and three times higher than that reported by Jackson et al. [33]. However, Jackson et al. [33] did not report which type of SEM was calculated (SEM$_{consistency}$ or SEM$_{agreement}$). Further reasons for their lower SEM could be having better image quality (plain film as opposed to fluoroscopic images) and/or more experienced observers.

Cervical lordosis in non-specific neck pain patients versus healthy volunteers
There was a non-statistically significant baseline difference (mean = 5.1°) in lordosis between patients and healthy volunteers, with the patients having the greater lordosis. However, this difference was not detectable in the current study. Based on a standard deviation of 14° (see Table 1, healthy volunteers), a sample size of at least 166 patients and 166 healthy volunteers would be required in order to detect a difference of 5° in lordosis with a statistical power of 90 % and significance level of 0.05. Thus, the non-significance for the difference may have been due to a type 2 error. Furthermore, while significant differences might be detected at the group-level with a sufficiently large sample size the large individual variability in cervical lordotic angles (–18–32° in patients and –22–36° in healthy volunteers) means that this is not a feasible technique for the evaluation of individual patients.

Cervical lordosis of patients at baseline and 4 week follow-up
The results from this study showed a mean increase in cervical lordosis in the patient group of 2.1° (SD 9.2°). This was not statistically significant and well below the natural variation in the healthy volunteers (MDC 13.5°). To attain a statistical power of 90 % with a 0.05 significance level, a sample size of at least 437 patients would be required to detect a mean difference of 2.1° in lordosis between baseline and follow-up, however this difference is not likely to be clinically meaningful. Two studies in the literature have attempted to measure change in cervical lordosis and have reported mean increases above 13.5°.

Harrison et al. found a 14.2° [11] and 17.9° [7] change in neck pain patients. In both of these studies the authors reported an increase in cervical lordosis coupled with a reduction in pain, but did not report the MDC or present a power calculation. The treatment groups received SMT for three weeks [11] and four weeks [7] and then a further traction period of nine weeks [11] and 14 weeks [7]. As the results from our study suggest that there is no association between cervical lordosis and pain it appears initially at odds with the Harrison studies. However, any changes in cervical lordosis that were achieved in those studies were perhaps due to traction rather than SMT [7] but that remains unknown. In the absence of randomisation or a control group there is also the possibility that these changes were due to natural variation (independent of treatment).

Strengths, limitations and suggestions for further research

A strength of this investigation lies in its use of prospective data of clinically presenting patients of all cervical sagittal alignments to be radiographically imaged under highly standardised conditions. In addition, the present study measured and reported both the measurement error and reliability of the method.

The MDC that was calculated from the healthy volunteers in this study, which provides information on the natural fluctuation of cervical lordosis over time, does not appear to have been previously reported. This suggests that small intervention effects on cervical lordosis will be difficult to detect. An MDC derived from a symptomatic cohort rather than asymptomatic subjects would give greater confidence in determining whether a change in treated symptomatic subjects could be attributed in part to the treatment, although this would present the ethical and practical challenges of recruiting patients who would consent to receiving no manual treatment.

While no significant difference in cervical lordosis was found between patients and healthy volunteers that does not preclude such a difference being detected in a study with a sufficiently large sample size. A further limitation of this study is that its design does not allow us to establish a causal relationship between cervical lordosis and pain, nor did it address other clinical outcomes. In addition, because six of the patients and two of the healthy volunteers had images where C7 could not be visualised, the study used C2-6 throughout, unlike previous studies [7]. However, this was thought not to be critical as the angle difference between C6 and C7 is considered to be very small [33].

Finally, it is noted that the width of the line drawn and decisions regarding accommodating osteophytes require interpretation and practice to develop consistency. This may be a further important source of variability in measurement.

Conclusions

This study found no difference in cervical lordosis (sagittal alignment) between patients with mild non-specific neck pain and matched healthy volunteers. Furthermore, there was no significant change in cervical lordosis in patients after 4 weeks of cervical SMT.

Consent

Written informed consent was obtained from the participant in Fig. 3 for the publication of this report and any accompanying images.

Competing interests

The authors declare they have no competing interests.

Authors' contributions

This article is based on a question generated by AB and JB. All fluoroscopic data were collected by JB assisted in part by AB and all cervical angles were measured by MS. Analysis was conducted by BPV and MS. All authors contributed to the paper. All authors read and approved the final manuscript.

Author details

[1]Anglo-European College of Chiropractic, 13-15 Parkwood Road, Bournemouth BH5 2DF, UK. [2]Faculty of Health and Social Sciences, Bournemouth University, Bournemouth House, Bournemouth BH1 3LH, UK. [3]Institute of Musculoskeletal Research and Clinical Implementation, Anglo-European College of Chiropractic, 13-15 Parkwood Road, Bournemouth BH5 2DF, UK.

References

1. Fejer R, Kyvik KO, Hartvigsen J. The prevalence of neck pain in the world population: a systematic critical review. Eur Spine J. 2006;15(6):834–48.
2. Hogg-Johnson S, van der Velde G, Carroll LJ, Holm LW, Cassidy JD, Guzman J, et al. The burden and determinants of neck pain in the general population: results of the Bone and Joint Decade 2000–2010 Task Force on Neck Pain and Its Associated Disorders. Spine. 2008;33(4 Suppl):S39–51.
3. Linton SJ, Hellsing AL, Hallden K. A population-based study of spinal pain among 35-45-year-old individuals. Prevalence, sick leave, and healthcare use. Spine. 1998;23(13):1457–63.
4. Cote P, van der Velde G, Cassidy JD, Carroll L, Hogg-Johnson S, Holm L, et al. The burden and determinants of neck pain in workers: results of the bone and joint decade 2000–2010 task force on neck pain and its associated disorders. Spine. 2008;33(4 Suppl):S60–74.
5. Cote P, Kristman V, Vidmar M, Van Eerd D, Hogg-Johnson S, Beaton D, et al. The prevalence and incidence of work absenteeism involving neck pain: a cohort of Ontario lost-time claimants. Spine. 2008;33(4 Suppl):S192–8.
6. Nordin M, Carragee EJ, Hogg-Johnson S, Weiner S, Hurwitz E, Peloso P, et al. Assessment of neck pain and its associated disorders: results of the Bone and Joint Decade 2000–2010 task force on neck pain and its associated disorders. J Manipulative Physiol Ther. 2009;32(2 Suppl):S117–40.
7. Harrison DE, Harrison DD, Betz JJ, Janik TJ, Holland B, Colloca CJ, et al. Increasing the cervical lordosis with chiropractic biophysics seated combined extension-compression and transverse load cervical traction with cervical manipulation: nonrandomized clinical control trial. J Manipulative Physiol Ther. 2003;26(3):139–51.
8. McAviney J, Schulz D, Bock R, Harrison DE, Holland B. Determining the relationship between cervical lordosis and neck complaints. J Manipulative Physiol Ther. 2005;28(3):187–93.
9. Hardacker JW, Shuford RF, Capicotto PN, Pryor PW. Radiographic standing cervical segmental alignment in adult controls without neck symptoms. Spine. 1997;22(13):1472–80.
10. Gore DR. Roentgenographic findings in the cervical spine in asymptomatic persons: a ten-year follow-up. Spine. 2001;26(22):2463–6.
11. Harrison DE, Cailliet R, Harrison DD, Janik TJ, Holland B. A new 3-point bending traction method for restoring cervical lordosis and cervical manipulation: a nonrandomized clinical controlled trial. Arch Phys Med Rehabil. 2002;83(4): 447–53.

12. Harrison DD, Harrison DE, Janik TJ, Caillet R, Ferrantelli JR, Haas JW, et al. Modeling of the sagittal cervical spine as a method to discriminate hypolordosis. Spine. 2004;29(22):2485–92.

13. Kumagai G, Ono A, Numasawa T, Wada K, Inoue R, Iwasaki H, et al. Association between roentgenographic findings of the cervical spine and neck symptoms in a Japanese community population. J Orth Sci. 2014;19(3): 390–7.

14. Grob D, Frauenfelder H, Mannion AF. The association between cervical spine curvature and neck pain. Eur Spine J. 2007;16(5):669–78.

15. Borden AG, Rechtman AM, Gershon-Cohen J. The normal cervical lordosis. Radiology. 1960;74:806–9.

16. Gay RE. The curve of the cervical spine: variations and significance. J Manipulative Physiol Ther. 1993;16(9):591–4.

17. Okada E, Matsumoto M, Ichihara D, Chiba K, Toyama Y, Fujiwara, et al. Does the sagittal alignment of the cervical spine have an impact on disk degeneration? Minimum 10-year follow-up of asymptomatic controls. Eur Spine J. 2009;18(11):1644–51.

18. Beltsios M, Savvidou O, Mitsiokapa EA, Mavrogenis AF, Kaspiris A, Efstathopoulos N, et al. Sagittal alignment of the cervical spine after neck injury. Eur J Orthop Surg Traumatol. 2013; 23 Suppl 1: S47–51.

19. Toftgaard ST, Hartvigsen J. Spinal curves and health: a systematic critical review of the epidemiological literature dealing with associations between sagittal spine curves and health. J Manipulative Physiol Ther. 2008;31(9):690–714.

20. Cooperstein R, Gleberzon B. Technique systems in chiropractic. Philadelphia: Churchill Livingstone; 2004.

21. Harrison DE, Harrison DD, Cailliet R, Troyanovich SJ, Janik TJ, Holland B. Cobb method or Harrison posterior tangent method: which to choose for lateral cervical radiographic analysis. Spine. 2000;25(16):2072–8.

22. Branney J, Breen AC. Does inter-vertebral range of motion increase after spinal manipulation? A prospective cohort study. Chiropr Man Therap. 2014; 22:24.

23. Field A. Discovering statistics using SPSS. 3rd ed. London: Sage; 2009.

24. de Vet HC, Terwee CB, Knol DL, Bouter LM. When to use agreement versus reliability measures. J Clin Epidemiol. 2006;59(10):1033–9.

25. Peterson DH, Bergmann TF. Chiropractic Technique: Principles and Procedures. 2nd ed. St Louis: Mosby Inc; 2002.

26. Bland JM, Altman DG. Measurement error. BMJ. 1996;313(7059):744.

27. Weir JP. Quantifying test-retest reliability using the intraclass correlation coefficient and the SEM. J Strength Cond Res. 2005;19(1):231–40.

28. Shrout PE, Fleiss JL. Intraclass correlations: uses in assessing rater reliability. Psychol Bull. 1979;86(2):420–8.

29. McGraw KO, Wong SP. Forming inferences about some intraclass correlation coefficients. Psychol Methods. 1996;1(1):30–46.

30. Katsuura A, Hukuda S, Saruhashi Y, Mori K. Kyphotic malalignment after anterior cervical fusion is one of the factors promoting the degenerative process in adjacent intervertebral levels. Eur Spine J. 2001;10(4):320–4.

31. Shrout PE. Measurement reliability and agreement in psychiatry. Stat Methods Med Res. 1998;7(3):301–17.

32. Gwinn DE, Iannotti CA, Benzel EC, Steinmetz MP. Effective lordosis: analysis of sagittal spinal canal alignment in cervical spondylotic myelopathy. J Neurosurg Spine. 2009;11(6):667–72.

33. Jackson BL, Harrison DD, Robertson GA, Barker WF. Chiropractic biophysics lateral cervical film analysis reliability. J Manipulative Physiol Ther. 1993;16(6):384–91.

21

Chiropractors' perception of occupational stress and its influencing factors: a qualitative study using responses to open-ended questions

Shawn Williams[1,2,3] ⓘ

Abstract

Background: Job stress and emotional exhaustion have been shown to have a negative impact on the helping professional. The development and causal relations of job stress and emotional exhaustion are rather unclear in the chiropractic profession. The objective of this study is to understand the main sources of occupational stress and emotional exhaustion among doctors of chiropractic.

Methods: Analysis of the written responses to web-based open-ended questionnaire was performed using an interpretive research methodology. Additionally, cross tabulation and Chi square statistical tests were conducted to match and couple the demographic data with the categorical themes.

Results: Fourteen professional stress categories emerged from the 970 completed surveys. "Managed Care Organization regulation", "Managed Care reimbursement" and "Scope of Practice Issues" were the most common stressors that negatively influenced chiropractors' professional and personal lives. The results of the categorical analysis suggests that age, marital status, number of years in practice and location of practice may have an influence on the category of stress reported by chiropractors.

Conclusions: The qualitative approach revealed common, conventional and culture-specific job stressors in doctors of chiropractic. Notably, these findings suggest an association between third-party payer influences (increased regulation/decreased reimbursement) with that of increased job stress. Further research will be undertaken to refine the stress and satisfaction parameters and address stress interventions.

Keywords: Chiropractic, Psychological stress, Occupational stress, Qualitative research, Burnout

Background

Occupational stress and emotional exhaustion (EE) are extensive problems for health-care workers [1–4]. Occupational stress refers to environmental conditions and situations that prompt an emotional response such as anger or anxiety [5]. Similarly, but operationally and conceptually distinctive, EE is a chronic state of physical and emotional depletion that results from excessive job demands, depletion of resources and continuous hassles [6–9]. The relationship between occupational stress and EE is outlined in a collection of theoretical models, such as the control-stress model [5] and job-demands control model [10, 11]. The conceptual framework underlying occupational stress models [4, 10, 11] provide insight to the disputable relationship between job-demands, job resources and perception [5].

Accumulated research on occupational stress has generated a wealth of knowledge about the stress process and how stress affects workers in a wide variety of jobs [12–15]. McManus et al. [16] suggest that EE and occupational stress may have reciprocal causation – that is, high levels of

Correspondence: swilliams2@york.cuny.edu
[1]CUNY York College – Department of Health Professions, 94 - 20 Guy R. Brewer Blvd, Jamaica, NY 11451, USA
[2]Department of Research, New York Chiropractic College, Seneca Falls, NY, USA
Full list of author information is available at the end of the article

EE may cause stress, and high levels of occupational stress caused may EE. Either way, the end-result of escalating occupational stressors in the health-care the arena is that the provider(s) experiences a shift from energy to exhaustion, engagement to cynicism and efficacy to infectiveness [1]. Similar processes have been observed in a comprehensive group of health professionals [2, 4, 17], and more recently in the chiropractic profession [18, 19]. A recent study [18] exploring burnout in the chiropractic profession suggests that although overall values of burnout are relatively low (~2 %), higher levels of EE (~21 %) remain workplace issues for this professional group.

As changes in the political sector of the health care arena continue to mount, and new socioeconomic trends occupy the environment of health care, the nature and construct of occupational stress and EE may continue to develop as a serious threat to workers' well-being [5, 10, 20–23]. As such, despite being common in health-care workers [2–4, 17], the development and causal relations of occupational stress and EE are rather unclear in the chiropractic profession, in part due to an absence of adequate exploratory qualitative studies. Thus, the current study attempted to understand chiropractors' perceptions of job-related stress and consequently EE (as per the symbiotic relationship that exist between the two constructs). The objective of this study was to explore the opinions and perceptions of occupational stress among Doctors of Chiropractic (DCs). In this study, the aim was to assess what reasons (if any) DCs give as their precursors of occupational stress. The use of qualitative methods to analyze the material derived from open-ended answers in a questionnaire was employed with the intent of creating occupational stress categories that could help increase an understanding of the phenomenon as it applies to the chiropractic profession. A greater understanding of the perceptions of occupational stress may, in turn, provide a means to understand and improve chiropractic services.

Methods

A demographic survey including six socio-demographic categorical questions and one open-ended question was emailed (July 2013) to a randomized and convenience sample of DCs whose email addresses were included in the database of a leading chiropractic-marketing agency [24]. The invitation letter included a description of the nature of the study, a notation guaranteeing anonymity, and an embedded hyperlink to the web-based survey (via Survey Monkey). Descriptions of the constructs (occupational stress and EE) were operationally defined in the instructional section of the invitation letter. Non-DCs and/or DCs that were not involved in chiropractic fieldwork were identified and excluded from the study via two qualification questions. The remaining participants were asked (in

open-ended format) to describe the occupational stressor(s) - if any - that they believed had a negative impact on their professional and personal life. The open-ended question (dependent variable) read as such: 'What factors do you feel influence the levels of occupational stress and emotional exhaustion in the chiropractic profession?'

A mixed methods approach was used to explore respondents' perceptions of occupational stress and EE. The qualitative portion of this research design used content analysis [25, 26], inductively, coupled with an epistemological assumption(s) and interpretational approach, as the foundation of analysis to the open ended responses. Moreover, the qualitative analytic strategy employed in this study relied on a general approach that involved interpretive description as a means of developing an understanding of occupational stress and EE endured by DCs. The aim was to generate categories of reason for occupational stress and EE by using content analysis [27, 28]. Each open-ended response was read thoroughly and organized into categories of reason. If the response included two or more different statements of reason – it was identified and categorized accordingly to form the separate responses. For example, a typical response like "...low fees, too much paperwork, too much government regulation, deny-minded IME interfering with care, staff training, high expenses" includes many items that could fall in one (Business & Administration) or more (MCO regulation and reimbursement) categories. Categories were not preconceived and were named using respondents' own terminology where possible. The principle investigator (PI) read all of the statements in the initial sample and carried out this analysis on two additional separate occasions. The initial analysis generated almost identical sets of categories. A set of 14 categories was composed based directly on the respondents' statements.

The quantitative analysis integrated summaries of the categorical themes that were obtained after the open-ended responses, with similar themes grouped together. Descriptive statistics involving the frequency and percentage summaries were conducted to determine the number of respondents that chose each of the categorical themes. Cross tabulation(s) were conducted to match the demographic data of gender, age, years in practice, marital status, current professional status, and location of practice with the categorical themes of the open-ended responses. Chi square statistical test(s) were conducted to determine if the demographic data was significantly related to, or differed with, the categorical themes of the open-ended responses. A level of significance of 0.05 was used in the statistical analysis. During the study, several methods were used to ensure the data trustworthiness (i.e. practices supporting credibility, transferability, dependability, confirmability) as outlined by Zhang [25]. All analyzes were conducted in SPSS. Ethics approval

Chiropractors' perception of occupational stress and its influencing factors: a qualitative...

197

for the study was obtained by Seton Hall University's IRB in January 2013.

Results
Descriptive statistics
Most of the respondents were solo-practitioners and practicing in the United States. Additionally, most of the respondents were male and were married. It was observed that the age of those that answered the open-ended questions were between 31 and 60 years old.

The open-ended question was examined for common themes. The most-common responses were Managed Care Organization (MCO) Regulation (33 %), MCO Reimbursement (26.8 %), and Scope of Practice Issues (21.3 %). There were also significant numbers of responses for Business and Administrative (16.4 %), Public Perception / Public Acceptance (16.1 %), Self–Perception / Purpose (11.2 %), and Economy / Money (10.3 %).

In the 14 categorical themes of response, it was observed that many of the respondents practiced chiropractic in California, Colorado, Connecticut, Florida, Georgia, Illinois, New Jersey, New York, North Carolina, Ohio, Pennsylvania, and Texas. The percentage distribution of gender, the number of years in the professions and the practice location found in this study was reflective of current industry data [29, 30].

Qualitative – content analysis
There were a total of 970 analyzed open-ended responses out of the 1149 total respondents (Table 1); thus resulting in an 84 % completing rate. Those remaining 179 surveys were deemed incomplete. The initial analysis of 2022 statements generated 14 subcategories that collectively described perceptions and/or potential sources of occupational stress and EE. A further grouping of these subcategories was executed reflecting the context of the healthcare system, at-large. This stage of analysis produced three main categories, which is also described in the literature as common, conventional, and cultural specific [27, 31]. For the purpose of understanding the causes of occupational stress in DCs the three main categories were observed as (1) Health Care System - Conventional, (2) Intra-professional conflict- Cultural Specific, (3) Personal / Individual attributes - Common. Table 2 represents the frequencies and a percentage for all subcategories found, and just equally as important reflects, the magnitude / impact of DCs perception(s) of occupational stress.

Conventional: deficiencies of the health care system
The statements expressing external sources of stress with the way health care services are organized were further compartmentalized into respective subcategories. One of the assumptions of such categorization is that many similar helping professions share similar sources of occupational

Table 1 Descriptive frequencies for open-ended factors

		Answered open ended response
Gender	Female	179
	Male	791
Total		970
Age	20–30	47
	31–40	177
	41–50	267
	51–60	329
	61–70	128
	70+	22
Total		970
Years of practice	0–5	70
	6–10	100
	11–15	168
	16–20	118
	20–25	143
	25–30	154
	30+	217
Total		970
Marital status	Married	784
	Widowed	6
	Divorced	90
	Separated	11
	Never married	79
Total		970
Current professional status	Associate	46
	Independent contractor	42
	Sole-Practitioner	651
	Group practice	197
	Not a direct care provider (academic and/ or administrative)	34
Total		970
State or U.S. territory practicing chiropractic	Australia or New Zealand	8
	Canada	31
	UK & Europe	10
	United States	672
Total		721

stress and EE. Globally, these statements reflect the respondents' dissatisfaction with the perceived dysfunction of the MCOs including perceived problems with regulation of the health care system, legislation and implementation of it or cost for services. These reasons were grouped into major distinctive groups, such as: MCO regulation and MCO reimbursement.

Table 2 Frequencies and percentages for open-ended factors

Factor	Number	Percent
Business and Administrative	190	16.4
MCO Reimbursement	311	26.8
Isolation	26	2.2
Lack of vacation	24	2.1
MCO Regulation	384	33
Intra-Professional Stress	151	13
Patients	112	9.6
Public Perception / Public Acceptance	187	16.1
Self–Perception / Purpose	130	11.2
Student loan debt	35	3
Economy / Money	120	10.3
Scope of Practice Issues	247	21.3
Physical demands	28	2.4
Working too hard (long hours)	77	6.6

Percentages may not total 100 due to rounding error

'Dealing with Insurance, third party administrators, insurance reviews.'
'Constant changes and dealing with/arguing with insurance companies. It's a constant fight to maintain a sustainable income due to constant decreases in reimbursement.'
'Uncertainty regarding the future of healthcare law and policy. Unfair reimbursement through the third party payer system and Medicare program.'

Cultural-specific: deficiencies of the chiropractic profession

The statement expressing intra-professional sources of stress and exhaustion with the way the chiropractic profession is organized. Globally, these statements reflect the respondents' sources of stress with the chiropractic profession as a unit. Further, the statements describe problems that appear to be unique to the chiropractic profession and/or may be reflective of the occupational stressors that other alternative medicine professions, at-large, experience. These reasons were grouped into distinctive groups: Opposing DC views, Public Acceptation/Perception, Scope of practice issues

'The lack of cultural authority along with divergence in clinical practice.'
'Persistent negative stereotypes/perception in the general public/media. Constant infighting within the profession. Atmosphere of competition among peer chiropractors, including dishonesty regarding the state of one's practice in talking with other chiropractors.'
'The insurance companies treating us as less than doctors and making our lives miserable by questioning our care. I want to help patients get well not spend all day on paperwork.'

'Lack of cultural authority, lack of solidarity, the fact that DC's don't have a common answer for what we do, too much infighting, lack of professionalism in the profession, allowing practice building groups taking advantage young practitioners.'

Deficiencies of the DCs attitudes, skills and work

These statements described perceived deficiencies of individual practitioners. Globally, the statements describe basically all aspects of practice: knowledge, skill, behaviors and attitudes. These reasons were grouped into distinctive groups: Self-Perception, Isolation, Working too hard and Business and Administrative.

'Having no goals, having a poor vision for the future and not willing to grow. Also, a long term view is necessary with goals to match and some risk taking make practice more interesting and exciting.'
'Unrealistic expectations upon entering profession. Inadequate communication skills. Poor business operation skills.'

Quantitative analysis
Cross tabulations

Both male and female DCs believed that the top two stressors that negatively influence their professional work were MCO Regulations (male 303; female 81) and MCO Reimbursement (male 252; female 59). Scope of Practice Issues (male 204; female 43) and Public Perception / Public Acceptance (male 143; female 44) and Business and Administrative (male 153; female 37) were also noted as significant stressors across both genders. The same trend was observed in those DCs that were currently married. The age of the participants and the number of years in their profession was spread fairly evenly. When investigating the top three stressors that influence their professional lives, those DCs aged 31 to 40, 41 to 50, and 51 to 60 years old respectively, believed that MCO Regulations (65, 101, 144), MCO Reimbursement (61, 89, 111), and Scope of Practice (49, 58, 85) had the most noteworthy negative impact. Interestingly, DCs that said MCO Regulations, MCO Reimbursement, and Scope of Practice Issues were the most influential stressors in practice – were also those that had most years in active practice (20 -30+ years in practice). Of the 311 respondents that noted MCO Reimbursement as a significant stressor, 208 were sole-practitioners and 69 were in group practice. Of the 384 respondents that noted MCO Regulations as a significant professional stressor, 262 were sole-practitioners and 74 were in group practice. Of the 247 DCs that noted Scope of Practice, 167 were sole-practitioners and 48 were in group practice.

Collectively, when investigating the top three stressors that influence their professional lives, DCs noted MCO Regulations, MCO Reimbursement, and Scope of Practice

Issues, the State or U.S. territory the respondents were practicing chiropractic was mostly from California, New York, and Pennsylvania. Of the 311 respondents that noted MCO Reimbursement, 37 were from Pennsylvania, 35 from California, and 33 from New York. Of the 384 respondents that noted MCO Regulations, 51 were from Pennsylvania, 41 from New York, and 35 from California. For the 247 respondents that noted Scope of Practice Issues, 33 were from California, 18 from New York, and 12 from Pennsylvania.

Chi-square test results

The results of the chi-square test showed that gender was significantly related with the responses of MCO Regulation (X^2 (1) = 3.93, $p = 0.05$), Patients (X^2 (1) = 35.35, $p = 0.02$), Public Perception / Public Acceptance (X^2 (1) = 4.76, $p = 0.03$), and Working too hard (X^2 (1) = 6.35, $p = 0.01$). Chi-square test also showed that age was significantly related with the responses of business and administrative (X^2 (5) = 11.68, $p = 0.04$), patients (X^2 (5) = 18.88, $p < 0.01$), self-perception (X^2 (5) = 15.99, $p = 0.01$), and working too hard (X^2 (5) = 16.90, $p = 0.01$). Additionally, chi-square test also showed that the number of years in practice was significantly related with the responses of MCO regulation (X^2 (6) = 12.68, $p = 0.05$), patients (X^2 (6) = 27.07, $p < 0.001$), other (X^2 (6) = 15.12, $p = 0.02$), and working too hard (X^2 (6) = 22.18, $p < 0.001$); and that marital status was significantly related with the responses of patients (X^2 (4) = 17.72, $p < 0.001$), economy (X^2 (4) = 13.04, $p = 0.01$), and working too hard (X^2 (4) = 11.60, $p = 0.02$). Collectively, this indicates that the two gender groups, the six age groups, the seven categories of years in practice and the five categories of marital status have significant different responses in the open-ended responses. As per the various DC working characteristics, the results of the chi-square test showed that current professional status was significantly related with the responses of Intra-Professional Stress (X^2 (4) = 14.94, $p = 0.01$), Patients (X^2 (4) = 26.11, $p < 0.001$), and Student Loan Debt (X^2 (4) = 12.40, $p = 0.02$). Additionally, location of practice (Table 3) was significantly related with the responses of insurance reimbursement (X^2 (3) = 9.77, $p = 0.02$), MCO regulation (X^2 (3) = 13.44, $p < 0.001$), and self-perception (X^2(3) = 9.89, $p = 0.02$). Collectively, this indicated that the five categories of current professional status and the four categories of location of practice have significant different responses in the open-ended responses of Intra-Professional Stress, Patients, and Student Loan Debt, and MCO Reimbursement, MCO Regulation, and Self-Perception / Purpose, respectively.

Discussion

The primary aim of the current study was to examine the perceptions of occupational stress among a representative

Table 3 Chi-square result of relationship between location of practice and categorical themes of response

	Value	df	Asymp. Sig. (2-sided)
Business and administrative	3.22	3	0.36
Insurance reimbursement	9.77	3	0.02[a]
Isolation	0.44	3	0.93
Lack of vacation	1.50	3	0.68
MCO regulation	13.44	3	0.00[a]
Opposing DC views (Identity) Intra-Professional Stress	4.48	3	0.21
Patients	1.31	3	0.73
Public perception (cultural authority)/ public acceptance	5.54	3	0.14
Self-perception (purpose)	9.89	3	0.02[a]
Student loan debt	0.78	3	0.86
Economy (money)	0.09	3	0.99
Other (scope)	1.67	3	0.64
Physical demands	1.50	3	0.68
Working too hard (long hours)	1.79	3	0.62

[a]Significant relationship at Level of Significance of 0.05

sample of chiropractors in the US. This mixed methods approach, with emphasis on the qualitative analysis, generated three main categories and 14 subcategories representing the perceived occupational stressors among DCs. Overall, the results showed that the most of the participants believed that MCO regulation, MCO reimbursement, and Scope of practice issues were the most common stressors that negatively influenced their professional and personal lives. Interestingly, scope of practice amongst DCs is highly variable [32–34] in the US, and when coupled with cost of living differences, a strong connection between these factors became apparent. The participants responses indicated their perception of a cause effect relationship between occupational stress, emotional exhaustion and *"cultural authority, government / Obama, education, long hours, time, tools, medical, competition for other professions, documentation, scope, expectations; overhead; risk; scope of practice; paperwork; State associations; college / school; unethical; pay; EHR/EMR; communicating; balance; respect; unity; reward; AMA; boredom"*. High student loans, the non-recognition by the medical community, and the administrative aspects of operating a business, also have a significant negative implication(s) on DCs' practice life; by means of reducing resources and increase demands, as outlined in the control-stress model [5] and job-demands control model [10, 11]. However, collectively it appeared that most significant stressor within the chiropractic profession is *"the frustration with the insurance companies"*. Complaints of constantly getting denied, the extremely low reimbursement (gets lower every year), the raising of co-pays to make patients not want to come in appear to be overwhelming the modern day DC. These findings are consistent with much of the current occupational stress research [10, 20–22, 27]; which lends the notion that major changes in the health care system have been driven by increase-regulation via third-party payer systems.

Similar precursors/processes to occupation stress and EE have been observed in a comprehensive group of health professionals [2, 4, 17, 35–37] – and while some stressors were consistent across occupations, others were more rare or occupation specific. Across health professions, it appears that healthcare workers suffer from occupational stress because of higher expectations, not enough time, lack of skills and social support at work [21, 35–37]. Notably, interpersonal conflict appears to be the most prevalent stressor across all occupations [20, 22] – organizational constraints and workload are just as commonly reported in the literature. Interpersonal conflict occurs when a person or group of people frustrates or interferes with another person's efforts at achieving a goal [38] – and may be reflective of the unique cultural-specific perceptions of stress that occur in the chiropractic profession.

As the content analysis progressed, a conceptual pattern amongst the participants began to unfold. It appears that many of the participants agreed – Chiropractic's lack of internal consensus and legitimacy (cultural authority) inhibits chiropractic's ability to keep up with rapidly changing events. Further, participants repeatedly noted/suggested that in order for the chiropractic profession to progress, that is keep up with external health care events, e.g., the Affordable Care Act, Health Care Education Reform Act, etc., the profession would needs to come to some modicum of internal consensus. Internal consensus will be needed if the profession is going to achieve cultural authority [39]. Keeping the profession rooted in metaphors — i.e., Universal Intelligence, Innate Intelligence, Subluxation, dis-ease, etc. — which for some have become unquestionable myths and dogma inhibits chiropractic's achievement of legitimacy, the other necessary ingredient of cultural authority [40].

Limitation of the analysis

The limitation of the categorical analysis involving determining the relationship between the demographics with the categorical themes of open-ended responses is that causality cannot be determined. Also, finding a significant relationship between two variables with a correlation coefficient does not take into account the possibility of other variables playing a part. In addition, the direction (positive or negative) of the relationship and the strength of the relationship (weak, moderate, and strong) cannot be determined with a chi-square test. The variables of demographic and categorical themes of open-ended responses are categorical variables. Thus, correlation test cannot be conducted. The analysis merely determined the relationship between variables by investigating whether there is significance different in the categorical responses according to the results of the chi-square analysis.

Conclusion

The findings from this current study add to a continuous dialog on the unique causes of stress, emotional exhaustion and occupational stress for chiropractic professionals. These findings in this study add to the notion of directional association between third party payer influences (increased regulation/decreased reimbursement) with that of increased job stress. Further research will be undertaken to refine the stress and satisfaction parameters and address stress interventions.

Competing interests
The author declares that he has no competing interests.

Authors' contributions
SW was the sole-principle investigator of study. SW conceived the study, performed all statistical analysis and was responsible for drafting the manuscript.

Acknowledgements
This work was originally presented at the Research Agenda Conference, Las Vegas, NV March 2015.

Author details
[1]CUNY York College – Department of Health Professions, 94 - 20 Guy R. Brewer Blvd, Jamaica, NY 11451, USA. [2]Department of Research, New York Chiropractic College, Seneca Falls, NY, USA. [3]Private Practice - Montclair Performance Health & Chiropractic, LLC, Montclair, NJ, USA.

References
1. Maslach C, Florian V. Burnout, job setting, and self-evaluation amoung rehabilitation counselors. Rehabil Psychol. 1988;33:85–93.
2. Schaufeli WB. Past performance and future perspectives of burnout research. SA J Ind Psychol. 2003;29(4):1–15.
3. Shanafelt TD, Boone S, Tan L, Dyrbye LN, Sotile W, Satele D, et al. Burnout and satisfaction with work-life balance among US Physicians Relative to the General US Population. Arch Intern Med. 2012;20:1–9.
4. Demerouti E, Bakker AB, Nachreiner F, Schaufeli WB. The job demands-resources model of burnout. J Appl Psychol. 2001;86(3):499–512.
5. Spector PE, Jex SM. Development of four self-report measures of job stressors and strain: interpersonal conflict at work scale, organizational constraints scale, quantitative workload inventory, and physical symptoms inventory. J Occup Health Psychol. 1998;3(4):356–67.
6. Gountas S, Gountas J. How the 'warped' relationships between nurses' emotions, attitudes, social support and perceived organizational conditions impact customer orientation. J Adv Nurs. 2015. doi:10.1111/jan.12833.
7. Seo JH, Kim HJ, Kim BJ, Lee SJ, Bae HO. Educational and relational stressors associated with burnout in Korean medical students. Psychiatry Investig. 2015;12(4):451–8.
8. Tijdink JK, Vergouwen AC, Smulders YM. Emotional exhaustion and burnout among medical professors; a nationwide survey. BMC Med Educ. 2014;14:183,6920-14-183.
9. Cropanzano R, Rupp DE, Byrne ZS. The relationship of emotional exhaustion to work attitudes, job performance, and organizational citizenship behaviors. J Appl Psychol. 2003;88(1):160–9.
10. Griep RH, Rotenberg L, Landsbergis P, Vasconcellos-Silva PR. Combined use of job stress models and self-rated health in nursing. Rev Saude Publica. 2011;45(1):145–52.

11. Karasek R, Brisson C, Kawakami N, Houtman I, Bongers P, Amick B. The Job Content Questionnaire (JCQ): an instrument for internationally comparative assessments of psychosocial job characteristics. J Occup Health Psychol. 1998;3(4):322–55.

12. Demerouti E. Strategies used by individuals to prevent burnout. Eur J Clin Invest. 2015;45(10):1106–12.

13. Karanikola M, Giannakopoulou M, Mpouzika M, Kaite CP, Tsiaousis GZ, Papathanassoglou ED. Dysfunctional psychological responses among Intensive Care Unit nurses: a systematic review of the literature. Rev Esc Enferm USP. 2015;49(5):847–57.

14. Singh P, Aulak DS, Mangat SS, Aulak MS. Systematic review: factors contributing to burnout in dentistry. Occup Med (Lond). 2016;66(1):27-31. doi:10.1093/occmed/kqv119.

15. Vijendren A, Yung M, Sanchez J. Occupational health issues amongst UK doctors: a literature review. Occup Med (Lond). 2015;65(7):519–28.

16. McManus IC, Winder BC, Gordon D. The causal links between stress and burnout in a longitudinal study of UK doctors. Lancet. 2002;359:2089–90.

17. Maslach C, Jackson SE. The measurement of experienced burnout. J Occup Behav. 1981;2(2):99–113.

18. Williams SP, Zipp GP. Prevalence and associated risk factors of burnout among US doctors of chiropractic. J Manipulative Physiol Ther. 2014;37(3):180–9.

19. Williams S, Pinto-Zipp G, Cahill T, Parasher RK. Prevalence of burnout among doctors of chiropractic in the northeastern United States. J Manip Physiol Ther. 2013;36(6):376–84.

20. Schonfeld IS, Mazzola JJ. A qualitative study of stress in individuals self-employed in solo businesses. J Occup Health Psychol. 2015;20(4):501–13.

21. Ruotsalainen JH, Verbeek JH, Marine A, Serra C. Preventing occupational stress in healthcare workers. Cochrane Database Syst Rev. 2014;11: CD002892.

22. Adib-Hajbaghery M, Khamechian M, Alavi NM. Nurses' perception of occupational stress and its influencing factors: a qualitative study. Iran J Nurs Midwifery Res. 2012;17(5):352–9.

23. Dickinson T, Wright KM. Stress and burnout in forensic mental health nursing: a literature review. Br J Nurs. 2008;17(2):82–7.

24. Chiropractic Research [Internet].; 2013 []. Available from: http://www.mpamedia.com/. Accessed Sep 2015.

25. Zhang Y, Wildemuth BM. Qualitative analysis of content. In: Wildemuth B, editor. Applications of Social Research Methods to Questions in Information and Library Science. Westport: Libraries Unlimited; 2008. p. 308–19.

26. Thorne S. Data analaysis in qualitative research. Evid Based Nurs. 2000;3(3):68–70.

27. Bankauskaite V, Saarelma O. Why are people dissatisfied with medical care services in Lithuania? A qualitative study using responses to open-ended questions. Int J Qual Health Care. 2003;15(1):23–9.

28. Graneheim UH, Lundman B. Qualitative content analysis in nursing research: concepts, procedures and measures to achieve trustworthiness. Nurse Educ Today. 2004;24(2):105–12.

29. Christensen MG, Kollasch MW, Hyland JK. Practic of chiropractic: a project report, survey analysis, and summary of the practice of chiropractic within the United States. Greeley: National Board of Chiropractic Examiners; 2010.

30. Licensure Statistics - U.S. [Internet].; 2012 []. Available from: http://www.fclb.org/. Accessed Sep 2015.

31. Cortese CG, Colombo L, Ghislieri C. Determinants of nurses' job satisfaction: the role of work-family conflict, job demand, emotional charge and social support. J Nurs Manag. 2010;18(1):35–43.

32. Chang M. The chiropractic scope of practice in the United States: a cross-sectional survey. J Manipulative Physiol Ther. 2014;37(6):363–76.

33. Copper R, McKee HJ. Chiropractic in the United States: trends and issues. Milbank Q. 2003;81(1):107–38.

34. DeVocht JW. History and overview of theories and methods of chiropractic: a counterpoint. Clin Orthop Relat Res. 2006;444:243–9.

35. Naumovska K, Gehl A, Friedrich P, Puschell K. Suicide among physicians–a current analysis for the City of Hamburg. Arch Kriminol. 2014;234(5–6):145–53.

36. Hatton C, Emerson E, Rivers M, Mason H, Mason L, Swarbrick R, et al. Factors associated with staff stress and work satisfaction in services for people with intellectual disability. J Intellect Disabil Res. 1999;43(Pt 4):253–67.

37. Smyth E, Healy O, Lydon S. An analysis of stress, burnout, and work commitment among disability support staff in the UK. Res Dev Disabil. 2015;47:297–305.

38. Graziano WG, Jensen-Campbell LA, Hair EC. Perceiving interpersonal conflict and reacting to it: the case for agreeableness. J Pers Soc Psychol. 1996;70(4):820–35.

39. Murphy DR, Schneider MJ, Seaman DR, Perle SM, Nelson CF. How can chiropractic become a respected mainstream profession? The example of podiatry. Chiropr Osteopat. 2008;16:10.

40. Establishing chiropractic cultural authority: Part one – setting the groundwork [Internet].; 2010 []. Available from: http://www.chiroweb.com/mpacms/dc_ca/article.php?id=52211&no_paginate=true&p_friendly=true&no_b=true. Accessed Sep 2015.

22

The simulated early learning of cervical spine manipulation technique utilising mannequins

Peter D Chapman[1], Norman J Stomski[2], Barrett Losco[3] and Bruce F Walker[3*]

Abstract

Background: Trivial pain or minor soreness commonly follows neck manipulation and has been estimated at one in three treatments. In addition, rare catastrophic events can occur. Some of these incidents have been ascribed to poor technique where the neck is rotated too far. The aims of this study were to design an instrument to measure competency of neck manipulation in beginning students when using a simulation mannequin, and then examine the suitability of using a simulation mannequin to teach the early psychomotor skills for neck chiropractic manipulative therapy.

Methods: We developed an initial set of questionnaire items and then used an expert panel to assess an instrument for neck manipulation competency among chiropractic students. The study sample comprised all 41 fourth year 2014 chiropractic students at Murdoch University. Students were randomly allocated into either a usual learning or mannequin group. All participants crossed over to undertake the alternative learning method after four weeks. A chi-square test was used to examine differences between groups in the proportion of students achieving an overall pass mark at baseline, four weeks, and eight weeks.

Results: This study was conducted between January and March 2014. We successfully developed an instrument of measurement to assess neck manipulation competency in chiropractic students. We then randomised 41 participants to first undertake either "usual learning" (n = 19) or "mannequin learning" (n = 22) for early neck manipulation training. There were no significant differences between groups in the overall pass rate at baseline ($x^2 = 0.10$, $p = 0.75$), four weeks ($x^2 = 0.40$, $p = 0.53$), and eight weeks ($x^2 = 0.07$, $p = 0.79$).

Conclusions: This study demonstrates that the use of a mannequin does not affect the manipulation competency grades of early learning students at short term follow up. Our findings have potentially important safety implications as the results indicate that students could initially gain competence in neck manipulation by using mannequins before proceeding to perform neck manipulation on each other.

Keywords: Chiropractic, Education, Neck manipulation, Randomised trial, Mannequin, Simulated learning

Background

Neck manipulation is a commonly used manual therapy for pain and stiffness and is likely to have been practised for centuries [1]. In more modern times it has become even more popular as a technique used by chiropractors and others; however it has been a source of controversy as to its risk/benefit ratio [2, 3]. Complications associated with neck manipulation have been estimated at a rate of one in three treatments but these adverse events are usually negligible causing minor soreness [4]. However, rare catastrophic events can occur. Over the past 30 years there has been a growing awareness of complications arising from the use of neck manipulation, in particular, stroke has become a prominent and worrying concern for practitioners of manual therapy and patients [5–10]. This adverse event may result in permanent impairment or more rarely death. Estimates of vertebral artery stroke (VAS) incidence following neck manipulation are likely to be between 1 in 400,000 cervical manipulations [11] and 1 in 100,000 patients receiving cervical spinal manipulative therapy (SMT) [5].

Some of these serious incidents have been ascribed to poor manipulative technique where the neck is excessively

* Correspondence: bruce.walker@murdoch.edu.au
[3]Discipline of Chiropractic, School of Health Professions, Murdoch University, 90 South St, Murdoch 6150, WA, Australia
Full list of author information is available at the end of the article

rotated. In a University setting where inexperienced students are learning manipulation it may be logical to speculate that these un-skilled operators may deliver a technique that contributes towards a greater complication risk.

The current method of teaching students the psychomotor skills of manipulation is to have students practice on each other. This is problematic for several reasons; a) the necessary skills (speed and accuracy) are not yet present in the student; b) a force that is not fully controlled is being put through the joints of fellow students and c) joints that do not need manipulation are being manipulated. In total this may lead to over stretching of the joint tissues with resulting soreness. To become proficient at the skill of neck manipulation a great amount of practice is needed and to obtain mastery a student has to practice many repetitive movements [12]. This usually means that over the course of an undergraduate chiropractic program the students may perform hundreds of manipulations on each other, with consequent increases in the risk of adverse reactions of varying severities. We found no evidence that stroke has occurred during neck manipulation training however it is intuitive that adverse events are more likely during this first phase of skills training. For example an epidemiological survey of chiropractic students enrolled in the chiropractic program offered at Parker College of Chiropractic in Dallas, Texas, USA revealed that 25 % (143/572) of respondents reported an injury as a result of manipulation being performed on them by other students during their studies [13]. These results are lower than those reported by an earlier study where 55 % of study participants experienced an injury as a result of learning to perform spinal manipulation [14].

Ndetan et al. (2009) reported that the most frequently injured region of the body as a result of students receiving spinal manipulation as part of their training was the neck and shoulder region [13]. However, Macanuel et al. (2005) differ slightly and suggest that this region is the second most commonly injured region, with the lumbopelvic region being the most commonly injured region, amongst chiropractic students when learning to perform spinal manipulative therapy [14].

It has been suggested that chiropractic students may be exposed to injuries to the cervical spine as a result of receiving "amateurish adjustments" or manipulations that deliver a substantial rotatory effect upon the cervical spine from other students [13].

It is therefore important in the early phases of training to search for innovative methods such as simulation to assist chiropractic students achieve a level of mastery of the manipulation techniques but with a low risk of adverse events. To this end we hypothesise that it may be useful to have students reach a level of proficiency by practicing on a mannequin with a flexible neck that approximates the resistance of a human cervical spine. To date very little research has been published on cervical manipulation mannequins and whether they assist the student with skill mastery or the effect upon student safety.

The teaching of spinal manipulative techniques at Murdoch University is consistent with that described by Harvey et al. [15]. Students are first introduced to the theoretical aspects of spinal manipulation by attending didactic lectures in areas such as anatomy, biomechanics and spinal manipulative technique, they then combine this knowledge with the subjective assessment of observing an instructor/expert perform spinal manipulative techniques. The students then progress to copy the demonstrated movements, which usually involves one student acting as a simulated patient while another student attempts to replicate the instructor's execution of the technique. This includes correct hand positions, patient pre-positioning, as well as the direction and magnitude of force required to perform the manipulative technique. Instructors then provide qualitative verbal feedback.

The aims of this study were first to design an instrument to measure competency of neck manipulation technique, and then to use this instrument to measure the suitability of using a simulation mannequin to teach the necessary psychomotor skills for chiropractic manipulative therapy of the neck.

Methods

Questionnaire development

We developed an initial set of questionnaire items in consultation with Murdoch staff members who taught cervical manipulation technique. An expert panel was then formed, who used a Content Validity Index (CVI) to ensure that the questionnaire was relevant to assess neck manipulation competency among chiropractic students [16, 17]. The expert panel consisted of seven chiropractors who teach neck manipulation at several Australian universities and one international university. The composition and size of this expert panel was congruent with guidelines that propose that the panel members' professional backgrounds reflect that of the target population, and that the ideal number is between six to twelve members [16, 17]. Every panel member evaluated each item using four categories: not relevant, unable to assess relevance without major revision, relevant but needs minor alteration, and very relevant. A value of one was assigned to the "very relevant" and "relevant but needs minor alteration" categories, whereas a value of zero was assigned to the other categories. The I-CVI for each item was derived by summing the values for each rater and then dividing by the number of raters. Items were retained if the CVI exceeded 0.79 [16, 17]. After the initial expert panel evaluation and feedback, the pilot version of the questionnaire was expanded considerably in the domains of rating expertise. In the second round of evaluation, the I-CVI for individual items ranged from 0.86-1.0 and all items were retained. The S-CVI, which is the proportion of items rated as either "relevant but needs minor alteration" or "very relevant" by all raters, was 0.94.

The final questionnaire comprised five assessment criteria, of which three contained several sub-criteria. The five assessment criteria were:

1) Patient and practitioner positioning
   • Is the patient positioned correctly?
   • Is the headrest in the correct position?
   • Is the practitioner positioned correctly?
2) Joint pre-tension
   • Has the joint been placed into the pre-manipulative tension position correctly?
3) Contact points
   • Is the contact point on the patient correct?
   • Has the correct side of the patient been contacted?
   • Is the contact on the practitioner's hand correct?
   • Is the practitioner's indifferent/stabilising hand correctly positioned?
4) Vector of correction/line of drive
   • Is the vector of correction correctly aligned with the presentation of the facet joints at the level manipulated?
5) Procedure
   • Is the amplitude of the thrust applied sufficient to address the fixation?
   • Is the speed of the thrust applied sufficient to address the fixation?
   • Was the demonstrated manipulation/adjustment executed safely?

Sample

All students enrolled in the fourth of the five year chiropractic program at Murdoch University during 2014 (N = 41) were invited to participate. Paper copy information notices were distributed in the first lecture of 2014, and a non-teaching staff member delivered an information session and provided an opportunity for students to raise questions about the study to inform the consent process. Students were informed that participation was entirely voluntary, and electing to participate or not participate, would not affect their relationship with University staff in any way. The Murdoch University Human Research Ethics Committee approval number was 2013/200. All 41 students initially invited to participate provided consent to have their results included in the final analysis.

Randomisation and blinding procedure

A staff member, not involved with group allocation, used a random number generator to generate a randomisation list. The group assignment was placed in sequentially numbered, opaque, sealed envelopes. After obtaining informed consent, staff not assessing neck manipulation competency opened the envelope and allocated students to one of two groups: usual learning or mannequin learning. Staff assessing neck manipulation competency, and undertaking data entry and analysis were blinded to group allocation.

Due to the nature of the study it was not possible to blind students to their group allocation, however at all times the assessor remained unaware of the group randomisation. Students are aware that under Australian Law, unless they are a registered practitioner with the Australian Health Professions Regulatory Authority, performing cervical spine manipulation outside of a recognised training program is prohibited [18]. Thus it is unlikely that students practised cervical spine manipulation outside of their usual teaching times.

The mannequin

The cervical mannequin is known as "Flexi-man" and is shown in Figs. 1 & 2. Fleximan has been developed and manufactured by Dr. Timothy Young, Chiropractor [19]. The mannequin consists of a flexible imitation of shoulders, neck and head made of a pliant "rubberised" material. The weight of the mannequin is 4.8 kgs with the specific head weight unknown, however a proxy head weight was 3.2 kgs. This proxy weight was established by laying the mannequin prone with the head recumbent on weight scales. The mannequin was designed to allow students to set up, place contacts and deliver a thrust in a line of drive of their choosing. It does not however allow for pre-manipulative tension. The mannequin is a stylised human facsimile and is not designed to mimic a human specimen. It does not have the variability of human subjects receiving manipulation, for example height, weight, and tissue compliance. The makers state that the mannequin is best used in the introductory phases of training [20].

Educational interventions

The usual learning group practised neck manipulation techniques on each other under supervision consistent with the description provided in the introduction to this article. This learning approach has been used since the inception of the Murdoch University chiropractic program in 2002. The mannequin learning group practiced the neck manipulation techniques on a mannequin with a flexible neck, once again under supervision. The mannequin learning approach was a novel method not previously used at Murdoch University. Each group received

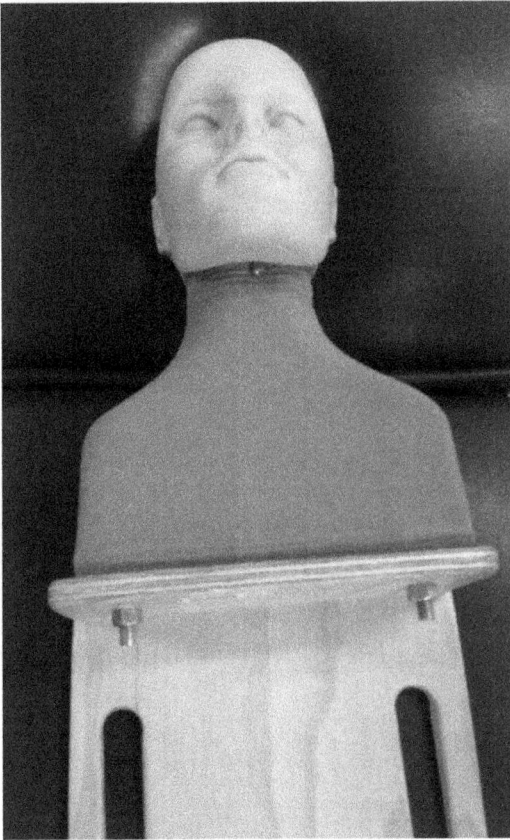

Fig. 1 The mannequin

three, two hour weekly training sessions in the performance of a commonly used cervical spine manipulation technique referred to as the index pillar push [21]. During the weekly training sessions and to ensure that the assessor remained blinded to group allocation students were supervised by academics not involved in the assessment of the students. The supervising academics provided each student with regular personalised feedback relating to their performance of the required technique during the weekly training sessions. After the third weekly training session, all members of each group crossed over and undertook three additional training sessions using the alternate method. The flow of the study is displayed in Fig. 3.

All fourth year students who participated in the study had already received training in neck manipulation in the third year of the program but there is a long summer break between third and fourth year so skills usually diminish. On the first week back at University, a staff member experienced in manipulation assessment who was blinded to group randomisation, assessed the student's performance of the index pillar push procedure at baseline on the mannequin (immediately before the first training session) and then again at four weeks, and eight weeks, by using the validated instrument of measurement.

Assessing student performance of the index pillar push technique involved the assessor requesting the student to perform the technique on both the left and the right hand side of the mannequin. Each student was allowed to perform the technique once on both sides, while the assessor graded their performance.

The maximum total score on the validated questionnaire is 100 %. In order to pass the assessment a student must achieve a minimum score of 69 % overall.

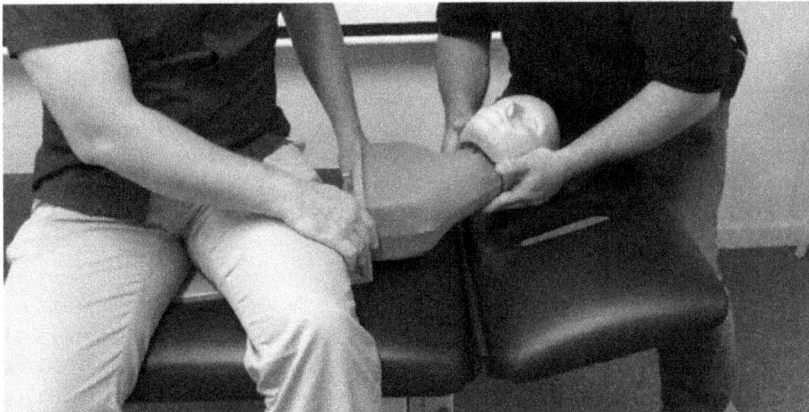

Fig. 2 Technique demonstration on the mannequin

Study Flow

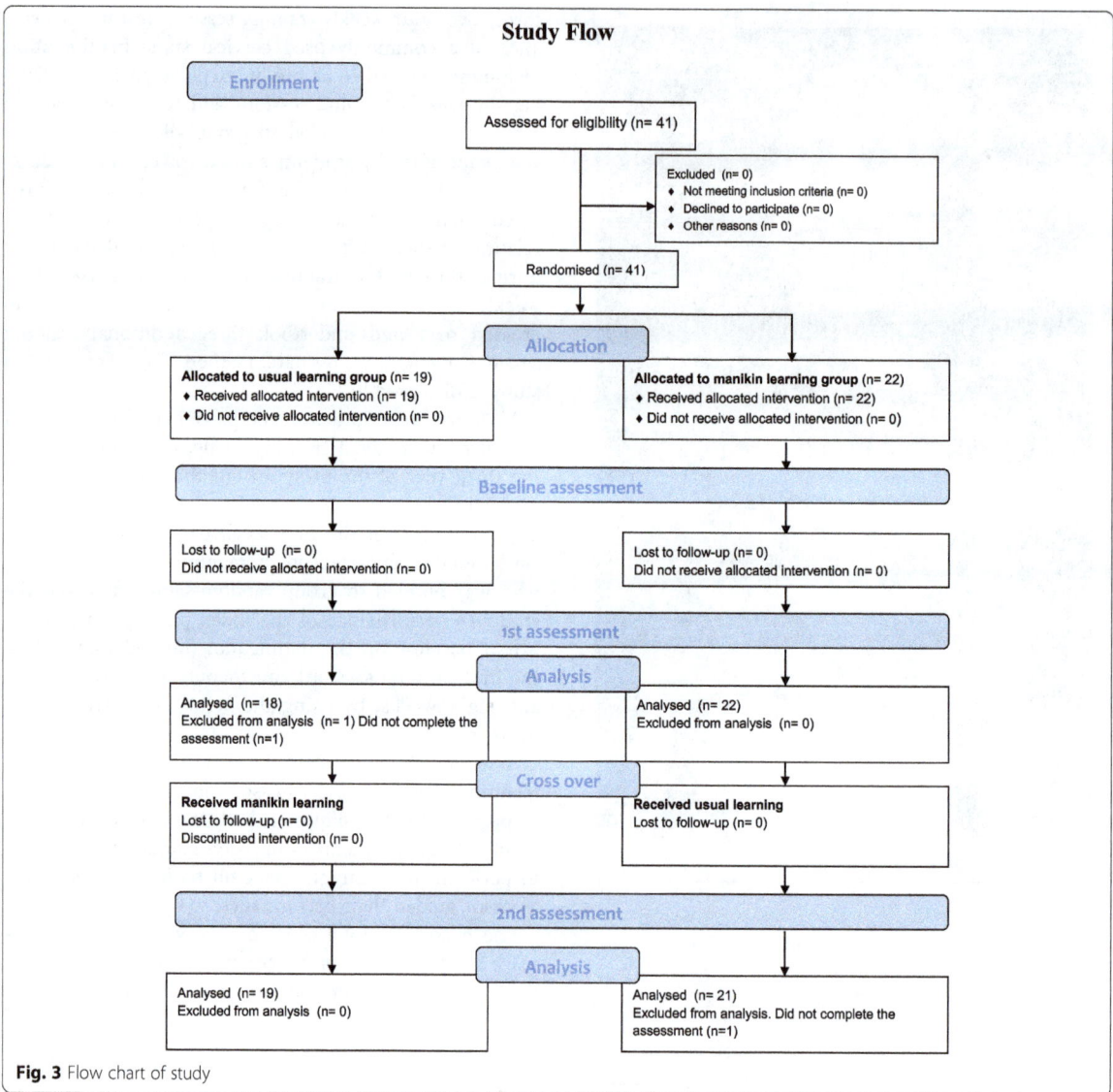

Fig. 3 Flow chart of study

Each of the five identified assessment criteria are considered critical to the successful performance of the required technique. If a student fails to perform one of these five assessment criteria adequately the student is awarded an overall score of 69 %. Should the student fail to perform two of the five assessment criteria adequately they are awarded a score of 49 %. Less than satisfactory performance of three criteria results in a score of 29 %. Inadequate performance of four assessment criteria results in a score of 19 % being awarded to the student. If all five assessment criteria are unsatisfactorily performed or the student is unable to perform the required technique, the student is awarded a score of zero.

Statistical analysis

All data were entered manually into SPSS v.21, cleaned and checked for implausibilities. A chi-square test was used to examine differences between groups for the proportion of students achieving an overall pass mark at baseline, four weeks, and eight weeks.

Results

This study was conducted between January and March 2014. We randomised 41 participants to first undertake either usual learning (n = 19) or mannequin (n = 22). The proportion of female participants was 36.8 % in the usual learning group, and 45.4 % in the mannequin group. The mean age was 23.3 (SD 4.7) years in the usual learning group, and 22.8 (SD 3.4) years in the mannequin group. All participants crossed over to undertake the alternative learning method after four weeks.

There were no significant differences between groups in the overall pass rate at baseline ($\chi^2 = 0.10$, p = 0.75), four weeks ($\chi^2 = 0.40$, p = 0.53), or at eight weeks ($\chi^2 = 0.07$, p = 0.79). The proportion of participants achieving an overall pass in each group at each time point is displayed in Table 1. There were no reported adverse events in the students' group from the therapy administered.

Discussion

Our findings show that mannequins can be used to teach cervical neck manipulation technique without affecting the grades for neck manipulation competency of chiropractic students. This result was consistent with a previous study examining the use of mannequins in teaching cervical manipulation [22]. These findings have important implications for the delivery of chiropractic curricula because the use of mannequins reduces the number of manipulations received by fellow students, which thereby improves the safety of chiropractic training.

In a previous study, differences in learning outcomes were examined by comparing students who undertook either practitioner-positioning training or complete practice training [15]. The practitioner-positioning approach involved students learning the components of spinal manipulation without ever delivering the thrust component. The complete practice approach incorporated the thrust component under instructor supervision and with proprioceptive feedback. This study was administered soon after students' commenced training in the first year of a Master's degree program at Macquarie University in Sydney, New South Wales, Australia which is the equivalent to the 4th year of Murdoch University's program. The study reported that the complete practice approach resulted in significantly higher peak force, and significantly lower time to peak force, both of which are thought to demonstrate higher proficiency in performing spinal manipulation [15]. So, although including the thrust component early in training may enhance the acquisition of manipulation competency, it could also potentially increase the likelihood of students experiencing

adverse events. Therefore, by introducing the mannequin into the early stages of students' training, students could experience enhanced learning outcomes without any risk of decreased competency or adverse events.

Several studies have suggested that quantitative assessment of spinal manipulation is superior to qualitative assessment for the acquisition of psychomotor skills [23–25]. Traditionally, students were provided qualitative spinal manipulation feedback by instructors who evaluated parameters such as thrust vector, preload force, amplitude, velocity, and body position. Indeed, these parameters comprised the assessment criteria we derived for the instrument used in this study. Qualitative assessment may be prone to feedback inconsistency due to instructor experience, differing opinions between instructors, and observational oversights, which all may impede the acquisition of psychomotor skills. However, these inconsistencies can be addressed by the use of quantitative feedback devices that measure peak force or force time histories [25–27]. Quantitative feedback has an immediate positive impact upon all parameters relating to the performance of lumbar spine manipulation including subjective patient ratings of task performance [28], and has been shown to be superior to qualitative feedback [29]. Timely quantitative feedback allows the student to make rapid changes to their performance of the required technique [28]. Given this, we recommend that as a next step further research examine how apparatus capable of producing quantitative feedback could be most effectively incorporated with the use of cervical mannequins.

A strength of this study was the use of an expert panel to evaluate the content validity of the neck manipulation competency questionnaire. This resulted in the development of a questionnaire that is appropriate to assess the skills of chiropractic students learning neck manipulation. However, we did not assess the test-retest reliability of the questionnaire, and its reliability should be further determined in other studies. Another limitation of this study was not evaluating intra-rater examiner reliability, so the extent to which this may have influenced the findings remains unclear. Finally, we used a convenience sample so the study may have been underpowered however the results for a reasonable class size allowed us to conclude equivalence between the methods of teaching.

Table 1 Overall pass rate for cervical manipulation

	Number of participants achieving overall pass at baseline	Number of participants achieving overall pass at four weeks	Number of participants achieving overall pass at eight weeks
Participants first undertaking usual learning (n = 19)	22.2 % (4/18)	44.4 % (8/18)	84.2 % (16/19)
Participants first undertaking mannequin training (n = 22)	18.2 % (4/22)	54.5 % (12/22)	81.0 % (17/21)

Conclusions

This study consolidates previous research concerning the use of mannequins to teach neck manipulation skills and confirms that the use of mannequins does not affect the manipulation competency grades of students. Our findings have potentially important safety implications as the results indicate that students could initially gain competence in neck spinal manipulation by using mannequins before proceeding to perform neck manipulation on each other, which is likely to lessen the risk of students experiencing adverse events.

Competing interests

The corresponding author (Walker) is the Editor-in-Chief of *Chiropractic & Manual Therapies*. Walker was blinded to all reviewers' identities and did not select the managing Associate Editor. No other authors had competing interests to declare.

Authors' contributions

PC was responsible for the concept development, design, data collection, literature search, writing of the article and the critical review. NS was responsible for design, literature search, data analysis, writing of the article and the critical review. BL was responsible for design, data collection, writing of the article and the critical review. BW was responsible for design, supervision, writing of the article and the critical review. All authors read and approved the final manuscript.

Authors' information

PC is in private practice but was a lecturer in clinical chiropractic at Murdoch University who taught chiropractic manipulative techniques.
BL is a senior lecturer in clinical chiropractic at Murdoch University and teaches chiropractic manipulative techniques.
NS is a senior health research officer in the School of Health Professions at Murdoch University.
BW is Head of Discipline for Chiropractic at Murdoch University.

Acknowledgments

This study was funded by a grant from the Clinical Simulation Support Unit, Health Department, Government of Western Australia.

Author details

[1]6 Claredon Court, Alexander Heights 6064, WA, Australia. [2]School of Health Professions, Murdoch University, 90 South St, Murdoch 6150, WA, Australia. [3]Discipline of Chiropractic, School of Health Professions, Murdoch University, 90 South St, Murdoch 6150, WA, Australia.

References

1. Burke GL. Backache: From Occiput to Coccyx. Richmond, Canada: Macdonald Publishing; 2008.
2. Gross A, Miller J, D'Sylva J, Burnie SJ, Goldsmith CH, Graham N, et al. Manipulation or mobilisation for neck pain: a Cochrane Review. Man Ther. 2010;15(4):315–33.
3. Hebert JJ, Stomski NJ, French SD, Rubinstein SM: Serious Adverse Events and Spinal Manipulative Therapy of the Low Back Region: A Systematic Review of Cases. *J Manipulative Physiol Ther* 2013.
4. Hurwitz EL, Morgenstern H, Harber P, Kominski GF, Yu F, Adams AH. A randomized trial of chiropractic manipulation and mobilization for patients with neck pain: clinical outcomes from the UCLA neck-pain study. Am J Public Health. 2002;92(10):1634–41.
5. Rothwell DM, Bondy SJ, Williams JI. Chiropractic manipulation and stroke: a population-based case-control study. Stroke. 2001;32(5):1054–60.
6. Smith WS, Johnston SC, Skalabrin EJ, Weaver M, Azari P, Albers GW, et al. Spinal manipulative therapy is an independent risk factor for vertebral artery dissection. Neurology. 2003;60(9):1424–8.
7. Dittrich R, Rohsbach D, Heidbreder A, Heuschmann P, Nassenstein I, Bachmann R, et al. Mild mechanical traumas are possible risk factors for cervical artery dissection. Cerebrovasc Dis. 2007;23(4):275–81.
8. Walker BF, Losco B, Clarke BR, Hebert J, French S, Stomski NJ. Outcomes of usual chiropractic, harm & efficacy, the ouch study: study protocol for a randomized controlled trial. Trials. 2011;12:235.
9. Cassidy JD, Boyle E, Cote P, He Y, Hogg-Johnson S, Silver FL, et al. Risk of vertebrobasilar stroke and chiropractic care: results of a population-based case-control and case-crossover study. Spine (Phila Pa 1976). 2008;33(4 Suppl):S176–183.
10. Walker BF, Hebert JJ, Stomski NJ, Clarke BR, Bowden RS, Losco B, French SD: Outcomes of usual chiropractic. The OUCH randomized controlled trial of adverse events. *Spine (Phila Pa 1976)* 2013, 38(20):1723-1729.
11. Klougart N, Leboeuf-Yde C, Rasmussen LR. Safety in chiropractic practice, Part I; The occurrence of cerebrovascular accidents after manipulation to the neck in Denmark from 1978-1988. J Manipulative Physiol Ther. 1996;19(6):371–7.
12. Kovacs G. Procedural skills in medicine: linking theory to practice. J Emerg Med. 1997;15(3):387–91.
13. Ndetan HT, Rupert RL, Bae S, Singh KP. Prevalence of musculoskeletal injuries sustained by students while attending a chiropractic college. J Manipulative Physiol Ther. 2009;32(2):140–8.
14. Macanuel K, Deconinck A, Sloma M, Ledoux M, Gleberzon BJ. Characterization of side effects sustained by chiropractic students during their undergraduate training in technique class at a chiropractic college: a preliminary retrospective study. J Can Chiropr Assoc. 2005;49(1):46–55.
15. Harvey MP, Wynd S, Richardson L, Dugas C, Descarreaux M. Learning spinal manipulation: a comparison of two teaching models. J Chiropr Educ. 2011;25(2):125–31.
16. Lynn MR. Determination and quantification of content validity. Nurs Res. 1986;35(6):382–5.
17. Polit DF, Beck CT. The content validity index: are you sure you know what's being reported? Critique and recommendations. Res Nurs Health. 2006;29(5):489–97.
18. Anon: Health Practitioner Regulation National Law (WA) Act 2010. URL: http://www.slp.wa.gov.au/legislation/statutes.nsf/main_mrtitle_12107_homepage.html
19. Young T: FLEXI-MAN. Cervical Manikin Version 4. Pacific Paradise, Queensland.: T&S Young; 2003.
20. Young T: Flexi-Man. Practice makes perfect. Pacific Paradise, Queensland.: T&S Young; 2003.
21. Bergmann T, Peterson D. Chiropractic Technique: Principles and Procedures. Missouri: Elsevier; 2011.
22. Young TJ, Hayek R, Philipson SA. A cervical manikin procedure for chiropractic skills development. J Manipulative Physiol Ther. 1998;21(4):241–5.
23. Triano JJ, Rogers CM, Combs S, Potts D, Sorrels K. Quantitative feedback versus standard training for cervical and thoracic manipulation. J Manipulative Physiol Ther. 2003;26(3):131–8.
24. Descarreaux M, Dugas C, Lalanne K, Vincelette M, Normand MC. Learning spinal manipulation: the importance of augmented feedback relating to various kinetic parameters. Spine J. 2006;6(2):138–45.
25. Descarreaux M, Dugas C. Learning spinal manipulation skills: assessment of biomechanical parameters in a 5-year longitudinal study. J Manipulative Physiol Ther. 2010;33(3):226–30.
26. Scaringe JG, Chen D, Ross D. The effects of augmented sensory feedback precision on the acquisition and retention of a simulated chiropractic task. J Manipulative Physiol Ther. 2002;25(1):34–41.
27. Rogers CM, Triano JJ. Biomechanical measure validation for spinal manipulation in clinical settings. J Manipulative Physiol Ther. 2003;26(9):539–48.
28. Triano JJ, Scaringe J, Bougie J, Rogers C. Effects of visual feedback on manipulation performance and patient ratings. J Manipulative Physiol Ther. 2006;29(5):378–85.
29. Downie AS, Vemulpad S, Bull PW. Quantifying the high-velocity, low-amplitude spinal manipulative thrust: a systematic review. J Manipulative Physiol Ther. 2010;33(7):542–53.

23

Spinal myxopapillary ependymoma in an adult male presenting with recurrent acute low back pain: a case report

Dean Petersen[1] and Reidar P. Lystad[2*] (iD)

Abstract

Background: Spinal intramedullary ependymomas are very rare and occur more commonly in the cervical and upper thoracic regions. These neoplasms tend to manifest in young adulthood, and patients typically present with mild clinical symptoms without objective evidence of neurologic deficits. The mean duration of symptoms is 40 months until the lesion is diagnosed.

Case Presentation: A 48-year-old male police officer was referred to a chiropractic clinic by a general practitioner for the evaluation of recurrent acute low back pain (LBP). Although the first episode of LBP was resolved, the clinical examination during the second episode revealed subtle changes that warranted referral to magnetic resonance imaging (MRI). The MRI revealed a spinal myxopapillary ependymoma.

Conclusion: Because the primary symptoms of spinal intramedullary ependymomas can mimic ordinary LBP presentations, in particular lumbar intervertebral disc herniations, clinicians need to be sensitive to subtle changes in the clinical presentation of LBP patients. Prompt referral to advanced medical imaging such as MRI and early neurosurgical intervention is key to achieve best possible outcomes for patients with spinal intramedullary ependymomas.

Keywords: Myxopapillary ependymoma, Spinal cord, Filum terminale, Neoplasm, Chiropractic

Background

Primary intraspinal neoplasms are rare, with an age-adjusted incidence rate of 0.5 in females and 0.3 in males per 100,000 population per annum [1]. Ependymoma is the most common intramedullary spinal neoplasm in adults, accounting for up to 60 % of all glial spinal cord tumors [2]. Spinal ependymomas occur most commonly in the cervical and upper thoracic regions, and only 6.5 % involve either the distal thoracic cord or the conus medullaris [2, 3]. Myxopapillary ependymoma, a benign special variant of ependymoma that is thought to arise from ependymocytes of the filum terminale, constitutes approximately 13 % of all spinal ependymomas in this region [4].

Spinal myxopapillary ependymomas tend to manifest in adulthood (mean age, 35 years) and is more commonly seen in male patients [2]. Patients typically present with mild clinical symptoms without objective evidence of neurologic deficits, which often results in a delay in diagnosis (mean duration of symptoms is 37 to 42 months) [2, 5]. At the time of diagnosis, patients typically have back or neck pain (67 %), sensory deficits (52 %), motor weakness (46 %), or bowel or bladder dysfunction (15 %) [2, 3]. Importantly, patients with a shorter duration of symptoms and less preoperative neurologic deficit tend to have better postoperative outcomes [2, 3].

Thus it becomes vital to promptly recognise important clues in the clinical presentation and evaluation that will lead to early diagnosis. Here we describe a rare case of an adult male with spinal myxopapillary ependymoma presenting as recurrent acute low back pain with subtle neurologic symptoms. The clinical presentation, chiropractic examination and management, imaging manifestations, and subsequent neurosurgical intervention and outcome are discussed below.

* Correspondence: reidar.lystad@mq.edu.au
[2]Department of Chiropractic, Macquarie University, Sydney, Australia
Full list of author information is available at the end of the article

Case presentation

Clinical history

A 48-year-old male police officer was referred to a chiropractic clinic by a general practitioner for the evaluation of acute low back pain (LBP) of two weeks duration. The patient reported that the LBP had come on after spending a 12-h night shift driving a patrol car. The LBP was described as diffuse and the patient reported sharp pain radiating down the left lateral thigh to the knee. The average pain intensity was rated as 6/10 on a visual analogue scale (VAS), but had progressed to 8/10 VAS at the time of presentation. The symptoms were aggravated by sitting, sleeping on the left side, and inactivity; while standing provided the most relief. The pain was worse in the morning, and improved only marginally during the day. Self-care with heat packs and over-the-counter non-steroidal anti-inflammatory drugs (6 × 200 mg ibuprofen tablets per day) provided only a 2-point reduction on the VAS. The patient denied the presence of any paraesthesia (e.g. pins or needles), saddle anaesthesia, loss or changes in bladder or bowel control, fever, or nocturnal pain. The patient reported an approximately 20 kg reduction in body weight over the past 10 months, which he attributed to dietary changes and uptake of a substantial exercise regimen.

The patient also complained of left-sided headaches in the suboccipital and temporal regions of three weeks duration. The headaches were accompanied by occasional dizziness (clarified to be a feeling of unease) that were aggravated by sustained awkward neck postures. He had a family history of hypertension, type 2 diabetes, and migraines. His grandmother had passed away from bowel cancer. The patient was currently being treated for haemochromotosis, for which he had been managed successfully for 8 years. The rest of the systems review was unremarkable.

Physical examination

The physical examination revealed a marked antalgic posture to the right with limited active lumbar range of motion (ROM) in left lateral flexion and flexion (finger-to-floor reach was noted to be 2 cm above the knees). Coughing, sneezing, and Valsalva manoeuvre reproduced the LBP, but not the leg pain. Straight leg raise was positive for leg and back pain at 40° on the left and negative at 70° on the right. Bragard's test was positive on the left, while slump test and well leg raise were negative. Deep tendon reflexes were normal (2+) in both upper and lower limbs, except for the patella reflex on the left which was slightly diminished (1+). There was no decreased sensation to pin prick or vibration sense in either the upper or lower limbs; however, sensation to light touch was slightly decreased in the left L4 dermatome. Motor and cranial nerve exams were unremarkable. Blood pressure was 152/92 mmHg and the resting heart rate was 75 bpm (measured in the sitting position).

The left temporal headache and dizziness (uneasiness) could be reproduced by combined flexion and 25° of rotation of the head to the right. The same manoeuvre on the contralateral side was pain free at 50° of rotation. There was marked tenderness to palpation over the left C2/3 zygapophysial joint and the lumbar spinous processes.

On the basis of the clinical presentation, history, and findings of the physical examination, a working diagnosis of posterolateral L3/4 intervertebral disc herniation affecting the left L4 nerve root was made, and a trial of conservative management was suggested to the patient. The patient also received a concurrent working diagnosis of cervicogenic headache. In addition, the patient was recommended to seek further evaluation of his blood pressure.

Case management and outcome

Conservative management consisted of cryotherapy (ice packs), high-velocity, low-amplitude spinal manipulation to the lumbar region, isometric stretching, and neurodynamic mobilisation techniques (neural flossing). This passive care was complemented by ergonomic advice and a prescribed back extension exercise program. The patient received a total of 6 treatments over a 4-week period. After this treatment regimen the patient reported the LBP to be 1-2/10 VAS, with no pain radiating down the left leg, and that he was able to perform all activities of daily living. Neurodynamic tension tests (e.g. straight leg raise and Bragard's test) were negative. Lumbar spine ROM was improved (finger-to-floor reach 34 cm below the knees during flexion) and pain free.

The patient was discharged with a 4-week core muscle strengthening program and asked to return for a follow-up consultation after its completion, or earlier if symptoms returned. The patient returned asymptomatic after 4 weeks, and was able to satisfactorily perform the functional core strength tests.

Second presentation

Two months after the last follow-up of the first episode of LBP, the patient presented to the chiropractic clinic with a new episode of acute LBP with pain radiating down the left leg. Similar to the first episode, the patient reported that the LBP had come on after an 8-h shift of driving a patrol car. However, this time the leg pain was radiating down the anterior aspect of the left thigh to the knee. He was taking prescription pain killers as directed by his general practitioner (1–2 tablets of 5 mg oxycodone [Endone, Aspen Pharamceuticals] per 6 h). However, the medication provided minimal relief and the pain was unrelenting, worse at night, and interfering with his sleep. Bladder and bowel function was normal. The physical examination mirrored the initial presentation but for two findings: (1) light touch was decreased in the left L3 and L4 dermatomes, and (2) slump test produced left anterior thigh pain radiating down to the left knee and lateral leg to the foot.

Because the patient now presented with indications of the possible involvement of multiple lumbar nerve roots, severe pain waking him up at night, and not responding to strong prescription pain medication, he was referred for magnetic resonance imaging (MRI) for an evaluation of possible compression of neurological structures at the L2 to L4 vertebral levels.

Imaging
The MRI revealed a substantial heterogeneous space-occupying lesion with an intramedullary orientation within the filum terminale at the L2/3 vertebral level (see Fig. 1). The lesion measured approximately 2.5 cm × 1.2 cm in the craniocaudal and anterior-posterior dimensions, respectively. It appeared predominantly cystic on T2-weighted sequences and contained several fine internal septations. On post-contrast imaging, there was a heterogeneous enhancement of the lesion (predominantly peripheral), with a non-enhancing central aspect indicating a possible haemorrhagic or calcific component. The remainder of the spinal cord and conus medullaris appeared normal. Because the observed lesion most likely represented a myxoapapillary ependymoma, the patient was promptly referred for a neurosurgical consultation.

Surgical intervention and outcome
The patient was scheduled for surgery the day after the neurosurgical consultation. A gross total resection was achieved and radiological adjunctive therapy was not pursued. Although the patient reported resolution of the neurological symptoms immediately after the surgery, low-grade LBP (3/10 VAS), described as a dull ache, still persisted for several weeks post-surgery. The patient received standard, post-surgical rehabilitation with a hospital-based physiotherapist for 6 months post-surgery. In long-term follow-ups at 6 and 12 months post-surgery, the patient reported no pain (0/10 VAS), with only a vague sensation of persistent numbness in the left anterior leg.

Discussion
The present case highlights a number of important points: (1) the primary symptoms of intramedullary ependymomas of the caudal spinal cord can mimic ordinary LBP presentations, in particular lumbar intervertebral disc herniations; (2) clinicians need to be sensitive to subtle changes in the clinical presentation of LBP patients; and (3) prompt referral to advanced medical imaging such as MRI and early surgical intervention is key to achieve best

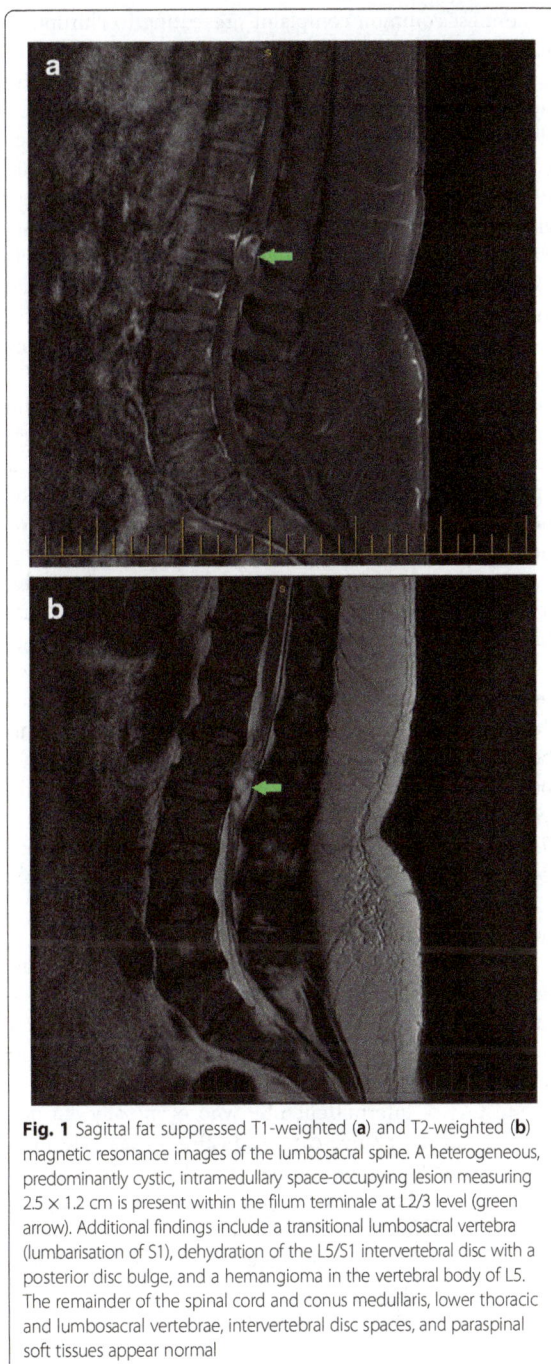

Fig. 1 Sagittal fat suppressed T1-weighted (**a**) and T2-weighted (**b**) magnetic resonance images of the lumbosacral spine. A heterogeneous, predominantly cystic, intramedullary space-occupying lesion measuring 2.5 × 1.2 cm is present within the filum terminale at L2/3 level (green arrow). Additional findings include a transitional lumbosacral vertebra (lumbarisation of S1), dehydration of the L5/S1 intervertebral disc with a posterior disc bulge, and a hemangioma in the vertebral body of L5. The remainder of the spinal cord and conus medullaris, lower thoracic and lumbosacral vertebrae, intervertebral disc spaces, and paraspinal soft tissues appear normal

possible outcomes for patients like the one described in the present case.

LBP is a very common health problem, and one of the leading causes of activity limitation and work absence worldwide [6, 7]. It is not surprising, therefore, that LBP is the most common complaint presenting to chiropractic clinics [8]. Although specific structural pathologies (e.g., intervertebral disk herniation or spinal stenosis) can be identified in a subset of patients presenting with LBP, the majority of cases (approximately 85 %) are referred to as nonspecific LBP [6, 9]. In the present case, the patient presented with typical LBP symptomatology with clinical findings indicative of a possible posterolateral L3/4 intervertebral disk herniation affecting the left L4 nerve root. Current evidence-based clinical practice guidelines recommend against the routine use of imaging in patients presenting with LBP [10, 11]. The patient was therefore offered conservative treatment consisting of a combination of passive and active care, to which he responded very well and was subsequently discharged.

At first glance the second episode appeared to be a typical recurrence of the first episode of LBP, with both the precipitating event and the clinical presentation of the second episode being very similar to the former. Furthermore, successful conservative management of the first episode could potentially lead to confirmation bias, that is, clinicians are likely to believe their working diagnoses are correct when their patients respond satisfactorily to care [12]. In the present case, however, a careful physical examination revealed subtle changes indicating the possible involvement of multiple lumbar spinal nerve roots. Moreover, the patient was not responding to strong prescription pain medication and the LBP would occasionally wake him up at night. Taken together, these were compelling reasons to suspect the presence of space-occupying pathologies such as spinal cord tumours and the patient was therefore referred to medical imaging.

It is difficult to estimate how often patients with an undiagnosed spinal ependymoma present to chiropractors with LBP because only a couple of cases have been reported in the literature to date. Lensgraf and Young described two cases: (1) a 46-year-old woman with 3–4 year history of intermittent LBP who eventually did not respond to conservative care; and (2) a 38-year-old man who presented with an unusual episode of LBP with leg pain [13]. In both cases the patient underwent surgical resection and was reported to be doing well at 12 months post-surgery [13]. Only the female patient received adjuvant radiation therapy [13].

In most jurisdictions, chiropractors can request advanced diagnostic imaging such as MRI. However, full government rebates for such referrals are only available in a few jurisdictions (e.g. Norway and Denmark). In Australia (the location of the present case), patients referred to MRI by chiropractors are not eligible for a Medicare rebate. Although the patient in the present case was both willing and able to pay for the MRI, this may of course not be true for all, or even the majority of, patients. It is, therefore, conceivable that such restrictions on advanced medical

imaging referrals can contribute to delayed diagnosis of some patients.

Early detection and treatment is key to achieve best possible patient outcomes for people with spinal intramedullary ependymoma. These neoplasms are best treated surgically and a complete resection indicates complete resolution for the vast majority of patients [14, 15]. Adjuvant radiation therapy is usually reserved for cases where only subtotal resection is possible, while chemotherapy is used more sparingly, for instance in young children who are more prone to negative side effects from radiation therapy [16]. Surgery should be performed early because patients with a shorter duration of symptoms and less preoperative neurologic deficit tend to have better postoperative outcomes [2, 3, 13, 15]. Although the mean duration of symptoms in patients with spinal ependymoma is more than 3 years [2, 5], the patient in the present case was diagnosed and referred for neurosurgical consultation within 6 months of onset of initial symptoms.

Conclusions

The primary symptoms of spinal intramedullary ependymomas can mimic ordinary LBP, in particular lumbar intervertebral disc herniations. Clinicians need to be sensitive to subtle changes in the clinical presentation of LBP patients. Prompt referral to advanced medical imaging such as MRI and early surgical intervention is key to achieve best possible outcomes for patients with spinal intramedullary ependymomas.

Ethics and consent

This study was approved by the Human Research Ethics Committee at Central Queensland University (ethics approval reference number: H15/08–194). Written informed consent was obtained from the patient for publication of this case report and any accompanying images. A copy of the written consent is available for review by the Editor-in-Chief of this journal.

Competing interests
The authors declare that they have no competing interests.

Authors' contributions
DP contributed to drafting the case presentation and discussion sections, and general editing of the manuscript. RPL contributed to the literature review, drafting the background and discussion sections, and general editing of the manuscript. All authors read and approved the final manuscript.

Author details
[1]Private practice, Mackay, QLD, Australia. [2]Department of Chiropractic, Macquarie University, Sydney, Australia.

References
1.   Helseth A, Mørk SJ. Primary intraspinal neoplasms in Norway, 1955–1986, a population-based survey of 467 patients. J Neurosurg. 1989;71:842–5.

2. Ferrante L, Mastronardi L, Celli P, Lunardi P, Acqui M, Fortuna A. Intramedullary spinal cord ependymomas: a study of 45 cases with long-term follow-up. Acta Neurochir. 1992;119:74–9.

3. Hoshimaru M, Koyama T, Hashimoto N, Kikuchi H. Results of microsurgical treatment for intramedullary spinal cord ependymomas: analysis of 36 cases. Neurosurgery. 1999;44:264–9.

4. Koeller KK, Rosenblum RS, Morrison AL. Neoplasms of the spinal cord and filum terminale: radiologic-pathologic correlation. Radiographics. 2000;20:1721–49.

5. Kucia EJ, Bambakidis NC, Chang SW, Spetzler RF. Surgical technique and outcomes in the treatment of spinal cord ependymomas, part 1: intramedullary ependymomas. Neurosurgery. 2011;68:57–63.

6. Hoy D, Brooks P, Blyth F, Buchbinder R. The Epidemiology of low back pain. Best Pract Res Clin Rheumatol. 2010;24:769–81.

7. Manchikanti L, Singh V, Falco FJ, Benyamin RM, Hirsch JA. Epidemiology of low back pain in adults. Neuromodulation. 2014;17 Suppl 2:3–10.

8. Lishchyna N, Mior S. Demographic and clinical characteristics of new patients presenting to a community teaching clinic. J Chiropr Educ. 2012;26:161–8.

9. da C Menezes Costa L, Maher CG, Hancock MJ, McAuley JH, Herbert RD, Costa LO. The prognosis of acute and persistent low-back pain: a meta-analysis. CMAJ. 2012;184:E613–24.

10. Koes BW, van Tulder M, Lin CW, Macedo LG, McAuley J, Maher C. An updated overview of clinical guidelines for the management of non-specific low back pain in primary care. Eur Spine J. 2010;19(12):2075–94.

11. Dagenais S, Tricco AC, Haldeman S. Synthesis of recommendations for the assessment and management of low back pain from recent clinical practice guidelines. Spine J. 2010;10(6):514–29.

12. Croskerry P. The importance of cognitive errors in diagnosis and strategies to minimize them. Acad Med. 2003;78(8):775–80.

13. Lensgraf AG, Young KJ. Ependymoma of the spinal cord presenting in a chiropractic practice: 2 case studies. J Manipulative Physiol Ther. 2006;29:676–81.

14. Klekamp J. Spinal ependymomas. Part 1: Intramedullary ependymomas. Neurosurg Focus. 2015;39(2):E6.

15. Tobin MK, Geraghty JR, Engelhard HH, Linninger AA, Mehta AI. Intramedullary spinal cord tumors: a review of current and future treatment strategies. Neurosurg Focus. 2015;39(2):E14.

16. Straus D, Tan LA, Takagi I, O'Toole JE. Disseminated spinal myxopapillary ependymoma in an adult at initial presentation: a case report and review of the literature. Br J Neurosurg. 2014;28(5):691–3.

24

Acute thoracolumbar pain due to cholecystitis: a case study

Chris T. Carter

Abstract

Background: This article describes and discusses the case of an adult female with cholecystitis characterized on initial presentation as acute thoracolumbar pain.

Case Presentation: A 34-year-old female presented for care with a complaint of acute right sided lower thoracic and upper lumbar pain with associated significant hyperalgesia and muscular hypertonicity. The patient was examined, referred, and later diagnosed by use of ultrasound imaging.

Conclusion: Despite many initial physical examination findings of musculoskeletal dysfunction, this case demonstrates the significance of visceral referred pain, viscerosomatic hyperalgesia & hypertonicity, and how these neurological processes can mimic mechanical pain syndromes. A clinical neurological discussion of cholecystitis visceral pain and referred viscerosomatic phenomena is included.

Background

Chiropractors are trained as primary contact providers and well positioned to provide initial assessment, diagnosis and treatment for patients with spinal pain in addition to assisting in referral to other practitioners [1]. The presentation of back pain is common to chiropractors and differentiating acute musculoskeletal (somatic) from visceral pain presentation may be difficult as they can present with a similar clinical pain picture. These challenging clinical presentations can lead to inappropriate and delayed patient care, serving as a reminder of the importance of performing a thorough history and physical examination.

Visceral pathology as a presenting complaint to chiropractors is generally considered rare, however a survey of American chiropractors indicated that 5.3 % of primary complaint presentations are non-musculoskeletal in origin [2]. It is estimated that up to 15 % of the American population have gallstones, 10-18 % of whom will develop biliary pain, and 7 % of which will require operative intervention [3]. With over 700,000 cholecystectomies performed annually in America, gallbladder disease is considered the most costly digestive disorder [3].

Although the majority of those with cholelithiasis will not develop acute cholecystitis, 1-3 % inevitably will. The transition of acute cholecystitis leading to a secondary bacterial infection of the gallbladder may occur in up to

50 % of cases. This increases the chance of complications such as the formation of an empyema, perforation, widespread peritonitis, sepsis and abdominal abscesses [4, 5]. Earlier intervention of acute cholecystitis has been increasingly recognized in a recent meta-analysis study that demonstrated performing early laparoscopic cholecystectomy (within 1–7 days of symptom onset) decreased incidence of complications including wound infections, provided shorter length of hospital stay and decreased costs versus delayed cholecystectomy. No difference in rates of mortality were noted. The authors advocated that early laparoscopic cholecystectomy is now considered best care and should be considered a routine in patients presenting with acute cholecystitis [6].

The statistics above provide evidence why early detection of acute cholecystitis by a primary contact practitioner may reduce risk of complications and help reduce costs. Unfortunately, there is no single clinical symptom or sign that carries sufficient weight to establish or exclude cholecystitis without right upper quadrant ultrasound testing [7]. Traditional cholecystitis symptoms (right upper quadrant pain, nausea, and emesis) and signs (Murphy, right upper quadrant tenderness and fever) have poor positive and negative likelihood ratios [7]. Further research into combining presenting signs and symptoms is needed as currently the use of clinical gestalt continues to be considered the most appropriate initial clinical management prior to obtaining more valid blood and imaging diagnostic tests [7].

Correspondence: c_carter88@hotmail.com
School of Health Professions, Murdoch University, 90 South Street, Murdoch, WA 6150, Australia

When back pain is the predominant or only clinical symptom of acute cholecystitis presentation, this may present a challenge to the practitioner. Firstly, being aware that cholecystitis visceral and referred pain can be perceived by patients in a variety of anatomical areas is important [8]. Pain may be perceived in such areas as the epigastrium, right hypogastrium, and lower areas of the right thoracic spine and posterior ribs [3, 9]. Pain perceived in the epigastrium and right hypogastrium may be true visceral pain, however pain felt in the back is referred viscerosomatic pain [8].

Distinguishing spine pain from somatic or visceral origin initially relies on a thorough history and physical examination. Pain of visceral origin tends to be characterised as sharp, cramping or achy, and is diffuse, poorly localized and perceived deep inside the body [9]. It usually starts insidiously, not relieved by rest or sleep, and may improve temporarily with short-term activity [10]. The physical examination for assessing cholecystitis will not only include checking for fever, abdominal tenderness and presence of Murphy sign, but should be aimed at using physical body movements and orthopaedic provocative tests to see if the back pain can be reproduced, worsened or relieved . This may help distinguish between visceral (no significant change with movement) and somatic back pain. Somatic pain is typically worsened or relieved with particularly range of motion movements or with provocative testing that stretch and/or compress somatic tissue [11].

The presence of somatic tissue hyperalgesia and muscle hypertonicity is a known common finding in somatic mechanical disorders of the spine [12]. However, cholecystitis referred pain to somatic structures also commonly presents with hyperalgesia and muscle hypertonicity in the somatic referred area [13]. This can make a more difficult differentiation between somatic and visceral pain during the physical examination as the patients back pain can theoretically be worsened with physical movements or palpation of somatic tissue in both presentations.

A thorough history should also inquire information on patient positive risk factor(s) for cholelithiasis. This is helpful in increasing the clinician's awareness that a pain presentation may be visceral in origin, and would be considered a part of the practitioner's clinical gestalt. Cholelithiasis development is multifactorial, however common risk factors include age over twenty years, female sex, history of pregnancy, parity, obesity, and ironically any recent rapid weight loss [3].

This case study describes an adult female presenting with cholecystitis characterized by acute right sided thoracolumbar pain. It highlights the challenges faced when visceral pathology creates viscerosomatic symptoms and signs that present similar to mechanical musculoskeletal clinical presentation. Prompt referral to the

appropriate medical health care provider is necessary to limit possible patient health complications and may improve management. A detailed clinical neurological discussion of cholecystitis visceral and referred pain, as well as the neurological phenomena of viscerosomatic hyperalgesia and muscular hypertonicity is included to assist the clinician in understanding how visceral pathology can mimic mechanical musculoskeletal syndromes.

Case presentation
Clinical history and examination
A 34 year-old female presented with two days of insidious onset right sided lower thoracic and upper lumbar pain. The pain was constant, worse with movement, and particularly increased with deep inspiration and laughing. No abdominal or limb pain, paraesthesia or numbness was noted. Her numerical rating scale (NRS) was 6/10, and she mentioned the pain felt slightly different yet no more severe than several previous episodes of lower lumbar pain. Characteristically, her pain was achy and deep, with no associated symptoms of nausea, malaise, fever, bloating, emesis, dysuria or haematuria. It was no worse or better around meals or alcohol intake. The patient was not in distress however appeared slightly more anxious as usually her back pain was not so constant.

The patient had presented several times over the preceding two years for chiropractic care for episodes of mechanical lower lumbar, neck, right hip and left shoulder pain. Her prior chiropractic treatments had consisted of spinal manipulation, mobilisation, myofascial release, rehabilitation and education. The patient's musculoskeletal complaints usually recovered successfully with conservative management. Static mechanical allodynia had been consistently noted axially and peripherally over the previous two years, however no other symptoms or signs indicating fibromyalgia diagnosis were noted. In fact, the patient's allodynia had been improving steadily in congruence with her increase in exercise over the preceding couple of years.

The youngest of her three children was two years old, and she had been increasing her frequency, duration and intensity of exercise over the preceding 1.5 years with regular jogging, boot-camp, and crossfit classes. Her increased exercise had resulted in reduction of weight from 92 kg to 85 kg, as well as a significant gain in strength and sense of well-being. Initial fear-avoidance behaviour to exercise post-partum due to chronic right hip pain of gluteal medius tendinopathy origin had taken several months to improve, and included education and graded progression of exercise.

Medical health history was significant for left sided Erb's palsy at parturition, and resection of 85 % of her pancreas at age five weeks due to intractable neonatal hypoglycemia. She had gestational diabetes during all three pregnancies and had current type 2 diabetes. No current medications were being consumed. Family history was unknown.

Physical examination revealed unremarkable lumbar neurological examination and lumbar nerve root stress tests. Active lumbar and thoracic range of motion caused increased right-sided back pain in all ranges along the T8-L2 segments in the area of the erector spinae muscles. Active and passive right lumbar lateral flexion and right lumbar Kemp's test particularly worsened her back pain. Using the Modified Ashworth Scale for grading hypertonia, this patient had Grade 2 muscle hypertonicity noted with palpation of the right sided lower thoracic and upper lumbar erector spinae and psoas muscles in contrast to Grade 0 on the left side. Palpation underneath the right costal margin elicited only mild tenderness without sharp pain or inspiratory arrest (i.e., negative Murphy sign).

Diagnosis and management
There were obvious signs of musculoskeletal involvement to her acute thoracolumbar back pain. However, due to the new, more constant pain presentation and positive cholecystitis risk factors in this patient that included pain location, female sex, age over twenty, parity (3 children), patient habitus, and significant weight-loss over the prior year, there was high suspicion of acute cholecystitis. Initial presentation was a weekend day and she was recommended and referred by letter to see her general practitioner on the following Monday for clinical opinion. She was also recommended to go to the hospital immediately if her pain worsened, began to affect the abdominopelvic region, or if she felt unwell. The patient consented to a trial treatment of myofascial release and spinal manipulation in hope that her symptoms and signs may just be of mechanical origin and some pain relief may be achieved. The patient felt slightly better immediately post treatment however interestingly pre- and post-treatment muscle hypertonicity was palpably unchanged.

Three days post initial presentation she had a diagnostic ultrasound which revealed clinical signs of acute cholecystitis including focal tenderness over the gallbladder, a 25 mm non-mobile stone at the body/fundal region, a moderate amount of sludge extending towards the gallbladder neck, slight thickening of the gallbladder wall, and no evidence of pericholecystic fluid. Phone discussion with the patient the day of the ultrasound revealed that she had recently developed right hypogastric pain which was severe post ingestion of fatty foods. Additionally, her back pain had increased in intensity to a NRS of 8/10.

She was diagnosed with acute cholecystitis by her General Practitioner, was prescribed antibiotics and

paracetamol and referred to a specialist. Within a week of medication introduction and restriction of high fatty meal intake, her back and abdominal pain had significantly decreased to a NRS of 1/10. Fifty-three days after initial presentation she had a successful laparoscopic cholecystectomy with no complications. Monthly follow-up over the next six months with this patient post-surgery revealed no current back or abdominal pain in the previously affected thoracolumbar area. She returned to exercise two month's post-surgery.

In this case, delayed cholecystectomy was decided by her specialist. Therefore, early referral to her general practitioner likely did not affect her temporal surgical outcome. However, early referral assisted in early diagnosis via ultrasound which may have reduced secondary bacterial complications and improved patient comfortability as she was prescribed antibiotics and paracetamol.

Discussion
Visceral pain of gallbladder origin
The majority of acute cholecystitis cases are due to the presence of cholelithiasis [5, 14]. The production of gallstones and sludge at or near the neck of the gallbladder can cause obstruction of bile into the cystic duct, causing a number of pathophysiological nociception contributors that result in the production of visceral pain [5]. Once obstructed, the continued production of gallbladder mucus has no outlet for drainage and causes distension of the gallbladder wall and ducts [15]. The subsequent increased peristalsis causing strong and sustained smooth muscle contraction results in increased intraluminal pressure. This activation of gallbladder nociceptors by distension can occur in the absence of visceral inflammation and may present clinically as episodic biliary colic [14, 16].

Biliary system nociception has two distinct types of peptidergic bare nerve-ending afferent sensory fibres that respond to noxious stimulation located in the mucosa, muscle and serosa [17, 18]. Two-thirds of these fibres have low-thresholds to biliary pressure and encode stimuli in both the innocuous and noxious range in addition to transmitting information related to autonomic phenomena. One-third respond only to high-threshold biliary stimuli in the noxious range and are functionally similar to cutaneous nociceptors [15, 19].

Initial painful contraction of the gallbladder appears to involve high-threshold receptors, whereas ischemia-induced hypoxic and inflammatory tissue environments that damage the mucosa peripherally sensitize both high and low threshold as well as visceral silent nociceptors [4, 19, 20]. Gallbladder nociceptors also release substance P and vasoactive intestinal peptide to induce a neurogenic inflammatory environment which appears to be a prominent contributor to cholecystitis development

[21]. Prostaglandins, in addition to their peripheral sensitization effects, also increase afferent nociceptive signalling by stimulating wall contraction and secretion of lumen fluid resulting in wall thickening, pericholecystic oedema, and peritonitis [4] Interestingly, the severity of visceral pathology is not well correlated with the severity of pain perceived, which attributes attention to unknown peripheral mechanisms as well as the role of spinal and higher brain centre mechanisms of pain perception [22].

Nociceptor afferents from the gallbladder are carried anatomically via vagal and splanchnic nerves, however the majority of nociception travels through the latter with their central terminations in dorsal and ventral horns of the spinal cord extending from T5 to L2 [11, 15, 22]. Therefore, the anatomical area of visceral pain perceived in acute cholecystitis significantly varies depending on which spinal segment second order neurons are stimulated over such a broad spinal cord distribution.

Visceral pain is characterised as sharp, cramping or achy, although tends to be diffuse, poorly localized and perceived deep inside [9]. This is due to the relative paucity of peripheral afferent nociceptor terminals in the viscera, central terminal arborisation, distinct absence of a separate visceral sensory pathway, and overall low proportion of visceral afferent nociceptors compared with those of somatic origin [19, 22]. The reality that such a low number of arriving visceral afferent signals can result in such a profound pain with possible additional autonomic phenomena (for example malaise and nausea) is likely due to the extensive arborisation and resultant functional divergence seen in the cord as well as the stimulation of so many cord levels at once [23].

Visceral nociceptor central terminals synapse with second-order neurons in lamina I, II, V, and X of the spinal cord [22]. Visceral nociception then projects to higher centres via several routes that lead to perceived pain as well as autonomic phenomena commonly associated with visceral pain. Stimulation of the spinomesencephalic, spinoreticular, and spinohypothalamic tracts mainly activate unconscious and/or automatic responses to visceral sensory input including alterations in behaviour and emotion [17]. The major pain perception pathways are the contralateral spinothalamic tract and more recently understood ipsilateral dorsal fasciculus that both project via nuclei of the thalamus to higher brain centres such as the somatosensory, anterior cingulate, prefrontal and insular cortices [17, 18]. The unique addition of strong emotional, behavioural and autonomic features commonly associated with heterogenous visceral pain presentation is likely due to the widespread distribution of afferent pathways to areas beyond those required for localisation alone [17]. Pre-existing affective and cognitive dysfunction may also play a role in acute visceral pain perception.

Gallbladder referred pain

Referred pain is commonly perceived in cholecystitis and can be an important clinical diagnostic measure [24]. The occurrence of referred pain is best explained by the convergence-projection model which postulates that the majority of dorsal horn second-order neurons that receive afferent nociceptive input from viscera also happen to receive input from somatic structures that share the same neuromeric field [13, 24]. In cholecystitis, referred pain to the back is explained by the dual synapsing of gallbladder afferents on the same viscerosomatic second-order neurons in the spinal cord that also receive innervation from somatic afferents coming from the right lower thoracic spine and ribs [16]. The convergence-projection model also involves overlapping visceral and somatic nociception signalling to similar higher brain centres involved in the perception of pain, however the brain likely attributes the origin of the sensation to the somatic domain because of pneumonic traces of previously experienced somatic pain [22].

Hyperalgesia and muscular hypertonicity

Cholecystitis referred pain to somatic structures commonly presents with hyperalgesia and muscle hypertonicity in the somatic referred area [13]. This hyperalgesia is likely due to 'convergence-facilitation' which is caused by neuroplastic central sensitization changes in the central nervous system due to the massive barrage of visceral afferent impulses from an algogenic inflamed and mechanically irritated gallbladder [13, 25]. Acute cholecystitis and biliary calculosis has been shown to cause mechanical and thermal hyperalgesia in superficial structures such as the subcutaneous tissue and skin, as well as efferent sympathetically induced trophic changes [24]. This can present as a diagnostic challenge when assessing patients such as this female who had shown previous long-term signs of static mechanical allodynia. Central sensitization hyperalgesic mechanisms may be involved in continual pain post cholecystectomy, however clinically this uncommonly occurs if adequate treatment is not delayed [26].

Muscle hypertonicity is a common finding in many mechanical musculoskeletal disorders. However, strong evidence exists for reflex efferent induced muscle contraction as a cause of the hyperalgesia seen in referred visceral pain syndromes [25]. Muscle contraction is commonly seen clinically in patients with acute visceral pain, and has been histologically shown in rats to involve significant microscopic changes in muscle fibre phenotype [27]. Referred pain to somatic structures is likely to involve not just central changes but also peripheral changes such as altered neurotransmitters and sensory terminals in the affected somatic tissue that affect tissue contractility [25].

Modulation of visceral pain

No discussion in pain presentation is complete without briefly mentioning the complex modulation that occurs in an individual's pain perception and the subsequent variable pain presentations that can ensue even in the acute patient. Similar to somatic pain, modulation of true and referred visceral pain occurs at both the spinal cord and the brain [25]. For example, in between biliary colic episodes, the nature of decreased perceived pain may be due to increased spinal cord neuron thresholds due to transient inhibition of transmission to higher centres [17]. Depending on the nature of the visceral stimulus, descending pathways from supraspinal structures can inhibit or facilitate spinal viscerosomatic neurons in both the dorsal and ventral horn [23].

The emotional state of individuals also appears to have a significant modulatory influence on visceral pain [17]. The final conscious and subconscious psychological processing and therefore perception of visceral pain in the higher pain matrix centres shares similarities but differs from that of somatic pain processing [23]. Visceral nociception likely plays a significant role in acute visceral pain perception, however the psychological influences of cognitions, mood and social setting are also likely to play an important role in pain perception and should never be under-appreciated.

Conclusion

Relatively uncommon in daily chiropractic practice, gallbladder pathology mimicking mechanical musculoskeletal back pain does occur and clinicians should be aware of its presentation due to it being one of the most frequent medically encountered gastrointestinal presentations. Similar clinical symptoms and signs may arise due to the anatomical areas of pain involved as well as the neurophysiological mechanisms of viscerosomatic hyperalgesia and muscular hypertonicity that commonly occur with biliary pain presentations. Timely differentiation of clinical pain is helpful in undertaking prompt referral to assist the patient in receiving appropriate medical care which may reduce complications and include advantageous early cholecystectomy.

Consent

Written informed consent was obtained from the patient for publication of this case report. A copy of the written consent is available for review by the Editor-in-Chief of this journal.

Competing interests
The author declares that there are no competing interests.

Author's contributions
CC cared for the patient, performed the literature review, and prepared the manuscript. The author read and reviewed the final manuscript.

References

1. Department of Health, Western Australia. Spinal Pain Model of Care. Perth: Health Networks Branch, Department of Health, Western Australia; 2009.
2. Christensen M, Kollasch M, Ward R, Webb K: Practice Analysis of Chiropractic 2010. Colorado. National Board of Chiropractic Examiners 2010, 95-120.
3. Knab L, Boller A-M, Mahvi D. Cholecystitis. Surg Clin N Am. 2014;94:455–70.
4. Elwood D. Cholecystitis. Surg Clin N Am. 2008;88:1241–52.
5. Strasberg S. Acute calculous cholecystitis. N Engl J Med. 2008;358:2804–11.
6. Cao A, Eslick G, Cox M. Early cholecystectomy is superior to delayed cholecystectomy for acute cholecystitis: a meta-analysis. J Gastrointest Surg. 2015;19:848–57.
7. Trowbridge R, Rutkowski N, Shojania K. Does this patient have acute cholecystitis? J Am Med Assoc. 2003;289(1):80–6.
8. Berhane T, Vetrhus M, Hausken T, Olafsson S, Sondenaa, K: Pain attacks in non-complicated and complicated gallstone disease have a characteristic pattern and are accompanied by dyspepsia in most patients: the results of a prospective study. Scand J Gastroenterol 2006;41:93–101.
9. Johnson C. Upper abdominal pain: Gall bladder. BMJ. 2001;323(7322):1170–3.
10. Mennell J. Differential diagnosis of visceral from somatic back pain. J Occup Med. 1966;8(9):477–80.
11. Rinkus K, Knaub M. Clinical and diagnostic evaluation of low back pain. Semin Spine Surg. 2008;20:93–101.
12. Walker BF, Williamson OD. Mechanical or inflammatory low back pain. What are the potential signs and symptoms. Man Ther. 2009;14:314–20.
13. Giamberardino M, Affaitati G, Lerza R, De Laurentis S. Neurophysiological basis of visceral pain. J Musculoskelet Pain 2002, 10(1/2):151-163.
14. Hennig R, Osman T, Berhane T, Vetrhus M, Sondenaa K, et al. Association between gallstone-evoked pain, inflammation and proliferation of nerves in the gallbladder: A possible explanation for clinical differences. Scand J Gastroenterol 2007, 42:878-884.
15. Cervero F. Sensory innervation of the viscera: Peripheral basis of visceral pain. Physiol Rev. 1994;74(1):95–129.
16. Sethi H, Johnson C. Gallstones. Medicine. 2011;39(10):624–9.
17. Knowles C, Aziz Q. Basic and clinical aspects of gastrointestinal pain. Pain. 2009;141:191–209.
18. Foreman R. Mechanisms of visceral pain: from nociception to targets. Drug Discov Today Dis Mech. 2004;1(4):457–63.
19. Cervero F, Laird J. Visceral pain. Lancet. 1999;353:2145–8.
20. Gebhart G. Pathobiology of visceral pain: Molecular mechanisms and therapeutic implications IV. Visceral afferent contributions to the pathobiology of visceral pain. Am J Physiol Gastrointest Liver Physiol. 2000;278:G834–8.
21. Prystowsky J, Rege R. Neurogenic inflammation in cholecystitis. Dig Dis Sci. 1997;42(7):1489–94.
22. Al-Chaer E, Traub R. Biological basis of visceral pain: recent developments. Pain. 2002;96:221–5.
23. Cervero F. Mechanisms of acute visceral pain. Br Med Bull. 1991;47(3):549–60.
24. Gerwin R. Myofascial and visceral pain syndromes: Visceral-somatic pain representations. J Musculoskelet Pain. 2002;10:165–75.
25. Giamberardino M, Affaitati G, Constantini R. Visceral referred pain. J Musculoskelet Pain. 2010;18(4):403–10.
26. Stawowy M, Bluhme C, Arendt-Nielsen L, Drewes A, Funch-Jensen P. Somatosensory changes in the referred pain area in patients with acute cholecystitis before and after treatment with laparoscopic or open cholecystectomy. Scand J Gastroenterol. 2004;10:990–3.
27. Aloisi A, Ceccarelli I, Affaitati G, Lerza R, Vecchiet L, Larenna D, et al: C-Fos expression in the spinal cord of female rats with artificial ureteric calculosis. Neurosci Lett 2004, 361:212-215.

Match injuries in amateur Rugby Union: a prospective cohort study - FICS Biennial Symposium Second Prize Research Award

Michael S. Swain[1,2*], Reidar P. Lystad[3], Nicholas Henschke[1,4], Christopher G. Maher[1] and Steven J. Kamper[1]

Abstract

Background: The majority of Rugby Union (rugby) players participate at the amateur level. Knowledge of player characteristics and injury risks is predominantly ascertained from studies on professional or junior athletes in rugby. The objectives of the current study are to: (1) describe the health-related quality of life (HRQoL) and physical characteristics of a cohort of amateur rugby players; (2) describe the incidence, severity and mechanism of match injuries in amateur rugby, and; (3) explore factors associated with rates of match injury in this population.

Methods: Participants ($n = 125$) from one amateur men's rugby club were followed in a one-season (2012) prospective cohort study. Match injury and match time exposure data were collected. A participant match exposure log was maintained. Baseline variables collected include: participant's age, playing experience, position of play, the SF-36v2 health survey, height and weight. Injury incidence rates (IIRs) per 1000 match-hours exposure were calculated. Injury sub-groups were compared by calculating rate ratios of two IIRs. Poisson mixed-effects generalised linear modelling was used to explore relationships between IIRs and baseline predictors.

Results: A total of 129 injuries occurred during a combined period of 2465 match-hours of exposure. The overall IIR was 52.3 (43.7–62.2) /1000 match-hours exposure. Moderate-severe injuries (>1 week time-loss from play) comprised 36 % of all injuries. Tackling was the most common mechanism of injury, the head/face was the most common body region of injury and sprain/ligament injuries were the most common injury type. Fewer years of rugby participation, lower BMI and lower SF-36v2 mental component summary score were associated with higher IIR in amateur rugby. Age, player position i.e., backs versus forwards and SF-36v2 physical component summary score were not associated with injury incidence.

Conclusion: Amateur rugby players report similar HRQoL as the general population. We found amateur players had a higher rate of injury and lower injury severity than previous amateur studies, but location, type, and mechanism were similar. In this study pre-season HRQoL and BMI were weakly associated with higher injury rate when controlling for other factors; a finding that should be interpreted with caution and clarified with future research.

Keywords: Sports, Football, Rugby Union, Athletic injuries, Epidemiology

* Correspondence: mswain@georgeinstitute.org.au
[1]The George Institute for Global Health, Sydney Medical School, University of Sydney, GPO Box 5389, Sydney, NSW 2001, Australia
[2]Department of Chiropractic, Faculty of Science and Engineering, Macquarie University, Sydney, Australia
Full list of author information is available at the end of the article

Background

Rugby Union (rugby) is a contact sport that is popular worldwide. Well known health benefits of sport and physical activity include improved cardiorespiratory and muscular fitness, bone health [1, 2] and reduced risk of non-communicable diseases such as obesity and depression [3]. Vigorous-intensity physical activity can further challenge aerobic fitness and muscle strength which is thought to provide additional improvements to health and wellbeing [4]. Rugby has been promoted in at least one public health campaign [5]. The stated benefits of rugby were not limited to physical health, but also included team participation, social interaction, communication skills and self-discipline.

The health benefits of sport participation should be weighed against inherent risks, which mostly exist as sport-related musculoskeletal injury. The risk of incurring an injury in rugby appears to be higher than in many other sports but comparable with other contact sports [6, 7] such as wrestling. Lee et al., [8] found approximately 10 % of participants stopped playing rugby completely as a result of injury. More than one-third of players report temporary or significant effects on education, employment, family life, or health and general fitness. For example, restriction or cessation of sporting activity, and continuing pain or stiffness [8]. Hence, the majority of rugby participants that incur an injury will experience minor health-related consequences. The need to put player's welfare first along with the rare occurrence of catastrophic injuries (e.g., spinal cord injury) [9] necessitates a greater understanding of both player's health and injury risks.

Factors that are thought to increase the risk of incurring a match injury in rugby include: increasing age [10] and more senior grade of play [11], high strenuous physical activity per week [10] and higher pre-season training attendance [12], playing while injured [10, 12], carrying an injury from the previous season [11, 12], and foul-play [10]. These reported increases in risk are typically small and are inconsistent between studies. While there has been some exploration on the influence of rugby injuries on players' subsequent health and lifestyle in amateur rugby, it is currently unclear whether health and wellbeing plays a role in the aetiology of sports injuries in amateur athletes. The New Zealand Rugby Injury and Performance Project undertaken by Quarrie et al., evaluated self-reported health status (response options: very good, good, not too good) and psychological wellbeing (measured using the General Health Questionnaire) as risk factors for injury in rugby. They found rugby players who reported negative health and psychological wellbeing did not differ significantly in the rate of injury compared to participants who reported positive health and wellbeing outcomes. Conversely, a large population-based study from New Zealand found a linear relationship between poorer health status and increasing injury risk, with the majority of injuries being sports-related [13].

Worldwide rugby participation continues to rise [14]. In Australia, recent statistics indicate that participation is slightly higher in junior age-groups [15] (juniors 50,000 vs. seniors 41,000) and the vast majority of rugby players participate at the amateur level [16]. Several prospective studies have investigated the epidemiology of sports injury in rugby [17, 18]; however these have largely consisted of cohorts of elite or junior athletes. There is a need to further explore health and injury in amateur rugby to better inform athletes of the potential benefits and harms as well as minimise risks associated with amateur participation.

The objectives of the current study are to: (1) describe health-related quality of life (HRQoL) and physical characteristics of a cohort of amateur rugby players; (2) describe the incidence, severity and mechanism of match injuries in amateur rugby, and; (3) explore factors associated with rates of injury in this population.

Methods

Ethics approval was received from the Ethics Review Committee (Human Research), Macquarie University, Sydney, Australia (reference number: 5201100183). Rugby players gave written consent to participate in the study. The study design was informed by the consensus statement on injury definitions and data collection procedures for studies of injuries in rugby [19].

Study population and sample

A prospective cohort study was conducted during the 2012 rugby season. Participants were recruited pre-season (March 2012) from one Australian amateur rugby club located in Sydney's northern suburbs. All participants were registered male amateur club players, aged 18 years and older.

Data collection

At recruitment, participants completed a self-reported questionnaire and underwent a physical assessment. The questionnaire gathered information regarding participant's age, playing experience, position of play and the SF-36v2 health-related quality of life survey. The physical assessment consisted of free-standing height (cm) and body mass (kg) measurements using a Seca digital column scale.

Injury was defined according to the Rugby Union consensus statement [20] as *any physical complaint, which was caused by a transfer of energy that exceeded the body's ability to maintain its structural and/or functional integrity, that was sustained by a player during a* rugby match or rugby training, irrespective of the need for medical attention or time-loss from rugby activities. In this study, only injuries that occurred during competition matches were recorded. A recurrent injury is defined as *an injury of the same type and at the same site as an index injury and which occurs after a player's return to full participation from the index injury.* Injury severity was reported as *the total number of days that have elapsed from the date of injury to the date of the player's return to full participation in team training or available for match selection* and injuries were categorised as slight (0–1 day), minimal (2–3 days), mild (4–7 days), moderate (8–28 days) and severe (>28 days). Actual time-loss was determined by conducting in-person or telephone follow-up of injured athletes. Finally, a non-fatal catastrophic injury was defined as *a brain or spinal cord injury that results in permanent (>12 months) severe functional disability.*

Match injuries were recorded by trained research assistants who were aligned with the rugby club's sports medicine personnel (a registered chiropractor). The research assistants attended all matches and tracked injured participants throughout the season.

Injury data were collected using the Injury Report Form for Rugby Union as outlined in the Rugby Union data collection consensus document [19]. Player grade was recorded at time of injury. Players were graded from 1st to 4th, with first grade players considered the highest level of play. In addition, a separate age-restricted grade; less than 21 years (Colts) was also followed. The time within the match that injury occurred was recorded as 1st quarter, 2nd quarter, 3rd quarter, 4th quarter or extra time. The position of play at the time of the injury was recorded, as was the injured body part, side of body and type of injury. The diagnosis of injury as identified by the club's sports medical personnel was coded according to the Orchard Sports Injury Classification System version 10.1 (OSICS-10.1) [21]. Details regarding whether their injury was recurrent, was caused by either overuse (repetitive strain) or single trauma and the type of contact were recorded. Details pertaining to whether the injury was a result of a violation of the laws of the game were recorded. The season for this cohort began on the 14th April and ended on the 25th August 2012, consisting of 17 rounds of competition.

Individual participant match-exposures were recorded over the course of the season. Each match typically lasted 60 min and exposure logs for each member were kept to the nearest half game, match-exposures were used to calculate the total match-hour exposure (MHE) during the 2012 season. Training exposure and training injuries were not recorded.

Data analysis

Injury incidence rates (IIRs) per 1000 h of match exposure were calculated by dividing the number of recorded injuries by the number of hours of match-play, multiplied by 1000. Player health-related quality of life (physical component summary [PCS] scores and mental component summary [MCS] scores), and physical characteristics (height, weight and BMI) were stratified by age-group and position of play, and expressed as means with standard deviations. SF-36v2 norm-based scores were calculated using gender/age-group matched Australian population data from The South Australian Health Omnibus Survey (SAHOS), 2008 [22]. PCS and MCS were calculated using Australian factor score coefficient weights [23]. In norm-based scoring, each scale is scored to have the same average (50) and the same standard deviation (10), meaning each point equals one-tenth of a standard deviation [24].

Regarding injuries, sub-groups were compared by calculating rate ratios (RR) of two IIRs. Ninety-five percent confidence intervals (95 % CIs) were calculated using standard formulae for Poisson rates [25]. The 95 % CIs for RRs were used to determine whether two rates or proportions differed significantly from one another, that is, two IIRs were deemed statistically different from one another if the 95 % CI for their RR did not include the number 1.

Poisson mixed-effects generalised linear modelling was also used to explore the multivariate relationships between IIRs and potential predictors as hypothesised a priori (age, participation years, playing position (forwards versus backs), BMI and SF-36v2 summary scores). The mixed-effects model used a random intercept for each athlete to account for the correlation induced by multiple observations of the same person. All analyses were performed using the statistical software R version 3.0.2 "(The R Foundation for Statistical Computing, Vienna, Austria).

Results

Data were collected from a cohort of 125 rugby players with a mean (SD) age of 24.3 (±4.9) years and 11.1 (±5.7) years of playing experience. Participants had mean (SD): SF-36v2 physical component score 47.2 (±9.8), SF-36v2 mental component score 50.0 (±9.3) and BMI 26.7 (±3.5). Participant characteristics as measured at baseline are listed in Table 1. The mean score of participants for each of the eight dimensions of health were generally within one standard-deviation of age-matched Australian males Fig. 1. Presented as supplementary material are the 0–100 and norm-based scores for the eight separate health domains of the SF-36v2 (Additional file 1: Tables S1 and S2).

A total of 129 injuries occurred during a combined period of 2465 match-hours of exposure. The overall IIR was 52.3 (95 % CI: 43.7–62.2) per 1000 match hours.

Table 1 Mean (SD) baseline SF-36v2 physical and mental component scores and physical characteristics

	PCS	MCS	Height (cm)	Weight (kg)	BMI
Age group					
18–24	46.2 (10.2)	49.9 (10.3)	184.4 (6.6)	87.4 (10.6)	25.8 (3.2)
25–34	49.5 (8.4)	50.3 (7.0)	181.2 (7.3)	93.5 (11.6)	28.5 (3.3)
>35	46.0 (12.8)	46.7 (8.5)	186.8 (2.4)	103.0 (15.7)	29.4 (4.0)
Position					
Forward	46.9 (10.0)	50.3 (8.4)	184.1 (7.3)	92.8 (11.3)	27.4 (3.3)
Back	47.6 (9.6)	49.5 (10.4)	182.8 (6.3)	86.0 (10.5)	25.8 (3.5)
All					
	47.2 (9.8)	50.0 (9.3)	183.5 (6.8)	89.6 (11.5)	26.7 (3.5)

PCS physical component summary score, *MCS* mental component summary, *BMI* body mass index

Table 2 Frequency distribution of injury severity as measured by time loss from play (days of absence) due to injuries and injury rate per 1000 match-hours of exposure (IIR_{MHE})

Time loss from play	N (%)	IIR_{MHE} (95 % CI)
Less than one-week		
Slight (0–1 day)	55 (42.6 %)	22.3 (16.8–29.1)
Minimal (2–3 days)	4 (3.1 %)	1.6 (0.4–4.2)
Mild (4–7 days)	23 (17.8 %)	9.3 (5.9–14.0)
Greater than one-week		
Moderate (8–28 days)	26 (20.2 %)	10.6 (6.9–15.5)
Severe (>28 days)	20 (15.5 %)	8.1 (5.0–12.5)

Excluding the severity of one injury lost to follow-up

Injuries were more frequently from trauma 46.7 (95 % CI: 38.5–56) than from overuse 5.7 (95 % CI: 3.1–9.5) The IIR for recurrent injuries was 3.2 (95 % CI: 1.4–6.9). Injury severity is presented in Table 2. The average injury severity was 9 (95 % CI: 7–12) days loss from play. Moderate and severe injuries (>1 week time-loss from play) comprised 36 % of all injuries. There were no fatal or catastrophic injuries.

The most common anatomical location of injury was the head and face (IIR 9.3 CI 5.9–14.0). Within the lower extremity, injuries at the knee were most frequent (IIR 7.3 CI 4.3–11.5); whereas the shoulder/clavicle was the most frequent injury location of upper extremity (IIR 7.3 CI 4.3–11.5). The most common injury types were ligament injuries (IIR 14.2 CI 9.9–19.7) followed by contusions (IIR 10.1 CI 6.6–15). Tackling was the most frequent mechanism of injury, followed by being tackled.

The vast majority of injuries were not a result of dangerous play. The lowest number of injuries occurred in first grade; however, the difference between grades was not statistically significant. The proportion of injuries did not vary according to the time of match. Table 3 lists the injury frequencies by anatomical location, injury type, phase of play, grade of play, time of match and dangerous play. Injury incidence rates were similar across categories of age-group, position of play and body mass index (Table 4). Visual inspection of Fig. 2 suggests the IIR was highest in the first two rounds of the season (not further evaluated via statistical analysis).

Age, years of participation, BMI and SF-36v2 summary scores were treated as continuous variables in the Poisson mixed-effects generalised linear modelling. Multivariate modelling found fewer years of rugby participation, lower BMI and lower SF-36v2 mental component summary score was associated with higher IIR in amateur rugby. Whereas age, player position i.e., backs versus forwards

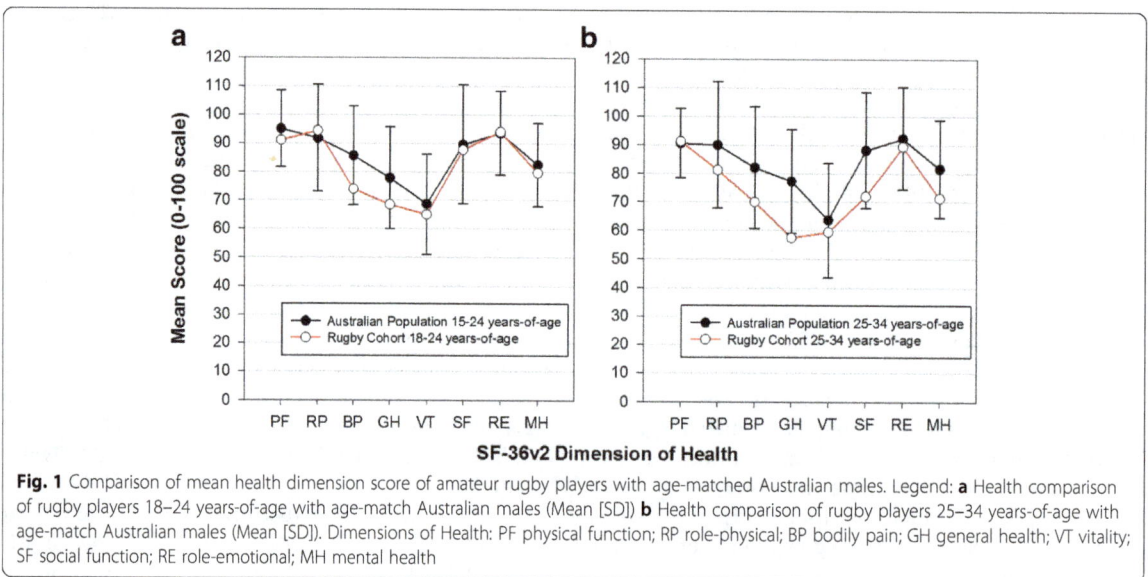

Fig. 1 Comparison of mean health dimension score of amateur rugby players with age-matched Australian males. Legend: **a** Health comparison of rugby players 18–24 years-of-age with age-match Australian males (Mean [SD]) **b** Health comparison of rugby players 25–34 years-of-age with age-match Australian males (Mean [SD]). Dimensions of Health: PF physical function; RP role-physical; BP bodily pain; GH general health; VT vitality; SF social function; RE role-emotional; MH mental health

Table 3 Frequency distribution of injuries by the anatomical location, type, phase of play, grade of play, time of match and dangerous play

	N	Percent % (95 % CI)
Anatomical location		
Head/face	23	17.8 (11.2–24.4)
Neck/cervical spine	6	4.7 (1.0–8.3)
Sternum/ribs/thorax	6	4.7 (1.0–8.3)
Abdomen	3	2.3 (0.0–4.9)
Low back	4	3.1 (0.1–6.1)
Sacrum/pelvis	1	0.8 (0.0–2.3)
Shoulder/clavicle	18	14 (8.0–19.9)
Upper arm	1	0.8 (0.0–2.3)
Elbow	4	3.1 (0.1–6.1)
Wrist	1	0.8 (0.0–2.3)
Hand/fingers/thumb	14	10.9 (5.5–16.2)
Hip/groin	2	1.6 (0.0–3.7)
Anterior thigh	2	1.6 (0.0–3.7)
Posterior thigh	8	6.2 (2.0–10.4)
Knee	18	14 (8.0–19.9)
Lower leg/achilles	6	4.7 (1.0–8.3)
Ankle	10	7.8 (3.1–12.4)
Other	2	1.6 (0.0–3.7)
Type of injury		
Ligament/sprain	35	27.1 % (19.5–34.8)
Hematoma/contusion/bruise	25	19.4 % (12.6–26.2)
Muscle	18	14 % (8.0–19.9)
Laceration	10	7.8 % (3.1–12.4)
Nerve	8	6.2 % (2.0–10.4)
Meniscus/cartilage/disc	7	5.4 % (1.5–9.3)
Concussion	6	4.7 % (1.8–3.0)
Other	6	4.7 % (1.0–8.3)
Dislocation/subluxation	4	3.1 % (0.1–6.1)
Tendon	4	3.1 % (0.1–6.1)
Fracture	3	2.3 % (0.0–4.9)
Abrasion	2	1.6 % (0.0–3.7)
Other bone	1	0.8 % (0.0–2.3)
Phase of play		
Tackling	44	34.6 (26.4–42.9)
Tackled	43	33.9 (25.6–42.1)
Ruck	13	10.2 (5.0–15.5)
Other	13	10.2 (25.6–15.5)
Collision	9	7.1 (2.6–11.5)
Maul	3	2.4 (0.0–5.0)
Scrum	2	1.6 (0.0–42.1)
Lineout	0	0 (0–0)

Table 3 Frequency distribution of injuries by the anatomical location, type, phase of play, grade of play, time of match and dangerous play (Continued)

Grade of play		
1st grade	16	12.5 (6.8–18.2)
2nd grade	25	19.5 (12.7–26.4)
3rd grade	33	25.8 (18.2–33.4)
4th grade	29	22.7 (15.4–29.9)
Colts (under 19-years)	25	19.5 (12.7–26.4)
Time of match		
1st quarter	22	17.2 (10.7–23.7)
2nd quarter	39	30.5 (22.5–38.4)
3rd quarter	31	24.2 (16.8–31.6)
4th quarter	36	28.1 (20.3–35.9)
Dangerous play		
No	127	99.2 (97.7–100.7)
Yes	1	0.8 (0.0–2.3)

and SF-36v2 physical component summary score were not associated with injury. Table 5 contains the results from the final Poisson mixed-effects generalised linear model.

Discussion

Amateur RU players report similar pre-season health-related quality of life characteristics as the general population. During the competitive season, the match injury rate for amateur rugby players was 52.3 /1000 match-hours exposure, with the head location, ligament tissue type, and tackling mechanism being the most common. Approximately one-third of injuries resulted in >1 week of time-loss from play. Factors associated with higher injury rates in this study were fewer years of playing, lower BMI and lower mental health, but the relationships were weak.

The study used standardised injury definition and data collection procedures, which allows for comparison of our findings with similar studies. We were also able to maintain an individual player exposure log for a more accurate estimate of exposure adjusted injury rate, which is a common limitation of larger (multiple-club observations) studies conducted over several seasons. Due to logistical constraints our study's hypothesis was explored with a cohort recruited from one amateur rugby club, followed over one-season and this limited sample size may have affected the precision of our estimates and the generalisability of our findings. Hence we likely identify moderate to strong associations. The notion that aspects of HRQoL may be associated with in-season sports injury is novel and adds to previous knowledge on the aetiology of sports injury in rugby.

Table 4 Injury rate and rate ratios by age, position of play and BMI

	N	Percent (95 % CI)	IIR$_{MHE}$ (95 % CI)	RR$_{MHE}$ (95 % CI)
Age				
18–24	89	69 (61–77)	52.6 (42.2–64.7)	ref.
25–34	36	27.9 (20.2–35.6)	51.8 (36.3–71.7)	0.99 (0.67–1.45)
≥35	4	3.1 (0.1–6.1)	51.4 (14.0–131.6)	0.98 (0.37–2.56)
Year of participation				
≤10 years	79	61.2 (52.8–69.6)	52.8 (41.8–65.8)	ref.
>10 years	50	38.8 (30.4–47.2)	51.6 (38.3–68.0)	0.69–1.39
Position				
Forward	67	51.9 (43.3–60.6)	52.2 (40.5–66.3)	ref.
Backs	62	48.1 (39.4–56.7)	52.4 (40.2–67.2)	1.00 (0.71–1.42)
BMI				
<25	48	39.3 (30.7–48)	58.7 (43.3–77.9)	ref.
25 to 30	58	47.5 (38.7–56.4)	50.4 (38.3–65.1)	0.86 (0.59–1.25)
>30	16	13.1 (7.1–19.1)	40.0 (22.8–64.9)	0.68 (0.39–1.19)
SF-36v2 PCS				
NBS <47	56	43.4 (34.9–52)	54.7 (41.3–71.1)	1.05 (0.70–1.58)
NBS 47–53	40	31 (23–39)	51.9 (37.1–70.7)	ref.
NBS >53	33	25.6 (18.1–33.1)	49.1 (33.8–69.0)	0.95 (0.60–1.49)
SF-36v2 MCS				
NBS <47	38	29.5 (21.6–37.3)	53.7 (38.0–73.7)	0.93 (0.57–1.50)
NBS 47–53	28	21.7 (14.6–28.8)	57.9 (38.5–83.7)	ref.
NBS >53	63	48.8 (40.2–57.5)	49.5 (38.0–63.3)	0.85 (0.55–1.33)

MHE /1000 match-hours exposure, *BMI* body mass index, *PCS* physical component summary, *MCS* mental component summary, *NBS* norm-based score

To the best of our knowledge this is this first time multiple dimensions of HRQoL have been evaluated in a cohort of amateur rugby players. On average both physical and mental component summary scores were similar in this cohort of amateur rugby players when compared to age-matched Australian males. There were however some small divergences below the population norm score in the health dimensions of bodily pain and general health perception. Presumably these lower average scores in bodily pain and general health are linked to

rugby related behaviours, such as physical contact in preseason training. Details about preseason injury status were not measured in this study, which limits us to speculation. Dimensions of health could also change with volume and type of rugby participation; consequently the temporal relationship between health, rugby exposure and injuries is an area for future research.

In this study, as expected, the overall match injury rate fell well below the high match injury rate of men's international and level-1-club professional rugby (52.3 vs.

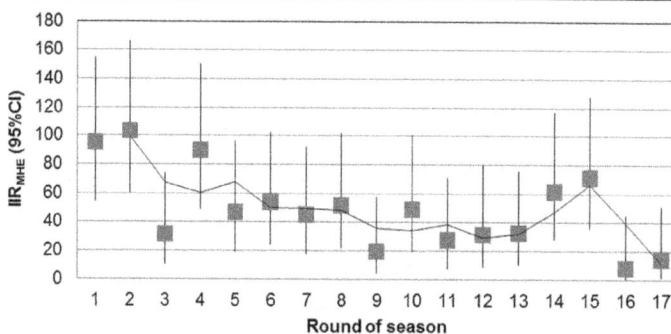

Fig. 2 Injury incidence rates per 1000 match-hours of exposure (IIR$_{MHE}$) with 95 % CI by round of season

Table 5 Rate ratio estimates per 1000 match hours of exposure (RR_{MHE}) with 95 % CIs using Poisson mixed-effects generalised linear modelling

Study factor	RR_{MHE} (95 % CI)	P-value
Age	0.98 (0.95–1.02)	0.329
Years of participation	0.93 (0.88–0.99)	0.017*
Backs (ref. forwards)	0.96 (0.42–2.17)	0.920
BMI	0.97 (0.95–1.00)	0.020*
SF-36v2 PCS	1.00 (0.99–1.01)	0.682
SF-36v2 MCS	0.98 (0.97–1.00)	0.012*

*$P < 0.05$

81.0 per 1000 match hours) [17]. However, the match injury rate in our cohort of amateur players was higher than level 2 professional rugby players (in Hong Kong and Japan) and a recent English cohort study of community rugby players (52.3 vs. 16.5–35.0 per 1000 match hours) [17, 26]. Also unexpected was the relatively low severity of injuries seen in this study (mean days of missed play 9 days); only around 16 % of injuries required more than one-month time loss from play. Results from a comparable study of community rugby players [26] report an average of 7.6 weeks missed per injury for all levels. The high proportion of slight injuries observed in our study may reflect a different risk profile in this cohort (i.e., a higher propensity for slight-mild injuries) or a greater sensitivity in our injury reporting.

Our description of match injuries was also similar to that seen in Scottish and English community rugby players in terms of location, mechanism, phase of play, player position and time of season [26, 27]. A point of difference from Roberts et al., [26] was that we found no difference in the rate of injury based on the time of the match or the grade of play. They, on the other hand, found injury incidence was lower in the first and second match quarters compared to the fourth and higher incidence in higher levels of competition. However, they observed a much larger sample and compared groups of clubs that play across wider levels of competitiveness, which likely accounts for the differences in injury rates across levels of play.

Previous studies have also measured rugby players' height and mass preseason to assess the relationship between BMI and injury incidence [10, 11]. These studies suggested that players with BMIs higher than 25 kg/m^2 are at greater risk of incurring an injury compared to players with BMIs less than 23 kg/m^2, though these findings were not statistically significant. We observed the opposite finding, that is, players with higher BMIs were less likely to incur an injury; however, this finding was only significant when BMI was included as a continuous variable in a multivariate analysis. Similarly, player experience (the number of years of rugby participation) has been previously been evaluated as a predictive factor

for injury occurrence in cohort studies [10, 11], but not found associated with injury rate. Unlike previous studies we did not categorise player experience and BMI in our model to avoid the known problems of loss of power and less precise estimation [28]. While our adjusted associations were significant the magnitude was small. At this time we believe inferences about the effects of BMI and experience on injury rate should be approached with caution, requiring further exploration in future research.

A simple yet commonly overlooked question in aetiological rugby studies is the impact of HRQoL of athletes on sport-related injury. The hypothesis for the current study follows work of Quarrie et al., [11] who, to the best of our knowledge, are the only group to have evaluated the potential role of a player's preseason health and psychological wellbeing on injury. To provide a more comprehensive evaluation of rugby player's overall health, HRQoL was measured with a robust measure that has been used with athletes [29, 30] and validated in patient populations [31]. A novel finding from our study was lower mental domain summary scores had a small association with higher rates of injury when controlling for other variables. Previous studies have found that rugby players who were injured in the previous season [12] or preseason [11] were more likely to be injured during the study season. It may be the case that previous injury adversely affects aspects of HRQoL such as physical functioning [29, 30]. Our model was established a priori with only a few potential predictors. A limitation of our study is that unaccounted for potential confounders such as previous injury may have distorted the prediction of HRQoL on injury incidence. Therefore further research is required to further evaluate the relationship between health and sports injury. Associations between health and rugby injury should be approached with caution at this time.

Conclusions

In this one-season and one-club cohort study, amateur Australian rugby players were on average overweight and report similar HRQoL as other Australian men of the same age. Australian amateur rugby players have a higher rate of injury and lower injury severity than English community rugby players. However, the location, type, and mechanism of injuries align with previous reports in the rugby literature. When questioned prior to the commencement of the season, rugby players who have lower mental components of health, BMI and years of participation may have a slightly higher injury rate when baseline other factors are accounted for. However, these associations are weak and should be interpreted with caution if applied to preseason screening and prevention programs. Future research should include health among other factors to clarify the magnitude of injury risk associated with rugby.

Additional file

Additional file 1: Table S1. SF-36v2 health domain scores: norm-based scores means and standard deviations. **Table S2.** SF-36v2 health domain scores: 0-100 means and standard deviations. (DOCX 21 kb)

Abbreviations
95 % CI: 95 % confidence interval; BMI: body mass index; HRQoL: health-related quality of life; IIR: injury incidence rate; MHE: match-hour of exposure; OSICS-10.1: orchard sports injury classification 10 version 1; RR: rate ratio; SF-36v2: short form 36 item health survey version 2 standard; PCS: physical component summary; MCS: mental component summary.

Competing interests
The authors declare that they have no competing interests.

Authors' contributions
MS conceived and designed the study, facilitated the acquisition of data, contributed to the analysis and interpretation of data, contributed to drafting and revising the manuscript critically for important intellectual content. RL, NH, CM and SK contributed to the analysis and interpretation of the data, drafting and revising the manuscript critically for important intellectual content. All authors read and approved the final manuscript.

Acknowledgements
The authors acknowledge the invaluable contribution of the research assistants and club chiropractor who assisted with data collection as well as the executive and participants from Lindfield Rugby Union who volunteered during the 2012 rugby season. The authors would like to thank the International Federation of Sports Chiropractic (FICS) (and their sponsor Life University) who awarded this paper second prize (US$5,000) at the 2015 FICS Symposium, Athens, Greece.

Author details
[1]The George Institute for Global Health, Sydney Medical School, University of Sydney, GPO Box 5389, Sydney, NSW 2001, Australia. [2]Department of Chiropractic, Faculty of Science and Engineering, Macquarie University, Sydney, Australia. [3]School of Medical and Applied Sciences, Central Queensland University, Sydney, Australia. [4]Institute of Public Health, University of Heidelberg, Heidelberg, Germany.

References
1. Garber CE, Blissmer B, Deschenes MR, Franklin BA, Lamonte MJ, Lee I-M, Nieman DC, Swain DP. Quantity and quality of exercise for developing and maintaining cardiorespiratory, musculoskeletal, and neuromotor fitness in apparently healthy adults: guidance for prescribing exercise. Med Sci Sports Exerc. 2011;43(7):1334–59.
2. Warburton DER, Nicol CW, Bredin SSD. Health benefits of physical activity: the evidence. CMAJ. 2006;174(6):801–9.
3. Lee IM, Shiroma EJ, Lobelo F, Puska P, Blair SN, Katzmarzyk PT. Effect of physical inactivity on major non-communicable diseases worldwide: an analysis of burden of disease and life expectancy. Lancet. 2012; 380(9838):219–29.
4. World Health Organization. Global recommendations on physical activity for health. Geneva: WHO Press; 2010.
5. Rugby codes - health benefits. http://www.healthtranslations.vic.gov.au/BHCV2/bhcpdf.nsf/ByPDF/Rugby_codes_-_health_benefits/$File/Rugby_codes_-_health_benefits.pdf. Accessed 7 Sept 2015.
6. Hootman JM, Dick R, Agel J. Epidemiology of collegiate injuries for 15 sports: summary and recommendations for injury prevention initiatives. J Athl Train. 2007;42(2):311–9.
7. Kerr HA, Curtis C, Micheli LJ, Kocher MS, Zurakowski D, Kemp SPT, Brooks JHM. Collegiate rugby union injury patterns in New England: a prospective cohort study. Br J Sports Med. 2008;42(7):595–603.
8. Lee AJ, Garraway WM, Hepburn W, Laidlaw R. Influence of rugby injuries on players' subsequent health and lifestyle: beginning a long term follow up. Br J Sports Med. 2001;35(1):38–42.
9. Brown JC, Lambert MI, Verhagen E, Readhead C, van Mechelen W, Viljoen W. The incidence of rugby-related catastrophic injuries (including cardiac events) in South Africa from 2008 to 2011: a cohort study. BMJ Open. 2013;3:2.
10. Chalmers DJ, Samaranayaka A, Gulliver P, McNoe B. Risk factors for injury in rugby union football in New Zealand: a cohort study. Br J Sports Med. 2012; 46(2):95–102.
11. Quarrie KL, Alsop JC, Waller AE, Bird YN, Marshall SW, Chalmers DJ. The New Zealand rugby injury and performance project. VI. A prospective cohort study of risk factors for injury in rugby union football. Br J Sports Med. 2001; 35(3):157–66.
12. Lee AJ, Garraway WM, Arneil DW. Influence of preseason training, fitness, and existing injury or subsequent rugby injury. Br J Sports Med. 2001;35(6):412–7.
13. Cunningham R, Carter K, Connor J, Fawcett J. Does health status matter for the risk of injury? New Zeal Med J. 2010;123(1327):35–46.
14. Chadwick S, Semens A, Schwarz EC, Zhang D. Economic impact report on global rugby. part III: strategic and emerging markets. Coventry, UK: Centre for International Business of Sport, Coventry University; 2010.
15. Australian Rugby Union. Annual report. 2012.
16. Brooks JHM, Kemp SPT. Recent trends in Rugby Union injuries. Clin Sports Med. 2008;27(1):51–73.
17. Williams S, Trewartha G, Kemp S, Stokes K. A meta-analysis of injuries in senior men's professional Rugby Union. Sports Med. 2013;43(10):1043–55.
18. Bleakley C, Tully M, O'Connor S. Epidemiology of adolescent rugby injuries: a systematic review. J Athl Train. 2011;46(5):555–65.
19. Fuller CW, Molloy MG, Bagate C, Bahr R, Brooks JHM, Donson H, Kemp SPT, McCrory P, McIntosh AS, Meeuwisse WH, Quarrie KL, Raftery M, Wiley P. Consensus statement on injury definitions and data collection procedures for studies of injuries in rugby union. Br J Sports Med. 2007;41(5):328–31.
20. Fuller CW, Laborde F, Leather RJ, Molloy MG. International Rugby Board Rugby World Cup 2007 injury surveillance study. Br J Sports Med. 2008; 42(6):452–9.
21. Rae K, Orchard J. The Orchard Sports Injury Classification System (OSICS) version 10. Clin J Sport Med. 2007;17(3):201–4.
22. Marin T, Taylor A, Gill T. A population profile of quality of life in South Australia - population norms for 2008 using the short form 36 version 2. 2009.
23. Hawthorne G, Osborne RH, Taylor A, Sansoni J. The SF36 version 2: critical analyses of population weights, scoring algorithms and population norms. Qual Life Res. 2007;16(4):661–73.
24. Ware JE. User's manual for the SF-36v2 health survey. Quality Metric; 2007.
25. Graham PL, Mengersen K, Morton AP. Confidence limits for the ratio of two rates based on likelihood scores: non-iterative method. Stat Med. 2003; 22(12):2071–83.
26. Roberts SP, Trewartha G, England M, Shaddick G, Stokes KA. Epidemiology of time-loss injuries in English community-level rugby union. BMJ Open. 2013;3:11.
27. Garraway M, Macleod D. Epidemiology of rugby football injuries. Lancet. 1995;345:1485–7.
28. Bennette C, Vickers A. Against quantiles: categorization of continuous variables in epidemiologic research, and its discontents. BMC Med Res Methodol. 2012;12(1):21.
29. McAllister DR, Motamedi AR, Hame SL, Shapiro MS, Dorey FJ. Quality of life assessment in elite collegiate athletes. Am J Sports Med. 2001;29(6):806–10.
30. Valovich McLeod TC, Bay RC, Parsons JT, Sauers EL, Snyder AR. Recent injury and health-related quality of life in adolescent athletes. J Athl Train. 2009; 44(6):603–10.
31. Brazier JE, Harper R, Jones NM, O'Cathain A, Thomas KJ, Usherwood T, Westlake L. Validating the SF-36 health survey questionnaire: new outcome measure for primary care. BMJ. 1992;305(6846):160–4.

PERMISSIONS

All chapters in this book were first published in CMT, by BioMed Central; hereby published with permission under the Creative Commons Attribution License or equivalent. Every chapter published in this book has been scrutinized by our experts. Their significance has been extensively debated. The topics covered herein carry significant findings which will fuel the growth of the discipline. They may even be implemented as practical applications or may be referred to as a beginning point for another development.

The contributors of this book come from diverse backgrounds, making this book a truly international effort. This book will bring forth new frontiers with its revolutionizing research information and detailed analysis of the nascent developments around the world.

We would like to thank all the contributing authors for lending their expertise to make the book truly unique. They have played a crucial role in the development of this book. Without their invaluable contributions this book wouldn't have been possible. They have made vital efforts to compile up to date information on the varied aspects of this subject to make this book a valuable addition to the collection of many professionals and students.

This book was conceptualized with the vision of imparting up-to-date information and advanced data in this field. To ensure the same, a matchless editorial board was set up. Every individual on the board went through rigorous rounds of assessment to prove their worth. After which they invested a large part of their time researching and compiling the most relevant data for our readers.

The editorial board has been involved in producing this book since its inception. They have spent rigorous hours researching and exploring the diverse topics which have resulted in the successful publishing of this book. They have passed on their knowledge of decades through this book. To expedite this challenging task, the publisher supported the team at every step. A small team of assistant editors was also appointed to further simplify the editing procedure and attain best results for the readers.

Apart from the editorial board, the designing team has also invested a significant amount of their time in understanding the subject and creating the most relevant covers. They scrutinized every image to scout for the most suitable representation of the subject and create an appropriate cover for the book.

The publishing team has been an ardent support to the editorial, designing and production team. Their endless efforts to recruit the best for this project, has resulted in the accomplishment of this book. They are a veteran in the field of academics and their pool of knowledge is as vast as their experience in printing. Their expertise and guidance has proved useful at every step. Their uncompromising quality standards have made this book an exceptional effort. Their encouragement from time to time has been an inspiration for everyone.

The publisher and the editorial board hope that this book will prove to be a valuable piece of knowledge for researchers, students, practitioners and scholars across the globe.

LIST OF CONTRIBUTORS

Robert Gordon
Cornerstone Professional Education, Inc, 4002 Streamlet Way, 28110 Monroe, NC, USA

Edward Cremata
Palmer College of Chiropractic West, San Jose, CA, USA
Fremont Chiropractic Group, Fremont, CA, USA

Cheryl Hawk
Logan University, 1851 Schoettler Rd 63017 Chesterfield, MO, USA

Iris Sun Rudy, Alexandra Poulos, Laura Owen, Ashlee Batters, Kasia Kieliszek, Jessica Willox and Hazel Jenkins
Macquarie University, Sydney, Australia

Peter Charles Emary
Master of Science (MSc) Candidate, MSc Advanced Professional Practice (Clinical Sciences), Anglo-European College of Chiropractic, 13-15 Parkwood Road, Bournemouth, Dorset, BH5 2DF, UK
Private Practice, 201C Preston Parkway, Cambridge, ON N3H 5E8, Canada

Kent Jason Stuber
Division of Graduate Education and Research, Canadian Memorial Chiropractic College, 6100 Leslie Street, Toronto, ON M2H 3J1, Canada

Corrie Vihstadt, Michele Maiers, Kristine Westrom and Craig Schulz
Northwestern Health Sciences University, Wolfe-Harris Center for Clinical Studies, 2501 W 84th Street, Bloomington, MN 55431, USA

Gert Bronfort and Roni Evans
University of Minnesota, Center for Spirituality and Healing, Mayo Memorial Building C592, 420 Delaware Street SE, Minneapolis, MN 55455, USA

Jan Hartvigsen
Institute of Sports Science and Clinical Biomechanics, University of Southern Denmark, Campusvej 55, Odense, M DK-5230, Denmark

Emiel van Trijffel
Department of Clinical Epidemiology, Biostatistics & Bioinformatics, Academic Medical Centre, University of Amsterdam, Amsterdam, the Netherlands
Institute for Master Education in Musculoskeletal Therapy, Amersfoort, the Netherlands

Robert Lindeboom, Patrick MM Bossuyt and Cees Lucas
Department of Clinical Epidemiology, Biostatistics & Bioinformatics, Academic Medical Centre, University of Amsterdam, Amsterdam, the Netherlands

Maarten A Schmitt
Institute for Master Education in Musculoskeletal Therapy, Amersfoort, the Netherlands

Bart W Koes
Department of General Practice, Erasmus MC University Medical Centre, Rotterdam, the Netherlands

Rob AB Oostendorp
Scientific Institute for Quality of Healthcare, Radboud University Nijmegen Medical Centre, Nijmegen, the Netherlands
Department of Rehabilitation, Physiotherapy and Manual Therapy, Faculty of Medicine and Pharmacology, Free University of Brussels, Brussels, Belgium

Patricia E Fikar
Private Practice, Vienna, Austria

Kent A Edlund and Dave Newell
AECC-Anglo-European College of Chiropractic, 13-15 Parkwood Road, Bournemouth, Dorset BH5 2DF, UK

Mattijs Clijsters and Francesco Fronzoni
Macquarie University Sydney, Sydney NSW 2109, Australia

Hazel Jenkins
Department of Chiropractic, Macquarie University Sydney, Sydney NSW 2109, Australia

Cecilia Bergström and Ingrid Mogren
Department of Clinical Sciences, Obstetrics and Gynecology, Umeå University, Umeå, Sweden

Margareta Persson
Department of Nursing, Umeå University, Umeå, Sweden

Stanley I Innes
Discipline of Chiropractic, Health Professions, Murdoch University, Murdoch, WA 6150, Australia

Peter D Werth
Private Practice, Australian Injury Management Consulting, 117 Hall Road, Carrum Downs, VIC 3201, Australia

Peter J Tuchin
Department of Chiropractic, Faculty of Science, Macquarie University, Sydney, NSW 2109, Australia

Petra L Graham
Department of Statistics, Faculty of Science, Macquarie University, Sydney, NSW 2109, Australia

Clinton J. Daniels
Chiropractic Clinic, VA St. Louis Healthcare System, Jefferson Barracks Rd, Saint Louis, MO, USA
Logan University, College of Chiropractic, 1851 Schoettler Rd, Chesterfield, MO, USA
811 Rowell St., Steilacoom, WA 98388, USA

Pamela J. Wakefield and Glenn A. Bub
Chiropractic Clinic, VA St. Louis Healthcare System, 1 Jefferson Barracks Rd, Saint Louis, MO, USA
Logan University, College of Chiropractic, 1851 Schoettler Rd, Chesterfield, MO, USA

Jordan A Gliedt
Private Practice, 725 S. Dobson Rd, Suite 100, Chandler, AZ 85224, USA

Cheryl Hawk and Michelle Anderson
Logan University College of Chiropractic, 1851 Schoettler Rd, Chesterfield, MO 63017, USA

Kashif Ahmad and Dinah Bunn
Northwestern University of Health Sciences, 2501 W. 84th St, Bloomington, MN 55431, USA

Jerrilyn Cambron
National University of Health Sciences, 200 E. Roosevelt Rd, Lombard, IL 60148, USA

Brian Gleberzon
Canadian Memorial College of Chiropractic, 6100 Leslie St, Toronto, Ontario, Canada

John Hart
Sherman College of Chiropractic, 2020 Springfield Rd, Boiling Springs, SC 29316, USA

Anupama Kizhakkeveettil
Southern California University of Health Sciences, 16200 E. Amber Valley Dr., Whittier, CA 90604, USA

Stephen M Perle
University of Bridgeport, Bridgeport, CT 06604, USA

Michael Ramcharan
Texas Chiropractic College, 5912 Spencer Highway, Pasadena, TX 77505, USA

Stephanie Sullivan
Life University, 1269 Barclay Circle, Marietta, GA 30060, USA

Liang Zhang
Palmer College of Chiropractic - Florida, 4777 City Center Parkway, Port Orange, FL 32129, USA

Hugh MacPherson and Ann Hopton
Department of Health Sciences, University of York, York, UK

Elizabeth Newbronner
Firefly Research & Evaluation and Visiting Fellow, Department of Health Sciences, University of York, York, UK

Ruth Chamberlain
Firefly Research & Evaluation, North Yorkshire, UK

Thomas M Kosloff and David Elton
Optum Health – Clinical Programs at United Health Group, 11000 Optum Circle, Eden Prairie MN 55344, USA

Jiang Tao and Wade M Bannister
Optum Health – Clinical Analytics at United Health Group, 11000 Optum Circle, Eden Prairie MN 55344, USA

Andreas Eklund, Irene Jensen and Malin Lohela-Karlsson
Unit of Intervention and Implementation Research, Karolinska Institutet, Institute of Environmental Medicine, Nobels v 13, S-171 77 Stockholm, Sweden

Charlotte Leboeuf-Yde
Research Department, Spine Center of Southern Denmark, Institute for Regional Health Research, Hospital Lillebælt, University of Southern Denmark, Østre Hougvej 55, DK-5500 Middelfart, Denmark

Iben Axén
Unit of Intervention and Implementation Research, Karolinska Institutet, Institute of Environmental Medicine, Nobels v 13, S-171 77 Stockholm, Sweden

Research Department, Spine Center of Southern Denmark, Institute for Regional Health Research, Hospital Lillebælt, University of Southern Denmark, Østre Hougvej 55, DK-5500 Middelfart, Denmark

Orla Lund Nielsen and Henrik Wulff Christensen
The Nordic Institute of Chiropractic and Clinical Biomechanics, Campusvej 55, DK-5230 Odense M, Denmark
Department of Sports Science and Clinical Biomechanics, University of Southern Denmark, Campusvej 55, 5230 Odense M, Denmark

Alice Kongsted
The Nordic Institute of Chiropractic and Clinical Biomechanics, Campusvej 55, DK-5230 Odense M, Denmark
Department of Sports Science and Clinical Biomechanics, University of Southern Denmark, Campusvej 55, 5230 Odense M, Denmark

Bas Penning de Vries and Michael Shilton
Anglo-European College of Chiropractic, 13-15 Parkwood Road, Bournemouth BH5 2DF, UK

Jonathan Branney
Faculty of Health and Social Sciences, Bournemouth University, Bournemouth House, Bournemouth BH1 3LH, UK
Institute of Musculoskeletal Research and Clinical Implementation, Anglo-European College of Chiropractic, 13-15 Parkwood Road, Bournemouth BH5 2DF, UK

Alan C. Breen
Institute of Musculoskeletal Research and Clinical Implementation, Anglo-European College of Chiropractic, 13-15 Parkwood Road, Bournemouth BH5 2DF, UK

Shawn Williams
CUNY York College – Department of Health Professions, 94 - 20 Guy R. Brewer Blvd, Jamaica, NY 11451, USA.
Department of Research, New York Chiropractic College, Seneca Falls, NY, USA Private Practice – Montclair Performance Health & Chiropractic, LLC, Montclair, NJ, USA

Peter D Chapman
6 Claredon Court, Alexander Heights 6064, WA, Australia

Norman J Stomski
School of Health Professions, Murdoch University, 90 South St, Murdoch 6150, WA, Australia

Barrett Losco and Bruce F Walker
Discipline of Chiropractic, School of Health Professions, Murdoch University, 90 South St, Murdoch 6150, WA, Australia

Dean Petersen
Private practice, Mackay, QLD, Australia

Reidar P. Lystad
Department of Chiropractic, Macquarie University, Sydney, Australia

Chris T. Carter
School of Health Professions, Murdoch University, 90 South Street, Murdoch, WA 6150, Australia

Michael S. Swain
The George Institute for Global Health, Sydney Medical School, University of Sydney, GPO Box 5389, Sydney, NSW 2001, Australia Department of Chiropractic, Faculty of Science and Engineering, Macquarie University, Sydney, Australia

Reidar P. Lystad
School of Medical and Applied Sciences, Central Queensland University, Sydney, Australia

Nicholas Henschke
The George Institute for Global Health, Sydney Medical School, University of Sydney, GPO Box 5389, Sydney, NSW 2001, Australia Institute of Public Health, University of Heidelberg, Heidelberg, Germany

Christopher G. Maher and Steven J. Kamper
The George Institute for Global Health, Sydney Medical School, University of Sydney, GPO Box 5389, Sydney, NSW 2001, Australia

Index

A

Acute Thoracolumbar Pain, 214-215, 217

Adverse Events, 31, 34, 40, 43, 161-162, 168-169, 203, 207-208

Attitudes and Beliefs, 28, 83, 95, 121-125, 127-128

B

Biennial Symposium, 219, 221, 223, 225

Biopsychosocial, 121-122, 124-125, 128, 173, 177

Bladder Cancer, 129-131, 133

Bladder Metastasis, 129, 131, 133

Bothersome Lbp, 171-173, 175

C

Catastrophic Injury, 221

Cervical Fluoroscopic Images, 186

Cervical Lordosis (sagittal Alignment), 186

Cervical Manipulation, 65, 161-162, 166, 168-169, 187, 193, 203, 207

Cervical Spine, 7, 11-14, 16-17, 65, 81, 129-130, 132-133, 169, 186-187, 192-194, 202-205, 207, 223

Chiropractic, 1, 3, 6, 8-9, 12-13, 18-21, 25-28, 42-43, 45, 47, 49, 54-55, 67-79, 81-97, 100, 102, 105-108, 112-114, 116, 118, 121, 123-130, 132-169, 171-187, 190, 193-204, 207-210, 212-213, 215, 218-219, 226

Chiropractic Manipulation, 55, 67, 76, 167, 169, 176, 208

Chiropractic Profession, 19, 27-28, 42, 69, 72-75, 83, 85-87, 90, 94, 134-135, 137-141, 146, 149, 178-179, 181-185, 195-196, 198, 200

Chiropractors' Perception, 24, 195, 197, 199, 201

Cholecystitis, 214-218

Comparative Effectiveness, 30-32, 46, 48

Complementary and Alternative Medicine, 85, 95-96

Complementary and Alternative Treatments, 108, 118

Cross-sectional Electronic Questionnaire, 134

Cross-sectional Survey, 18, 69, 75-77, 79, 81, 83, 86, 120, 136, 151, 153, 155, 157, 159, 201

D

Danish Chiropractic Association (dca), 178

Degenerative Joint Disease, 11-16

Demarcation, 171-172, 174

Descriptive Statistical Analysis, 134

Diagnostic Coding, 142-149

Dissemination, 85-86, 95, 124

Drug Prescription, 18-21, 23-29

E

Encompassed Demographics, 135

Evidence-based Medicine, 85, 95-96

Exercise Therapy, 31, 42, 45-47, 54

F

Filum Terminale, 209, 211, 213

Fitness to Practice, 151-152, 155

G

Goal-setting, 68, 70-73

H

Headache or Migraine, 162

Health Consumers, 108, 110, 119

Health Prevention, 68

Health Promotion, 68-69, 71-73, 95-96

Health-related Quality of Life (hrqol), 219-220

Hyperalgesia, 214-215, 217

I

Influencing Factors, 195, 197, 199, 201

Information Search, 108-111, 113, 115, 117-120

Injury Incidence Rates (iirs), 219, 221

Intraclass Correlation Coefficients (icc), 191

K

Knowledge Translation, 85

M

Magnetic Resonance Imaging (mri), 209, 211

Manipulation Under Anesthesia, 1, 3-5, 7, 9-10

Mannequin, 202-207

Manual Therapy, 1-2, 30-31, 47, 53, 55, 57-59, 62, 64-66, 75, 96, 122, 169, 202
Motion Assessment, 57, 63, 65
Muscular Hypertonicity, 214-215, 217-218
Musculoskeletal Dysfunction, 78, 214
Myxopapillary Ependymoma, 209, 211, 213

N
Neck Disability, 30-32, 37, 43, 59, 191
Neck Manipulation, 169, 202-205, 207-208
Neck Stiffness, 11-16
Non-specific Neck Pain, 65, 186-187, 189, 191-193
Numerical Rating Scale (nrs), 215

O
Occupational Stress, 195-197, 199-201
Ontario Chiropractors, 18-21, 23-27, 29
Osteoarthritis, 11, 13, 17, 42, 65, 107

P
Patients' Expectations, 151, 159-160
Patients' Experiences, 151, 153, 155, 157, 159
Posterior Tangents, 186
Postpartum Period, 97
Pregnancy Complications, 97
Pregnancy Related Low Back Pain, 97-99, 101, 103, 105, 107
Prevalence, 12, 17, 42, 57, 60, 63-64, 66-67, 69, 74, 82, 97-98, 100, 102, 105-106, 129, 162-163, 167, 171-174, 176, 180, 183, 186, 193, 201, 208
Prevalent Condition, 172

Primary Intraspinal Neoplasms, 209, 212
Prostaglandins, 217
Psychological Stress, 103, 195

Q
Qualitative Research, 19, 110, 120, 150, 159, 195, 201

R
Range of Motion (rom), 210
Right Sided Lower Thoracic, 214-215

S
Simulated Learning, 202
Spinal Cord, 133, 209, 211-213, 217-218
Spinal Joint Mobilisations, 57-59, 61, 63, 65, 67
Spine-related Pain, 1-2
Static Mechanical Allodynia, 217
Survey Research, 85

T
Technique Systems, 75-76, 78, 82-83, 194
Thorax Pain, 129, 131-133
Transitional Cell Carcinoma, 129, 133
Treatment Modalities, 58, 78, 132, 178, 181, 184
Trivial Pain, 202

U
Upper Lumbar Pain, 214

V
Victorian Chiropractors, 121, 125, 127

www.ingramcontent.com/pod-product-compliance
Lightning Source LLC
Chambersburg PA
CBHW061946190326
41458CB00009B/2795